Systemic
Cardiac
Embolism

FUNDAMENTAL AND CLINICAL CARDIOLOGY

Editor-in-Chief
Samuel Z. Goldhaber, M.D.
*Harvard Medical School
and Brigham and Women's Hospital
Boston, Massachusetts*

Associate Editor, Europe
Henri Bounameaux, M.D.
*University Hospital of Geneva
Geneva, Switzerland*

Additional Volumes in Preparation

Valvular Heart Diseases, edited by Muayed Al Zaibag and Carlos G. Duran

Automatic Implantable Cardioverter-Defibrillators: A Comprehensive Text, edited by Paul J. Wang, N. A. Mark Estes III, and Antonis Manolis

Systemic
Cardiac
Embolism

edited by

Michael D. Ezekowitz

Yale University School of Medicine
West Haven Veterans Affairs
and Cardiovascular Thrombosis Research Laboratory
New Haven, Connecticut

Marcel Dekker, Inc.   **New York•Basel•Hong Kong**

Systemic cardiac embolism/edited by Michael D. Ezekowitz.
    p.   cm.—(Fundamental and clinical cardiology; 18)
    Includes bibliographical references and index.
    ISBN: 0-8247-9151-7 (alk. paper)
    1. Embolism.   2. Thromboembolism.   I. Ezekowitz, M. D. (Michael
D.)   II. Series: Fundamental and clinical cardiology; v. 18.
    [DNLM: 1. Blood Coagulation—physiology.   2. Thrombolytic Therapy—
methods.   3. Thromboembolism—diagnosis.   4. Thromboembolism—
therapy.   5. Cardiovascular Diseases—etiology.   6. Cardiovascular
System—physiopathology.   W1 FU538TD v. 18 1994/WG 540 S995 1994]
RC691.S97   1994
616.1′35—dc20
DNLM/DLC   93-37225
for Library of Congress   CIP

The publisher offers discounts on this book when ordered in bulk quantities. For more information, write to Special Sales/Professional Marketing at the address below.

This book is printed on acid-free paper.

Marcel Dekker, Inc.
270 Madison Avenue, New York, New York 10016

Current printing (last digit):
10 9 8 7 6 5 4 3 2 1

PRINTED IN THE UNITED STATES OF AMERICA

To My Family

Series Introduction

Marcel Dekker, Inc., has focused on the development of various series of beautifully produced books in different branches of medicine. These series have facilitated the integration of rapidly advancing information for both the clinical specialist and the researcher.

My goal as editor of the Fundamental and Clinical Cardiology series is to assemble the talents of world-renowned authorities to discuss virtually every area of cardiovascular medicine. In the current monograph, *Systemic Cardiac Embolism*, Dr. Michael D. Ezekowitz has edited a much needed and timely book. Future contributions to this series will include books on molecular biology, interventional cardiology, and clinical management of such problems as coronary artery disease and ventricular arrhythmias.

Samuel Z. Goldhaber

Foreword

Thrombotic and thromboembolic arterial disease are important, and possibly the major contributors to the most common causes of death in the western world, i.e., myocardial infarction and stroke. Unfortunately, in spite of their importance in clinical practice, these disorders are often not clearly understood by the practicing physician. This is probably due to the fact that the unifying process, thrombosis, does not constitute a single discipline, but rather is included in the practice of most doctors, whether general practitioners, cardiologists, neurologists, surgeons, or, of course, hematologists. It is therefore not surprising that with the exception of investigators that deal with disorders of coagulation, most physicians are uncomfortable with this complex field.

Three aspects of Dr. Ezekowitz's book are of special interest. First of all, contemporary books dealing with cardiovascular thrombosis often focus on coronary artery disease; this is the first book that focuses on systemic embolization. Second, using a unified approach, this book has assembled contributors who bridge the various disciplines of cardiology, hematology, molecular biology, neurology, and clinical medicine and thus provides the reader with a complete overview. Third, concerns about the complexity of the field of coagulation are overcome in Part I, with outstanding and relevant chapters on the fundamental issues from renowned specialists in their respective fields. This book, therefore, is indeed an important and much needed addition to the cardiovascular literature.

Dr. Ezekowitz, the editor, has a unique background and perspective. He emerges from the British-inspired medical tradition that emphasizes clinical excellence and bedside evaluation of patients. At the same time, he has an investigational mind that is an outgrowth of his scientific training at the Imperial College in London and his experience with an outstanding cardiovascular group in thrombosis at the University of Oklahoma and, most recently, with an equally outstanding group at Yale University School of Medicine. Dr. Ezekowitz's broad clinical research training is clearly evident throughout the entire book.

Part I deals with the physiology of coagulation and the pharmacology of the drugs used to treat these disorders; it clearly presents and updates a very complex field in a manner that is comprehensive, yet understandable, to the clinician. Part II deals with the technology utilized in the diagnosis and treatment of patients with systemic cardiac embolism, a field in which Dr. Ezekowitz has made perhaps the most outstanding contribution. This glimpse at the emerging state of technology is quite stimulating for the reader. It successfully defines the role of this technology in clinical practice but also emphasizes its limitations. Finally, Part III is devoted to treatment options, an area of investigation where Dr. Ezekowitz has been particularly prominent, and is unique in its focus on understanding the various anatomical regions that serve as potential sources of embolism. There is particular emphasis on recent knowledge of pathophysiology as well as recently completed clinical trials and future directions.

I believe that this volume will prove invaluable to all investigators of thromboembolic disorders, as well as to cardiologists, hematologists, neurologists, internists, and students who wish to make informed clinical decisions when dealing with thromboembolic problems in their daily practice.

Valentin Fuster, M.D., Ph.D.
Mallinckrodt Professor of Medicine
Harvard Medical School
Chief of Cardiac Unit
Massachusetts General Hospital
Boston, MA

Preface

Two factors were significant in the work that led up to this book. The first was my long-standing interest in thrombosis and vascular disease. The second, and most significant, was my introduction to the pioneering work of Thakur and McAfee. Working at Hammersmith Hospital in 1975, these investigators successfully labeled platelets with indium-111, making it theoretically possible for the first time to noninvasively image thrombosis in humans. Our priority for implementation of this technology was directed toward the coronary circulation. Unfortunately, my initial attempts to image coronary thrombi with indium-111 were futile. This early experience led to a redirection of the thrombus imaging project toward the identification of left ventricular thrombi. My own preliminary work, incorporating Thakur and McAfee's invaluable technique, was conducted at Johns Hopkins Medical School with Ursula Scheffel and Pat McIntyre and then as a faculty member at the University of Oklahoma. Our first positive cardiac image was obtained in 1979 at the University of Oklahoma. This success led to a systematic comparison of indium-111 platelet scintigraphy with the then evolving technology of two-dimensional ultrasound for the diagnosis of left ventricular thrombi, which was published in the *New England Journal of Medicine* in 1982. We now had tools to identify sources of systemic embolization. The research interests of the Oklahoma group evolved into investigations of new techniques for identifying intracardiac masses in other locations.

In 1981, we performed probably the first outpatient transesophageal echocardiography in the United States and, later that year, identified a patient with left atrial myxoma using this technique. It was apparent that this technique would be useful for identifying masses in the left atrium. Our work increased in scope with the design of a Veterans Administration Cooperative Study, with Dr. Sam Bridges, a neurologist, as co-principal investigator and Dr. Ken James as the statistician. This study evaluated low doses of warfarin in patients with atrial fibrillation as a means of preventing stroke. Clearcut benefit of treatment was shown.

These events, together with important advances in the field of thromboembolism, motivated the writing of this book. Although many questions remain unresolved, the decade has seen clarification of many important issues.

ACKNOWLEDGMENTS

Several mentors and collaborators played critical roles in the projects contained within this book and I gratefully acknowledge their contributions. Both Dr. Pat MacIntyre and Dr. Henry N. Wagner, Jr., from the Nuclear Medicine Department at Johns Hopkins Hospital, played a major role in helping me formulate my ideas and in supporting me in those difficult early years in my newly adopted country. Numerous colleagues at the University of Oklahoma were also instrumental in the success of these projects. Dr. Fletcher Taylor, especially, helped me write my first NIH grant. His advice and support were always invaluable. Eileen Smith, my first technician, played a critical role in those early patient projects. She was joined by Terry Streits. Cielo Martinez and Francesca Migliaccio were her successors. Dr. Daniel Deykin, Director of the Veterans Administration Co-operative Study program, has been a particularly important mentor and colleague. Collaborators, research fellows, technicians, and administrative assistants too numerous to name individually have been involved in these studies. I thank them collectively. Special thanks to Paulette Trent, Sutton Teeple, Juliette Mitchell, and Thuy Ai Dinh for their administrative assistance in compiling this book.

This book has been written in three parts. Part I deals with the physiology of coagulation and the pharmacology of the drugs used in the treatment of thromboembolic disorders. Part II deals with the technology utilized in the investigation of these patients, and Part III covers treatment options.

PART I: FUNDAMENTAL ISSUES

Chapter 1: Introduction

Clinical trials play a central role in guiding health care providers to optimal care. There is no area in medicine where this is better exemplified than in guiding treatment in patients who have thromboembolic disease, and this book relies heavily on data collected from such trials.

Chapter 2: Physiology of Coagulation

Normal hemostasis is a complex process dependent upon the coordinated interaction of three major components: humoral plasma proteins, which promote and modulate blood coagulation; platelets, which initiate and promote hemostasis; and vascular endothelial cells, which synthesize, store, and release vasoactive substances, adhesive proteins, and activators and inhibitors of coagulation, platelet function, and fibrinolysis. This sequential and orchestrated process is designed to preserve the integrity of the closed circulatory system and to minimize blood loss following injury to the vascular framework while simultaneously maintaining the fluidity and uninterrupted flow of blood.

The physiology of normal coagulation is extremely complex and its orchestration is profoundly dependent on the optimal functioning of each of the separate components. Even slight alterations in the integrity of endothelial cells, the activation of coagulation proteins and their inhibitors and modulators, and platelet function can result in disordered coagulation producing clinical symptoms of either bleeding or thrombosis.

Chapter 3:   Biochemistry of Vitamin K: Implications for Warfarin Therapy

Over the past decade, clinical studies have demonstrated the efficacy of progressively lower doses of warfarin with fewer hemorrhagic complications. The clinical use of lower warfarin doses has challenged the traditional prothrombin time-based methods of monitoring anticoagulant therapy. For example, at the lowest doses of warfarin, little or no effect is observed on the prothrombin time and, at higher doses, the prothrombin time demonstrates considerable variability due to differences in the reagents used in the test systems.

Progress in understanding the biochemical mechanisms of vitamin K metabolism and vitamin K-dependent hemostasis has created new and promising methods for monitoring oral anticoagulant therapy. Most of these new approaches are undergoing aggressive evaluation, although none is fully validated for clinical use at the present time. In the meantime, the prothrombin time ratio or the international normalized ratio (INR) remains the mainstay of clinical monitoring. The development of more sensitive thromboplastins and their standardization by the INR should improve the therapeutic utility of this time-tested clinical tool.

Chapter 4:   Mechanisms of Thrombolysis

This chapter is written in the context of the concept of coagulant balance, which, briefly stated, refers to the ongoing, linked processes of procoagulation and profibrinolysis, each held in check by appropriate inhibitory activities. The key to this process is the generation of thrombin, which is important not only for fibrin generation, but also for platelet activation. In the process of profibrinolysis, the ultimate enzyme is plasmin. This chapter focuses on the mechanisms of thrombolysis as well as its inhibition. There is much current interest in a newly described lipid fraction, lipoprotein (a), also called Lp(a). This lipid particle is very similar to the low density lipoprotein (LDL) particle, with the exception that the protein moiety, instead of being composed of apolipoprotein B alone, also contains the apo (a) protein structure. The apo (a) moiety bears a striking resemblance to plasminogen: it contains a large, but variable, number of Kringle domains, each of which is homologous to Kringle 4 from plasminogen, and it contains a sequence similar to the active site of plasmin, although the arginine residue associated with the active site-generating cleavage has been replaced with a serine. As a consequence of this alteration, the generation of an active enzyme cannot occur by the known serine protease activating mechanism, and enzymatic activity is not possible. Because of the multiple Kringle structures it has been proposed that Lp(a) might compete with plasminogen for fibrin or endothelial cell binding sites, thereby limiting plasmin generation. Whether this hypothesis is true remains to be proven, but this mechanism has tremendous potential as a long-term regulator of plasminogen activation, especially since plasma Lp(a) levels appear to be tightly controlled genetically. There is considerable epidemiological evidence that Lp(a) is an independent risk factor for cardiovascular disease and, with elements of both the lipid factors (the LDL-like particle structure) and the thrombotic factors (plasminogen Kringle homology), Lp(a) has the potential to be involved with cardiovascular disease in several ways.

Chapter 5:   Heparin: Biochemistry, Pharmacology, Pharmacokinetics, and Dose-Response Relationships

In this chapter, the biochemistry of heparin and its interaction with AT-III is described. The physiological role of heparin and related compounds, therapeutic action, pharmacokinetics, and dose response relationships as well as side effects has been reviewed in detail. A new class of heparins, the low molecular weight heparins, are discussed in detail and compared to standard therapy.

Chapter 6:   Pharmacological Strategies for Antithrombotic Therapy

Thromboembolic disease in its various forms remains a primary cause of morbidity and mortality in the most developed countries. The pharmacological strategies currently available for the treatment of both venous and arterial thrombosis are limited, and innovative new approaches are urgently required. This need has fostered intensive basic research aimed at understanding the process of vascular repair and thrombus formation. From such research, a highly complex system involving an intimate interaction and communication between the vascular wall and components of the blood is emerging. This system is characterized by positive feedback mechanisms that permit a fast response to vascular damage, as well as negative feedback mechanisms to prevent inappropriate and dangerous thrombus development. Such a complex and highly regulated process offers numerous therapeutic possibilities to effect change in the system to protect the patient from harmful thrombus formation, and a variety of these promising strategies have been outlined. Despite the variety of therapeutic approaches that might be successfully exploited, it is certain that only those approaches which account for (and possibly take advantage of) the feedback mechanisms of blood-vessel–wall interaction have the best chance of making significant inroads in the treatment of thromboembolic disease.

PART II: TECHNOLOGY

Chapter 7:   Cardiac and Peripheral Ultrasound

Ultrasound has wide application in the study of both cardiac and peripheral arterial and venous disease. To date, the use of ultrasound for medical imaging is without known biologic adverse effects. In general, the objectives of the ultrasound examination are to define anatomy and characterize blood flow patterns and velocities. By so doing, it is possible to identify disease processes in the heart that are associated with embolic potential and also identify atherosclerotic disease in the aortic arch and carotid vessels. For the diagnosis of venous disease, it is particularly accurate for proximal vein thrombosis.

Chapter 8:   Radionuclide-Based Imaging Techniques for Thrombus Detection

Indium-111 labeled platelets are the prototypic thrombus imaging method. The promise for the future for radionuclide imaging of thrombosis rests with the use of monoclonal antibodies that are directed against components of the coagulation process, bind tightly to their target, and are cleared rapidly from the circulation.

Chapter 9: Magnetic Resonance Imaging

Although in its infancy, MRI has expanded our diagnostic armamentarium in the detection of intracardiac and intravascular masses of embolic potential. It is best considered as a complementary modality to echocardiography. The well-rounded clinician must have some familiarity with the technology, because in certain circumstances it provides diagnostically unique information. This information may be important in guiding appropriate medical or surgical therapy.

Chapter 10: Comprehensive Cardiac Evaluation with Cine Computed Tomography

Cine computed tomography is one of a new generation of cardiac imaging techniques potentially useful in the evaluation of patients who are at risk for thromboembolic disease. Early experience suggests that this modality can provide a highly accurate and comprehensive cardiac assessment with consistently excellent image quality.

Chapter 11: Miscellaneous Techniques

This chapter covers the radiocontrast techniques, as well as impedance plethysmography. Angiographic examinations are generally performed to confirm an anatomic abnormality suggested by noninvasive tests or as a primary imaging technique for determination of anatomic detail. Traditionally, radio contrast techniques have been considered the "gold standard" for diagnosis. For many areas, this technology has been superseded by noninvasive tests. Impedance plethysmography is a technique that measures changes in blood volume and is usually applied to the diagnosis of deep vein thrombosis. This test is accurate for proximal vein thrombosis.

PART III: MANAGEMENT CONSIDERATIONS

Chapter 12: The Left Ventricle

With the demonstration of reliable techniques for the identification of left ventricular thrombi, important questions have emerged concerning the value of these tests not only for diagnosis, but also for stratifying risk for embolization and identifying patients who would benefit most from treatment. This chapter critically reviews each technique and attempts to define a rational approach to the diagnosis of left ventricular thrombi in the setting of an acute myocardial infarction, chronic left ventricular aneurysms, and patients with poor ventricular function. Each of these entities has either global or regional left ventricular dysfunction, a prerequisite for the development of ventricular thrombi. Much rarer intraventricular masses that might embolize are tumors. Following the discussion of the diagnostic approaches, strategies for treatment are developed.

Chapter 13: Cardiac Valves: Native and Prosthetic

Cardiac valves, native and prosthetic, are important sources of embolization. For bioprosthetic valves, it is recommended that paitents with valves in the mitral position, who are also in sinus rhythm, be treated for the first 3 months after valve insertion with warfarin at an INR of 2.0–3.0. Bioprosthetic valves in the aortic position, for patients in sinus rhythm, do not require anticoagulation. Patients with bioprosthetic valves in atrial fibrillation require anticoagulation with warfarin at an INR of between 2.0–3.0. This recommendation is extrapolated from the five atrial fibrillation studies that have recently been completed and which are discussed in detail in Chapter 14. Patients with mechanical valves should be anticoagulated at INRs of 2.0–3.0.

Thromboembolism is most common in patients with isolated mitral stenosis, less common in mitral regurgitation. Other conditions associated with systemic embolization are mitral valve prolapse and aortic valve disease. Infective causes of embolization are discussed in detail.

Chapter 14:   The Left Atrium

As in any other part of the body, the formation of thrombi in the left atrium is related to blood stasis. Factors contributing to left atrial stasis are left atrial enlargement and reduced atrial flow velocities due to atrial fibrillation, mitral stenosis, or low cardiac output state. The peripheral position of the left atrial appendage makes it particularly prone to low blood flow velocities. Recently, a new echocardiographic finding—spontaneous echocardiographic contrast (SEC) or "smoke"—has been associated with the presence of left atrial thrombus and/or embolization. It appears to be a marker of low velocity blood flow as well as of red cell rouleaux formation (clumping) and requires the presence of fibrinogen.

In addition to thrombi in the left atrium, myxomas and aneurysms of the atrial septum may constitute sources of systemic embolization. The major source of embolization, however, remains those patients with atrial fibrillation. It is strongly recommended that long-term warfarin therapy (INR 1.8–3) be used in patients with nonrheumatic atrial fibrillation who are eligible for anticoagulation. Patients with lone atrial fibrillation, irrespective of age, probably should not be treated. Patients with atrial fibrillation, younger than 65 with no history of hypertension, previous stroke, TIA, or diabetes, are at low risk of stroke and should not be anticoagulated. Patients with thyrotoxicosis, rheumatic heart disease, or congenital heart disease should be anticoagulated but may be considered for aspirin therapy. All other patients without a contraindication to warfarin therapy should be treated with warfarin. Patients who have a contraindication to warfarin therapy, but who otherwise could be treated with aspirin, should be treated at a dose of 325 mg daily, the only dose of aspirin shown to be better than placebo.

Chapter 15:   Paradoxical Embolization: Diagnosis and Management

The preponderance of systemic emboli probably arises from sources in the left-sided cardiac chambers or from systemic arterial embolization. These common causes of systemic embolization are covered in other chapters of this book. Sources of systemic embolization may also arise from the venous circulation, or the right heart chambers, and this phenomenon is termed *paradoxical embolization*. The gist of the paradox lies in the fact that the embolized material is not filtered from the circulation by the pulmonary capillaries; instead it transits to the systemic arterial circulation by an occult (e.g., patent foramen ovale) or manifest (e.g., atrial septal defect, ventricular septal defect, patent ductus arteriosus, pulmonary arteriovenous malformation) right to left shunt. In most clinical circumstances there is insufficient data to make a definitive diagnosis of paradoxical systemic embolization. The clinician must make a presumptive diagnosis based on four cardinal findings: (1) an identifiable embolic source; (2) a potential or manifest communication between the systemic venous and systemic arterial circulations; (3) appropriate physiological conditions favoring right to left shunting across this communication; and (4) a systemic arterial embolic event.

Chapter 16: The Aorta and Carotid Arteries

Historically, the aorta has received little attention as a possible source of unexplained embolic stroke or other embolic phenomena. The aortic arch is usually not visualized in detail during routine transthoracic echocardiography. With the introduction of trans-esophageal echocardiography it can now be seen with high resolution. Using this technique, large, protrusive plaques in the aortic arch and descending aorta, which have mobile projections that move freely with the blood flow, have been identified in patients with embolic events. The curious vulnerability of the carotid bifurcation to plaque formation has been ascribed to the local dynamics of flow. Flow studies of model bifurcations have demonstrated heterogeneous regions of high and low flow velocity, high and low shear stress, boundary layer separation, stagnation points, and secondary flow motions such as vortex and eddy formations. Medical management in symptomatic carotid disease is derived from contemporary understanding of the phathophysiology of the disease process. Treatment spans from risk factor management to platelet antiaggregation therapy to systemic anticoagulation to thrombolytic therapy. Modification of risk factors alone is appropriate only for asymptomatic patients who fall into high-risk categories. Once symptoms develop, modification of risk factors should be combined with other measures.

Chapter 17: Ventricular Assist Devices and the Total Artificial Heart: Clinical Uses and Thromboembolic Complications

Further advances in mechanical circulatory support are dependent upon the elimination of device-related complications such as infection and thromboembolic events that are particularly devastating in this critically ill patient population. The development of biocompatible materials that are resistant to infection and thrombosis is key to the realization of this goal. When gelatin glue becomes available for clinical use in the United States, a more aggressive antithrombotic approach may be possible. Endothelialized prosthetic materials may also provide a thromboresistant surface. Each of these developments will benefit the growing number of patients who require mechanical circulatory support by minimizing thrombo-embolic complications.

Michael D. Ezekowitz

Contents

Contributors

Gerald G. Blackwell, M.D.   Director, Clinical Cardiovascular Magnetic Resonance Imaging and Assistant Professor, Department of Medicine, Division of Cardiovascular Disease, University of Alabama, Birmingham, Alabama

Edwin G. Bovill, M.D.   Professor and Chairman, Department of Pathology, University of Vermont College of Medicine, Burlington, Vermont

Catherine M. Broome, M.D.   Assistant Clinical Professor of Medicine, Department of Hematology/Oncology, George Washington University Medical Center, Washington, D.C.

Terence L. Chen, M.D.   Diablo Neurosurgery Medical Group, Inc., Walnut Creek, California

Douglas Chyatte, M.D.   Assistant Professor of Neurosurgery and Head, Cerebrovascular Neurosurgeon, Division of Neurosurgery, Northwestern University Medical School, Chicago, Illinois

Ira S. Cohen, M.D.   Associate Professor of Medicine (Cardiovascular), Yale University School of Medicine, and Director, Noninvasive Cardiovascular Laboratories, West Haven Veterans Affairs, New Haven, Connecticut

Michael L. Dewar, M.D.   Assistant Professor of Surgery (Cardiothoracic), Yale University School of Medicine, New Haven, Connecticut

Holley M. Dey, M.D.   Associate Professor of Diagnostic Radiology, Yale University School of Medicine and Assistant Chief, Nuclear Medicine/PET, West Haven Veterans Affairs, New Haven, Connecticut

Michael D. Ezekowitz, M.D., Ph.D.   Professor of Medicine (Cardiovascular), Yale University School of Medicine, Chief, Cardiovascular Division, West Haven Veterans Affairs, and Director, Cardiovascular Thrombosis Research Laboratory, New Haven, Connecticut

Kenneth L. Franco, M.D.   Assistant Professor of Surgery, Department of Cardiothoracic Surgery, Yale University School of Medicine, New Haven, Connecticut

Charles C. Gornick, M.D.   Associate Professor of Medicine and Director, Pacing and Electrophysiology, Department of Medicine, VAMC and University of Minnesota, Minneapolis, Minnesota

Brian D. Guth, Ph.D.   Department of Pharmacological Research, Dr. Karl Thomae GmbH, Biberach, Germany

Lynwood W. Hammers, D.O.   Associate Professor, Department of Diagnostic Imaging, and Clinical Director of Ultrasound, Yale University School of Medicine, New Haven, Connecticut

Robert S. D. Higgins, M.D.   Surgical Director of Thoracic Organ Transplant Program, Division of Cardiac Surgery, Henry Ford Hospital, Detroit, Michigan

Jack Hirsh, M.D.   Director, Hamilton Civic Hospitals Research Centre, Henderson General Hospital, and Professor, Department of Medicine, McMaster University, Hamilton, Ontario, Canada

Clive Kearon, M.B., F.R.C.P.(C) , Ph.D.   Assistant Professor, Department of Medicine, McMaster University, Hamilton, Ontario, Canada

Craig Martin Kessler, M.D.   Professor of Medicine, Division of Hematology and Oncology, George Washington University Medical Center, Washington, D.C.

Jeffrey H. Lawson, M.D., Ph.D.   Resident, General and Thoracic Surgery, Department of Surgery, Duke University Medical Center, Durham, North Carolina

Eric K. Louie, M.D.   Associate Professor, Division of Cardiology, Department of Medicine, Loyola University Medical Center, Stritch School of Medicine, Maywood, Illinois

Kenneth G. Mann, Ph.D.   Professor and Chair, Department of Biochemistry, University of Vermont College of Medicine, Burlington, Vermont

Patrick H. McNulty, M.D.   Assistant Professor of Medicine, Section of Cardiovascular Medicine, Yale University School of Medicine, New Haven, Connecticut

Thomas H. Müller, M.D., Ph.D. Department of Pharmacological Research, Dr. Karl Thomae GmbH, Biberach, Germany

James A. Sadowski, Ph.D Professor, Scientist I, USDA Human Nutrition Research Center on Aging, Tufts University School of Nutrition, Boston, Massachusetts

William Stanford, M.D. Professor and Chief, Cardiovascular Radiology, Department of Radiology, University of Iowa College of Medicine, Iowa City, Iowa

Mathew L. Thakur, Ph.D. Professor and Director, Radiopharmaceutical Reseach and Professor of Diagnostic Radiology, Division of Nuclear Medicine, Department of Radiation Therapy, Thomas Jefferson University Hospital, Philadelphia, Pennsylvania

Russell P. Tracy, Ph.D. Associate Professor, Departments of Pathology and Biochemistry, University of Vermont College of Medicine, Burlington, Vermont

Robert M. Weiss, M.D. Assistant Professor, Department of Internal Medicine, Cardiovascular Division, University of Iowa College of Medicine, Iowa City, Iowa

I

FUNDAMENTAL ISSUES

1

Introduction

Michael D. Ezekowitz
*Yale University School of Medicine, West Haven Veterans Affairs,
and Cardiovascular Thrombosis Research Laboratory,
New Haven, Connecticut*

I. PREAMBLE

Until recently, the direct recognition of intracardiac thrombi was not possible. In most situations the diagnosis was inferred from the occurrence of an event consistent with a systemic embolus in a clinical setting in which the source was most likely cardiac. Thus, there has been considerable impetus to evaluate diagnostic modalities suitable for the detection of intracardiac thrombi. As a result, several techniques are now available, and strategies for treatment have followed. This book is based on the supposition that a thrombus may form in one location, dislodge, and be transported by the blood stream to a second location where it produces its adverse effect (embolization). For the most part in the chapters that follow, the origin of the thrombus is the heart and its final resting place is the brain. This book will emphasize prevention of systemic embolization rather than improved management of patients once embolic events have occurred. There are three sections. The first provides fundamental information regarding thrombosis and agents used to influence this process. The second will deal with tests used in evaluating patients with thrombotic disease, and the third discusses management.

II. DEVELOPMENT OF THE CONCEPT OF EMBOLIZATION

The first monograph discussing the relationship between the heart and stroke was published by Sir George Burrows in 1846 and was entitled "On disorders of the cerebral circulation; and the connections between affections of the brain and diseases of the heart" (1). It is difficult to determine with certainty, however, to whom the credit for the recognition of the phenomenon of thromboembolism should be given. Vesalius, according to Virchow, recognized the relationship between gangrene of an extremity and "unnatural depositions in the left atrium" (2). Lancisi, also according to Virchow, reported a case of heart disease in which the right hand suddenly was deprived of blood (2).

However, it is clear that Virchow, in 1847, made the greatest initial experimental contribution in furthering the concept of thromboembolism. In an autopsy study in 1846, he found clots in both the veins of the extremities and the pulmonary artery and deduced that intravascular coagula might be transported from the venous blood stream to the lungs. In 1847 he demonstrated the same phenomenon on the arterial side of the vascular system when he described seven cases of obstruction to the cerebral, splenic, renal, hepatic, and peripheral vessels by clots that appeared to have originated in the left atrium or on the heart valves. To further substantiate these findings, Virchow performed experiments showing that coagula and foreign bodies could be transported by the arterial blood stream.

It is intriguing to consider that the major obstacle to the evolution of the concept of thromboembolism was the controversy over whether intravascular clots could form during life. Kerkring, in 1670, and Pastas, in 1786, both argued that all intravascular clots occurred after death. Haller and Morgagni in the late 18th century developed the theory that most clots occurred post mortem but that it was possible for an intravascular clot to develop during life (3). Matthew Baillie, in 1793 (4), used the example of clots forming after a ligature as evidence that intravascular thrombosis is possible. In the same year, John Hunter (5) noted the occurrence of "inflammation of veins after surgery." Hunter believed that venous clots, if not adherent to the wall, could be swept into the general circulation and carried to distant parts of the body.

III. OVERVIEW

Today we are aware that thrombi occur most commonly within the left ventricle and the left atrium (Table 1). Less commonly, they are found in the right atrium and right ventricle.

Table 1 Causes of Cardiac Sources of Systemic Embolization

Left ventricle
    acute anterior transmural myocardial infarction
    acute inferior transmural myocardial infarction with apical involvement
    left ventricular aneurysm
    cardiomyopathy
    ventricular tumors
Valves
    endocarditis, infective and noninfective
    prosthetic valve dysfunction
    mitral prolapse
    rheumatic heart disease
Left atrium
    atrial fibrillation
    left atrial tumors (myxoma)
    atrial septal aneurysms
Paradoxical
Complications of cardiac manipulation
    cardiac catheterization
    cardiac surgery

Prosthetic valves, particularly of the nonbiological variety, are an important source of intracardiac thrombosis and systemic embolization. This is true also of native heart valves, especially in the setting of endocarditis, degenerative disorders, and mitral valve prolapse. Because thrombi at each of these locations provide different diagnostic challenges, have different clinical implications, and are diagnosed with varying degrees of accuracy, each will be considered separately. To complete the overall picture, chapters have been included that deal with paradoxical embolization (thrombi originating in the venous circulation or right side of the heart that traverse a defect, usually in the atrial septum, and then lodge in the systemic circulation) and emboli originating from the aorta and great vessels. Finally, emboli that complicate cardiac catheterization and bypass surgery are considered.

IV. THE USE OF STROKE AS A MARKER OF EMBOLIZATION

The most easily recognized and thus the most extensively studied manifestation and most commonly used marker of systemic embolization is stroke. This condition is multifactorial in etiology. In spite of an age-adjusted decline since the turn of the century, stroke remains the third leading cause of death in the United States (6,7). In this introductory chapter the nature and etiology of this decline will be discussed, as will the changing picture of stroke etiology, with emphasis on the declining role of hypertension and increasing importance of cardiac sources of embolization. Of the cardiac causes of systemic embolization, nonrheumatic atrial fibrillation is the most important.

Stroke mortality has been falling rapidly in the United States since the turn of the century (Fig. 1). The rate of decline accelerated after 1973 both in the United States (6,7) and in most Western nations (8), and this has been attributed to improvement in treatment and control of hypertension (7,9–12). Between 1973 and 1981 more than 200,000 fewer deaths were observed than would have been expected without the accelerated decline in stroke mortality (13). The accelerated decline since 1973 was seen in all age groups (Fig. 1) and races studied and in both sexes (6). Within each race and sex group the rate of decline increases with increasing age. The lowest rate of decline, 3.5 deaths per 100,000 per year, was seen among 55- to 64-year-old white women; the greatest, 69.7 deaths per 100,000 per year, among 75- to 84-year-old white men. With the exception of the latter groups, blacks had greater rates of decline than whites. Overall, stroke mortality between 1973 and 1981 fell approximately 7% per year, compared with approximately 2% per year between 1950 and 1972 (6).

That more than 200,000 fatal strokes were prevented between 1973 and 1981 in the United States is impressive. Moreover, if one assumes that only about one-third of strokes are fatal, approximately 400,000 nonfatal strokes, with considerable associated morbidity, also were prevented. It has been suggested (14) that data reflecting declining mortality rates related to stroke may be artifacts of changes in death certification or diagnostic practices, or of improved treatment. However, data collected from Olmstead County, Minnesota, in a population that has been evaluated with uniform methods over time, confirm that the national statistics (15,16) are likely to reflect a genuine declining trend in stroke-related mortality.

The decline of stroke is attributable to antihypertensive therapy. The national high blood pressure education program was instituted in 1973, coincident with the beginning of the period of rapid decline in stroke mortality. Clinical trials have demonstrated the efficacy of

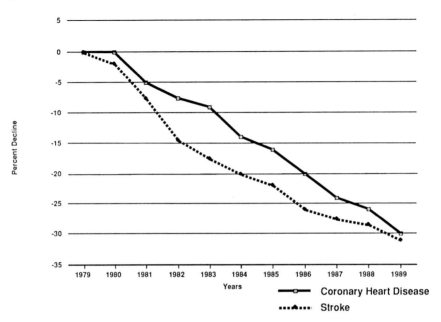

Figure 1 Cumulative percent decline in age-adjusted death rates for coronary heart disease and stroke, 1979–1989.

antihypertensive therapy in preventing approximately 40% of strokes within a relatively brief time after starting therapy (17).

Research by Klag et al. (8), however, does not entirely support an association between treatment and control of hypertension and the decline in stroke mortality. Their work is consistent with studies from New Zealand that attribute only 10% of the reduction in stroke mortality to the treatment of hypertension (18). Klag and colleagues (13) suggest that if control of hypertension does not entirely explain this decline, some widespread environmental agent may be a major factor in stroke etiology. They acknowledge that hypertension is the main risk factor for stroke and that other major risk factors such as age, sex, preexisting coronary disease, ventricular hypertrophy, cigarette smoking, elevated hematocrit, oral contraceptive use, and diabetes mellitus may contribute further. Mortality due to coronary heart disease has decreased since 1968, and the lower prevalence of heart disease may explain some of the decline in stroke mortality.

Several studies have demonstrated an increased risk of stroke among cigarette smokers (19–22). In fact, the risk of stroke attributable to cigarette smoking has been claimed to be higher than that associated with hypertension (20). Furthermore, persons who stop smoking have a lower risk of stroke than persons who continue to smoke (19,21,22). From 1965 to 1980 the number of ex-smokers in the United States rose among men and women, whites and blacks, and those aged 45 to 64 years and more than 64 years. Since persons with hypertension have been targeted for encouragement of smoking cessation, it is conceivable that smoking cessation either among hypertensives or in the general population could have accounted for some of the large decline in stroke mortality (13).

It is unlikely that changes in the formulation of oral contraceptives have played a role in the recent decline in strokes, since the decline is seen among both men and women.

Alcohol consumption also has been shown to be a risk factor for stroke (23,24). However, per-capita consumption of alcohol increased between 1950 and 1981 (23), while stroke rate declined. Thus, alcohol is an unlikely independent contributor to the current decline in stroke mortality. Other factors such as low potassium intake (24) and declining lead exposure (25) also have been implicated.

While national statistics have consistently shown an increased risk of death from stroke among blacks, few studies have addressed the etiology of this difference. Kittner (26) concluded that the higher prevalence of hypertension and diabetes among blacks may not account entirely for their higher stroke risk. Thus, a more complete understanding of the determinants of stroke may be required to account for the excess stroke risk experienced by blacks.

From the above, it seems clear that the declining incidence of stroke is largely attributable to the improved treatment of hypertension. Cardioembolic mechanisms have been implicated with increasing frequency as a cause of stroke (27). In spite of the increased understanding of the heart-brain relationship and the development of very sophisticated diagnostic technologies, establishing a cardiac cause of systemic embolization remains a diagnosis of inference. The diagnosis is made after considering both the neurological and the cardiovascular aspects of the presentation and after review of appropriately selected diagnostic studies. These will be discussed in more detail in subsequent chapters. In general, however, the diagnostic approach to a patient suspected of cardioembolic stroke is to determine from the clinical presentation whether there are features that suggest a cardioembolic mechanism or other mechanisms and also whether a cardiac condition is present that predisposes to systemic embolization. The diagnostic evaluation is then designed to identify the mechanism of cerebral infarction and also to determine whether a cardiac cause is present. A number of clinical features of cardioembolic brain infarction have been suggested by Mohr (27) and Easton (28). These are its sudden onset in 79% of cases and lack of history of antecedent transient ischemic attacks in 89% of cases. Alteration in level of consciousness, the presence of seizures at onset, and headache are generally infrequent and nondiscriminating.

Additional clinical features useful in suggesting cardioembolic mechanisms are related to the distribution of the infarction. The middle cerebral artery distribution is the most common site, implicated in about 75% of cases, with the posterior cerebral artery and basilar artery each accounting for an additional 10%. The anterior cerebral artery distribution is a very uncommon site for embolization. The age of the patient also may be significant. Younger patients have less atherosclerotic vascular disease, and thus, if a cardiac mechanism is identified, it is most likely the etiology. Evidence of systemic embolizations to other locations within the brain or elsewhere in the body is highly suggestive of a cardioembolic mechanism. Negative findings such as the absence of extracranial carotid artery disease ipsilateral to the site of the ischemic event increases the likelihood of a cardiac source. The presence of a cardiac condition known to be associated with systemic embolization increases the possibility of a cardiac source of systemic embolization.

Given that the diagnosis of cardiac causes of systemic embolization is at best imperfect, there is mounting evidence that, although the incidence of ischemic stroke has declined and continues to do so, the proportion of strokes attributable to cardiogenic causes is increasing. This may, in part, be due to the introduction and development of noninvasive diagnostic modalities such as echocardiography, which have allowed the improved detection of cardioembolic sources. It is estimated that about 20% of ischemic strokes are related to cardiac emboli (27).

Among the causes of stroke attributable to the heart (Table 1), nonrheumatic atrial fibrillation is gaining in importance. It is accepted that the prevalence of nonrheumatic atrial fibrillation increases with age, and this prevalence estimated to be between 2% and 5% among persons over the age of 60 (30,31). As the population of the United States and other developed countries ages, the prevalence of atrial fibrillation will increase substantially. The embolism rate among untreated patients with atrial fibrillation is between 3.8% and 7.2% per year (31–34). Most patients with nonrheumatic atrial fibrillation have intrinsic heart disease and associated disease in other vascular beds. There is a smaller subset of patients with isolated atrial fibrillation. These are apparently at lower risk for systemic embolization than patients with associated disease (31–35).

In contrast to the situation with patients who have nonrheumatic atrial fibrillation, the proportional decline of ischemic heart disease and the dramatic role that thrombolytic agents have played in the treatment of the hyperacute phase of myocardial infarction support the contention that myocardial infarction will play a declining role as a potential source of systemic embolization. This is largely because improved therapy serves to reduce the extent of left ventricular dysfunction, thereby reducing stasis and low-flow situations in the ventricle, both of which lead to thrombosis and ultimately to embolization.

V. CLINICAL TRIALS

Clinical trials play a central role in guiding health care providers to optimal care. There is no area in medicine where this is better exemplified than in treatment of patients who have thromboembolic disease, and this book will rely heavily on data collected from such trials. The modern era of randomized clinical trials began in the early 1950s with the evaluation of streptomycin in patients with tuberculosis (36,37). Mechanisms have been established to safeguard the interests of the individual patient who elects to participate in one of these trials. Passamani, in an editorial in the *New England Journal of Medicine* (37), made several important points concerning the validity of clinical trials. Randomization tends to produce treatment and control that are equally balanced. Clinical trials strengthen or refute many common therapies so as to better guide physicians in the optimal care of patients and to protect patients enrolled in clinical studies.

REFERENCES

1. Burrows G. Disorders of the cerebral circulation; and on the connection between affections of the heart. Philadelphia: Lea & Blanchard, 1848.
2. Virchow R. Ueber die akut Entzundung der Arterien. Virchows Arch Pathol Anat 1847; 1: 272–378.
3. Furlan AJ, ed. The heart and stroke—exploring mutual cerebrovascular and cardiovascular issues. Berlin: Springer-Verlag, 1987.
4. Baillie M. Trans Soc Improv Med Chir Knowl (London) 1793; 1:119–137.
5. Hunter J. Observations on the inflammation of the internal coats of veins. Trans Soc Improv Med Chir Knowl (London) 1793; 1:18–29.
6. Whelton PK. Declining mortality from hypertension and stroke. South Med J 1982; 75:33–8.
7. Baum HM, Goldstein M. Cerebrovascular disease type specific mortality: 1968–1977. Stroke 1982; 13:810–7.
8. Whelton PK, Klag MJ. Recent trends in the epidemiology of stroke: What accounts for the stroke decline in Western nations? Curr Opin Cardiol 1987; 2:741–7.
9. Why has stroke mortality declined? (editorial). Lancet 1983; 1:1195–6.

10. Garraway WM, Whisnant JP, Furlan AJ, Phillips LH, Kurland LT, O'Fallon WM. The declining incidence of stroke. N Engl J Med 1979; 300:449–52.

11. Tuomilheto J, Nissinen A, Wolf E, Geboers J, Piha T, Puska P. Effectiveness of treatment with antihypertensive drugs and trends in mortality from stroke in the community. Br Med J 1985; 219:857–61.

12. Ostfelt AM. A review of stroke epidemiology. Epidemiol Rev 1980; 2:136–52.

13. Klag MJ, Whelton PK, Seidler AJ. Decline in US stroke mortality—demographic trends and antihypertensive treatment. Stroke 1989; 20:14–21.

14. Wolf PA, Kannel WB, Cupples LA, D'Agostino RB. Risk factor interaction in cardiovascular and cerebrovascular disease. In: Furlan AJ, ed. The heart and stroke—exploring mutual cerebrovascular and cardiovascular issues. Berlin: Springer-Verlag, 1987:331–56.

15. Anderson GL, Whisnant JP. A comparison of trends in mortality from stroke in the United States and Rochester, Minnesota. Stroke 1982; 13:804–9.

16. Garraway WM, Whisnant JP, Drury I. The continuing decline in the incidence of stroke. Mayo Clin Proc 1983; 58:520–3.

17. MacMahon SW, Cutler JA, Furberg CD, Payne GH. The effects of drug treatment for hypertension on morbidity and mortality from cardiovascular disease: a review of randomized controlled trials. Prog Cardiovasc Dis 1986; 29(suppl 1):99–118.

18. Bonita R, Beaglehole R. Does treatment of hypertension explain the decline in mortality from stroke? Br Med J 1986; 292:191–2.

19. Abbott RD, Yin Y, Reed DM, Yano K. Risk of stroke in male cigarette smokers. N Engl J Med 1986; 315:717–20.

20. Bonita R, Scragg R, Stewart A, Jackson R, Beaglehole R. Cigarette smoking and risk of premature stroke in men and women. Br Med J 1986; 293:6338–40.

21. Colditz GA, Bonita R, Stampfer MJ, Willett WC, Rosner B, Speizer FE, Hennekens CH. Cigarette smoking and risk of stroke in middle-aged women. N Engl J Med 1988; 318:937–41.

22. Wolf PA, D'Agostino RB, Kannel WB, Bonita R, Belanger AJ. Cigarette smoking as a risk factor for stroke. JAMA 1988; 259:1025–9.

23. Doernberg D, Stinson F. US alcohol epidemiologic data reference manual, vol 1. US apparent consumption of alcoholic beverages based on state sales, taxation, or receipt data. NTIS PB 86-147576/AS. Washington, DC: US Government Printing Office, 1985.

24. Khaw KT, Barrett-Connor E. Dietary potassium and stroke-associated mortality: a 12-year prospective population study. N Engl J Med 1986; 316:235–40.

25. Roberts J, Mahaffey KR, Annest JL. Blood lead levels in general populations, In: Mahaffey KR, ed. Dietary environmental lead: human health effects. New York: Elsevier, 1985:355–72.

26. Kittner SJ, White LR, Katalin GL, Wolf PA, Hebel R. Black–white differences in stroke incidence in a national sample. JAMA 1990: 264:1267–1270.

27. Mohr J, Caplan LR, Melski JW, Goldstein RJ, Duncan GW, Kistler JP, Pessin MS, Bleich HL. The Harvard Cooperative Stroke Registry: a prospective registry. Neurology 1978; 28:754–62.

28. Easton JD, Sherman DG. Management of cerebral embolism of cardiac origin. Stroke 1980; 11:433–42.

29. Hart RG, Sherman DJ, Miller VT, Easton JD. Diagnosis and management of ischemic stroke, part II, selected controversies. Curr Prob Cardiol 1983; 8:53–9.

30. Wolf PA, Dawber TR, Thomas HE, Jr., Kannel WB. Epidemiologic assessment of chronic atrial fibrillation and risk of stroke: the Framingham Study. Neurology 1978; 28:973–7.

31. The Boston Area Anticoagulation Trial for Atrial Fibrillation Investigators. The effect of low-dose warfarin on the risk of stroke in patients with nonrheumatic atrial fibrillation. N Engl J Med 1990; 323:1505–11.

32. Ezekowitz MD, Bridgers SL, James KE, Carliner NH, Colling CL, Gornick CC, Krause-Steinrauf H, Kurtzke JF, Nazarian SM, Radford MJ, Rickles FR, Shabetai R, Deykin D, for the VA SPINAF Investigators. Warfarin in the prevention of stroke associated with nonrheumatic atrial fibrillation. N Engl J Med 1992; 327:1406–12.

33. Petersen P, Godtfredsen J, Bovsen G, Anderson ED, Andersen B. Placebo-controlled, randomized trial of warfarin and aspirin for prevention of thromboembolic complications in chronic atrial fibrillation. The Copenhagen AFASAK Study. Lancet 1989; 1:175–9.
34. Singer DE. Randomized trials of warfarin for atrial fibrillation (editorial). N Engl J Med 1992; 327:1451–3.
35. Brand FN, Abbott RD, Kannel WB, Wolf PA. Characteristics and prognosis of lone atrial fibrillation: 30 year follow-up in the Framingham study. JAMA 1985; 254:3449–53.
36. Streptomycin and Tuberculosis Trial Committee, Medical Research Council. Streptomycin treatment of pulmonary tuberculosis: a Medical Research Council investigation. Br Med J 1948; 2:769–82.
37. Passamani E. Clinical trials—are they ethical? N Engl J Med 1991; 324:1589–91.

2

Physiology of Coagulation

Craig Martin Kessler and Catherine M. Broome
George Washington University Medical Center,
Washington, D.C.

I. INTRODUCTION

Normal hemostasis is a complex process dependent on the coordinated interaction of three major components: humoral plasma proteins, which promote and modulate blood coagulation; the platelets, which initiate and promote hemostasis; and the vascular endothelial cells, which synthesize, store, and release vasoactive substances, adhesive proteins, and activators and inhibitors of coagulation, platelet function, and fibrinolysis. This sequential and orchestrated process is designed to preserve the integrity of the closed circulatory system and to minimize blood loss following injury to the vascular framework while simultaneously maintaining the fluidity and uninterrupted flow of blood.

II. ENDOTHELIAL CELLS

The endothelial cells lining the luminal surfaces of the vasculature provide the primary barrier against hemorrhage and possess the capacity to influence thrombus formation by serving as a surface on which certain molecular interactions can proceed. They also elaborate a variety of substances that interact with vascular smooth muscle cells, circulating coagulation proteins, and platelets. The endothelial cell monolayer is supported by a selectively impermeable subendothelial matrix, which functions as a secondary protective membrane against hemorrhage in the event of endothelial cell injury. Many of the interstitial components of the subendothelial matrix are synthesized and secreted by endothelial cells; these components predominantly include collagen, elastin, microfibrils, mucopolysaccharides such as heparan sulfate, laminin, fibronectin, von Willebrand factor (vWf), vitronectin, thrombospondin, and fibrin (1), each of which participates to various degrees of physiologic significance in the process of normal hemostasis. Intact endothelium primarily maintains blood fluidity; however, vascular injury denudes the protective endothelium and

Table 1   The Endothelium and Hemostasis

	Location	Function
Thrombogenic Mediators		
Collagen	Subendothelial matrix	Endothelial cell and platelet adhesion
		Platelet aggregation
		Platelet activation
von Willebrand factor	Subendothelial matrix	Platelet adhesion
	Endothelial cell–synthesized	Platelet aggregation
		Platelet activation
Vitronectin	Subendothelial matrix	Platelet adhesion
Fibronectin	Subendothelial matrix	Platelet adhesion
Thrombospondin	Subendothelial matrix	Platelet adhesion
		Platelet aggregation
Platelet activating factor	Endothelial cell–associated	Platelet adhesion
		Platelet activation
Tissue factor	Endothelial cell–associated	Activates factor VII
Factor V	Endothelial cell–associated	Accelerates activation of prothrombin by factor Xa
Endothelin	Endothelial cell–associated	Vasoconstriction
Antithrombogenic Mediators		
Endothelial cells	Overlying subendothelium	Intrinsically nonthrombogenic
Prostacyclin	Endothelial cell–synthesized	Vasodilitation
		Inhibitor of platelet activation
Endothelium-derived relaxing factor (nitric oxide)	Endothelial cell–synthesized	Vasodilitation
		Inhibitor of platelet adhesion
		Inhibitor of platelet aggregation
Heparan sulfate	Endothelial cell	Potentiator of antithrombin III
	Extracellular matrix	Inhibition of serine proteases
	Endothelial cell–synthesized	
13-Hydroxyoctadecadienoic acid	Endothelial cell–synthesized	Inhibitor of platelet adhesion
		Inhibitor of platelet aggregation
Thrombomodulin	Endothelial cell–associated	Binds thrombin

exposes the constituents of the subendothelial matrix, which ultimately function as templates for the localized generation of coagulation enzyme activity, the binding of adhesive glycoproteins, and the binding of signal-inducing ligands that promote vasoconstriction or vasodilatation and amplify platelet recruitment and activation at the site of vessel injury (2).

A.   Prothrombotic Reactions: The Endothelium and Subendothelial Matrix

Although endothelial cells cultured in vitro synthesize five major types of collagen (designated I, III, IV, V, and VIII) (3), the subendothelial matrix contains primarily collagen types IV and V. Each type of collagen is capable of supporting platelet adhesion. Collagen types IV and V also promote endothelial cell adhesion and chemotaxis (4), with the VLA-2 integrin-related protein (homologous with glycoprotein Ia/IIa on the platelet membrane) serving as the type I and IV collagen receptor on the surface of endothelial cells (5). Collagen types IV and V induce platelet aggregation and thromboxane A_2 release in a nonrandom fashion (6) at the site of vascular injury. Collagen types I and III also support the adhesion and aggregation of platelets but, in addition, provide the negatively charged surface necessary to activate coagulation factor XII (FXII), which initiates the intrinsic pathway of thrombin (FIIa) generation and fibrin formation. Increased amounts of collagen types I and IV have been observed in diabetic vascular disease and in atherosclerosis, but while this finding is provocative, cause-effect relationships have yet to be established.

Circulating platelets interact with the exposed collagen components of the subendothelial matrix directly through specific collagen receptors on the platelet membrane, or indirectly by binding to bridging proteins attached to collagen. The former process is facilitated by the glycoprotein Ia-IIa complex on the platelet surface. The congenital deficiency of this integrin receptor has been associated with defective collagen-induced platelet aggregation in vitro and a hemorrhagic diathesis in vivo. The latter mechanism of platelet-collagen interaction is mediated by the bridging protein vWf. The importance of this adhesive protein has been confirmed in numerous in vivo and in vitro experiments employing immobilized collagen on glass bead surfaces (7) or de-endothelialized rabbit aorta (8) (Baumgartner model), demonstrating the critical bridging properties of vWf between platelets and collagen. Von Willebrand factor is synthesized by megakaryocytes and endothelial cells and stored in Weibel-Palade bodies of endothelial cells and the alpha granules of platelets. It is secreted into plasma and the surrounding subendothelial matrix. Von Willebrand factor circulates in plasma as an extremely large glycoprotein with variable molecular weights up to 20 million daltons, depending on the degree of multimeric composition (8). The multimers of vWf protein with the largest molecular weight possess the most potent biological potential to support platelet collagen interactions (adhesion) and platelet-platelet interactions (aggregation) (9). Under pathologic conditions such as exposure of the type I collagen contained in ruptured atherosclerotic plaques (10,11) to circulating platelets and coagulation proteins, the high-molecular-weight multimers of vWf protein have been shown to play a vital role in the generation and propagation of thrombus. The bridging property of vWf protein between platelets and collagen occurs most efficiently at high shear rates, such as would be encountered in atherosclerotic, stenotic, or small-diameter vessels (12), and is achieved through the binding of separate distinct vWf domains to collagen and to the glycoprotein Ib receptor on the platelet surface. In contrast, when vWf mediates platelet-platelet interactions during platelet activation and aggregation, it interacts along with various other adhesive proteins (fibrinogen [FI], fibronectin, thrombospondin, vitronectin, etc.) with the glycoprotein IIb-IIIa complex on the platelet membrane. Von Willebrand factor circulates in plasma stoichiometrically complexed to the FVIII coagulant (FVIII:C) protein and probably stabilizes FVIII:C activity, protecting it from in vivo proteolysis and prolonging its circulation time in the intravascular space.

Additional constitutive proteins present in the subendothelial matrix include vitronectin, thrombospondin, and fibronectin (13). Each of these "adhesins" appears capable of supporting platelet adhesion by binding to the glycoprotein IIb-IIIa complex on the platelet surface, and all are released from the platelet alpha granule upon platelet activation. Vitronectin also mediates the attachment of endothelial cells to the subendothelium (14) and complexes to plasminogen activator inhibitor (PAI-1), possibly modulating fibrinolytic activity induced by urokinase and tissue plasminogen activator.

No hereditary deficiency of vitronectin has been reported to corroborate its physiologic significance. Fibronectin and thrombospondin bind to receptors on endothelial cells to affect endothelial cell attachment and growth. Thrombospondin may modulate atheromatous plaque formation at sites of vascular injury by regulating smooth muscle cell proliferation. The single reported case of thrombospondin deficiency manifested subtle abnormalities in collagen-induced platelet aggregation in vitro. Similar platelet dysfunction has been associated with a congenital qualitative fibronectin abnormality. Both fibronectin and thrombospondin bind to heparan sulfate, the predominant anticoagulant mucopolysaccharide on the endothelial cell surface. The significance of these interactions remains to be determined.

Once platelets adhere to subendothelial matrix components, they may be activated through interactions with vWf protein, fibrin complexes, and/or collagen. This process involves an initial shape change, which exposes membrane phospholipids and induces phospholipase A_2, subsequently releasing arachidonic acid from the platelet membrane. Arachidonic acid is then converted by the enzyme cyclooxygenase to prostaglandin G_2 (PGG_2) and PGH2, prostaglandin endoperoxide intermediates, and subsequently to thromboxane A_2 via the enzyme thromboxane synthetase. An additional but minor pathway for the release of arachidonic acid involves the cleavage of phosphatidylinositol by phospholipase C into inositol phosphates and diacylglycerol (15). A mono- and di-aglyceride lipase then removes arachidonic acid from diacylglycerol (Fig. 1). Thromboxane A_2 and the intermediate endoperoxides are secreted from the platelet and function as potent vasoconstrictors and platelet agonists, potentiating platelet recruitment and aggregation. Platelets bound to collagen also can release adenosine diphosphate (ADP) from the dense granules, and ADP serves as an additional agonist for platelet aggregation. Platelet aggregation is an irreversible reaction that is associated with the local release of numerous coagulation factors, vWf protein, and modulators of coagulation and fibrinolysis. Endothelial cells synthesize an additional prothrombotic substance termed platelet-activating factor (PAF), which induces platelet adhesion to endothelial cells. Because of its simultaneous capacity to promote

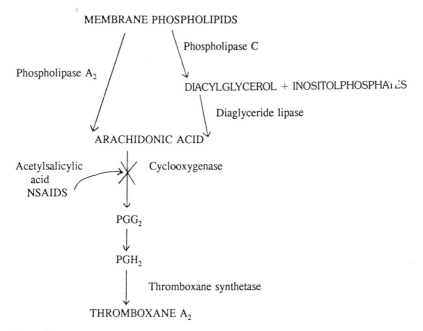

Figure 1 Platelet arachidonic acid metabolism.

monocyte adherence and polymorphonuclear leukocyte chemotaxis, PAF may be particularly important in stimulating hemostasis in areas of inflammation (16).

In resting endothelial cells, minimal tissue factor activity is expressed (17). However, when the endothelial cell is exposed to thrombin, endotoxin, interferon, or tissue necrosis factor, the activity of this transmembrane protein is increased up to 40-fold (18). Tissue factor then supports thrombin generation and fibrin formation predominantly through the extrinsic pathway, but there is considerable activation of factor IX (FIX) in the intrinsic pathway by FVIIa (19). Factor V also is synthesized by endothelial cells (20) and is activated by a membrane-associated protease, the expression of which is up-regulated by endothelial cell injury (21). Factor V functions in the common pathway of the coagulation system as a cofactor in the enzymatic cleavage of prothrombin (FII) by factor Xa (FXa) in the presence of calcium.

The vascular endothelium plays an important role in the localization of the coagulation process by providing binding sites on its membrane surface for several coagulation proteins. These include both the native and the active forms of coagulation factors IX and X, as well as high-molecular-weight kininogen (HMWK), fibrinogen, and fibrin (22,23). Not only do endothelial cells bind coagulation proteins but, through a specific endothelial cell membrane–bound protease, rabbit endothelial cells have been shown to activate FXII directly via proteolytic cleavage (24), thus further localizing the activation of the intrinsic pathway of thrombin generation and fibrin formation. Binding of FIX and FX may also provide an efficient clearance mechanism to reduce circulating activated coagulation proteins, thus reducing hypercoagulable potential. Endothelial cells also synthesize, store, and upon injury or perturbation release plasminogen activator inhibitors, which prevent plasmin formation and fibrinolysis by urokinase and tissue plasminogen activator; PAF, a potent agonist of platelet aggregation; and tissue factor, which complexes with coagulation FVII to enhance activation of FX and FIX.

B. Antithrombotic Properties of the Endothelial Cell and Subendothelial Matrix

The endothelial cell is naturally antithrombogenic by virtue of its antiplatelet and anticoagulant properties. Antiplatelet activities of endothelial cells are accomplished in part by the synthesis, storage, and secretion of prostacyclin (PGI$_2$), a very potent vasodilator and inhibitor of platelet function that stimulates adenylate cyclase activity (25). The subsequent increase in intraplatelet cyclic AMP inhibits platelet shape change, platelet aggregation and the secretion of granule contents (26). Prostacyclin also acts to prevent platelet adhesion to the subendothelial matrix. This direct inhibition of adhesion is most pronounced under conditions of high shear rates (27). Endothelium-derived relaxing factor (EDRF), which acts synergistically with PGI$_2$ to inhibit platelet adhesion and aggregation (28), is identical to nitric oxide and is synthesized predominantly by vascular endothelial cells but also by neutrophils, monocytes, and cytokine-treated smooth muscle cells. Endothelium-derived relaxing factor is the product of the enzymatic action of nitric oxide synthase on L-arginine (29) and mediates vasodilatation and platelet inhibition by increasing the intracellular concentration of cyclic guanosine monophosphate (GMP) (30) in smooth muscle cells and platelets. Cyclic GMP levels can be enhanced pharmacologically by nitrosothiols and organic nitrates, frequently given to cardiac patients. Reduced thiols such as N-acetylcysteine induce guanylate synthetase and potentiate the antiplatelet effects of EDRF by enhancing cyclic GMP levels. Significantly decreased levels of EDRF production have been observed in isolated atherosclerotic blood vessels from experimental animals and may be implicated in pathologic platelet activation with subsequent coronary artery vasospasm in humans. 13-Hydroxyoctadecadienoic acid (13-HODE) is a less well understood prostaglandin produced by endothelial cells from linoleic acid (31). It is located on the subendothelial basement membrane in vivo and is believed to function there to inhibit platelet adhesion to the subendothelium (16).

Endothelial cells are coated by a mucopolysaccharide layer consisting predominantly of the proteoglycan heparan sulfate, a potent anticoagulant (32) that is synthesized and released by the endothelial cell into the subendothelial matrix. When circulating antithrombin III interacts with the highly negatively charged heparan sulfate, a conformational alteration occurs and exposes a binding site for activated serine proteases, including FXa, FXIa, and thrombin. Once the serine protease–antithrombin III complex forms, the activated clotting factors are neutralized (33,34) and fibrin formation is inhibited on the endothelial cell surface. (Hereditary or acquired deficiency of antithrombin III results in the recurrent formation of clinically important venous and, less commonly, arterial thrombosis.)

Thrombomodulin is a large adhesin glycoprotein (35) that conveys antithrombotic activity by binding to thrombin and preventing thrombin from converting fibrinogen to fibrin, from activating platelets, and also by activating protein C. Thrombomodulin is contained and secreted by platelets, macrophages, endothelial cells, and smooth muscle cells and is predominantly a surface-bound protein, providing 50–60% of the thrombin-binding sites on endothelial cells (36) and the subendothelial matrix. Thrombomodulin interacts with the glycoprotein IIb-IIIa complex on the platelet membrane. Thrombomodulin is therefore strategically located to mediate platelet adhesion and aggregation and to modulate fibrin formation. No cases of thrombomodulin deficiency have been documented.

Protein C, a vitamin K–dependent protein synthesized in the liver, modulates thrombin generation by inactivating clotting factors Va and VIIIa and complexes with plasminogen activator inhibitor type 1 (PAI-1) to enhance fibrinolysis via plasmin generation induced by tissue plasminogen activator. The anticoagulant activity of protein C, which can be achieved only after activation by thrombin (a process modulated by thrombomodulin), is markedly enhanced by interacting with another vitamin K–dependent protein, protein S (37). Protein S binds to the endothelial cell membrane and then binds protein C, creating a cell surface–bound complex (16) that inactivates FVa and FVIIIa. Inherited or acquired deficiencies of protein C and/or protein S are associated with hypercoagulability manifested as recurrent venous and/or arterial thromboses (38). Protein S is contained in and released from endothelial cells and the alpha granules of platelets.

Additional antithrombotic potential is promoted by the endothelial cell synthesis, storage, and release of tissue plasminogen activator and urokinase plasminogen activator, both of which enhance plasmin generation and fibrinolysis. The synthesis and secretion of tissue plasminogen activator are stimulated after endothelial cell activation by the unique pathogenic plasma lipoprotein lipoprotein (a) [Lp(a)], which is atherogenic, antifibrinolytic, and prothrombotic. Increased levels of Lp(a) are associated with an increased risk of coronary atherosclerosis, cerebrovascular disease, and stenosis of coronary artery bypass grafts. Because the protein has marked homology with plasminogen, thrombogenesis may be promoted by the competitive inhibition of the two proteins for plasminogen binding sites on fibrin, endothelial cell surfaces, and platelet membranes, resulting in impaired plasminogen activation by tissue plasminogen activator. In the presence of normal Lp(a) levels, plasminogen activation is enhanced on these surfaces. These observations provide a new focus for development of antiatherogenic drugs that possess the capability of lowering Lp(a) levels or reversing their effects.

III. PLASMA COAGULATION PROTEINS

The plasma coagulation proteins play a vital role in normal hemostasis via a series of sequential enzymatic reactions culminating in the generation of thrombin, which then proteolytically cleaves fibrinogen to form fibrin, the framework of a stable clot. Most of the coagulation proteins function in this system as enzymes and circulate in the plasma as inactive proenzymes, or zymogens, which are activated via the proteolytic cleavage of peptide bonds by the preceding activated clotting factor protein—thus the term "coagulation cascade" (39). Other coagulation proteins such as FVIII (procoagulant protein FVIII:C) and FV function as coenzymes for pivotal enzymatic reactions. Because these cofactors require the presence of a phospholipid template and calcium ions, they participate in localizing reactions to platelet and/or endothelial cell membrane surfaces, thus decreasing the propensity for uncontrolled diffuse activation of the coagulation system.

The coagulation system has been traditionally divided into the intrinsic pathway of coagulation, which is activated by components intrinsic to the blood vessel itself, i.e., negatively charged collagen within the subendothelial matrix exposed after endothelial cell injury, and the extrinsic pathway of coagulation, which depends on elements extrinsic to the blood vessel for activation, i.e., tissue factor or tissue thromboplastin in the interstitium. This separation has continued to provide a valid clinical approach to the laboratory detection of coagulation deficiencies; however, in vitro evidence indicates that extensive biochemical interactions occur among components of the two pathways and that these reactions are physiologically significant.

The activation of coagulation through the intrinsic pathway can be accomplished through multiple mechanisms of activation of factor XII (FXII), or Hageman factor, named for the propositus patient described with FXII deficiency. The most physiologically important process of FXII activation involves interactions of the circulating plasma FXII zymogen with negatively charged surfaces such as the exposed collagen in the denuded subendothelial matrix of damaged vessels. Factor XII circulates in plasma complexed to HMWK. In vitro, this reaction may be initiated by contact with a glass surface—thus, the term "contact phase" of coagulation. Deficiency of FXII does not produce any clinical bleeding problems, even with surgical trauma. The fact that the propositus, Mr. Hageman, and numerous others since have experienced fatal or life-threatening thromboembolic events suggests a role for FXII as a plasminogen activator to initiate fibrinolysis; however, this remains unproven. Factor XIIa (activated FXII) in turn enzymatically facilitates the conversion of FXI to FXIa.

Other components of the contact phase of coagulation include HMWK and prekallikrein (PK), which mediate inflammatory responses and enhance the activation of FXI by FXIIa. Hereditary deficiencies of HMWK (Williams, Fleaujeac, Fitzgerald factor) and PK (Fletcher factor) produce no hemorrhagic complications. The diagnosis of deficiencies in the contact phase of coagulation is suggested by isolated prolongation of the partial thromboplastin time (PTT), which normalizes in mixing studies with normal plasma.

Factor XIa in the presence of calcium ions activates FIX to FIXa. Deficiency of FXI occurs most commonly in Ashkenazi Jewish kindreds, and the severity of associated bleeding manifestations does not always correlate with the decreased FXI levels measured in the laboratory. This discrepancy may be related to the presence of normal levels of FXI in circulating platelets.

Factor IXa complexes with FVIIIa and calcium on the phospholipid template provided by the endothelial cell or platelet membrane to form tenase (40–42), which proteolytically cleaves the proenzyme FX to form the enzyme FXa. The sex-linked recessive inherited deficiencies of clotting FVIII:C protein and FIX are the most commonly encountered congenital coagulopathies in clinical practice, occurring in approximately one per 5000 live male births for FVIII (hemophilia A) versus one per 25,000 to 30,000 live male births for FIX (hemophilia B, Christmas disease). Factor IX is characteristic of all of the vitamin K–dependent coagulation proteins (FII, FVII, FIX, and FX) in that it is synthesized in the hepatocyte and requires postribosomal modification (mediated by a vitamin K–dependent carboxylase enzyme) and carboxylation of glutamic acid residues in order to participate in calcium-dependent phospholipid template binding for expression of clotting activity; and these proteins have considerable amino acid sequence homology, with multiple epidermal growth factor–like domains, activation peptide regions, and catalytic domains typical of serine proteases (serpins). The activation of FIX by FXIa generated in the intrinsic pathway appears to proceed less rapidly and efficiently than FIX activation by FVIIa generated in the extrinsic pathway. This "crossover" activation step may explain the mild nature of the bleeding problems seen in many FXI-deficient patients. Factor VIII:C also is synthesized in hepatocytes and possesses structural homology with FV and ceruloplasmin. Factor VIII:C circulates in plasma complexed to vWf protein, which stabilizes FVIII:C activity by protecting the molecule from proteolysis and preventing it from leaving the intravascular space. The expression of FVIII:C activity is enhanced in the presence of vWf complex; the adhesion qualities of vWf probably juxtapose FVIII:C with the phospholipid membranes of activated platelet aggregates and injured endothelial cells and thus localize the coagulation process. Factor VIII:C activation occurs by thrombin cleavage; subsequent inactivation of FVIIIa occurs in the presence of larger amounts of thrombin as well as by FXa and activated protein C. Deficiencies of FVIII:C and FIX typically produce isolated prolongations in the activated partial thromboplastin time (aPTT).

The vWf protein is an extremely large multimeric protein that is synthesized in the endothelial cells and megakaryocytes and stored within endothelial cell Weibel-Palade bodies and the alpha granules of platelets and megakaryocytes. Von Willebrand factor is critical in mediating platelet adhesion to collagen contained in the subendothelial matrix, especially at high shear rates, promotes platelet-platelet interaction and aggregation, and complexes with and stabilizes FVIII:C to maximize its circulation time and coagulation activity in plasma. Von Willebrand factor is an adhesive protein (adhesin or integrin), and its structure-function relationship is conveyed by its multimeric composition. The largest-molecular-weight multimers are the most effective in bridging platelets to subendothelial collagen with the glycoprotein Ib receptor on the platelet membrane to mediate adhesion and in interacting with the membrane glycoprotein IIb-IIIa complex on adjacent platelets to achieve aggregation. Quantitative deficiencies and qualitative abnormalities of vWf are associated with von Willebrand disease (vWd), characterized predominantly by mucocutaneous bleeding problems, such as epistaxis, gastrointestinal bleeding, and menorrhagia. Except for the very unusual and severe autosomal recessive type III form of vWd, all other forms of vWd, including the classical type and variants, are inherited in an autosomal dominant pattern and therefore affect both sexes, with a prevalence estimated at around 1% of the population. Animal studies suggest that vWf protein may be involved in atherogenesis in vivo, since severely vWf-deficient pigs do not develop atherosclerotic vascular disease despite being fed atherogenic diets.

The laboratory diagnosis of vWd is based on the presence of a prolonged bleeding time, decreased functional (vWf activity and ristocetin cofactor activity) and immunologic (vWf antigen) levels of vWf in plasma, and the analysis of the multimeric composition of plasma vWf protein on SDS-agarose electrophoresis. Factor VIII:C activity levels are variably decreased as well, reflecting vWf-FVIII:C interactions, and this may prolong the aPTT and exacerbate the bleeding potential of vWd. Because of decreased FVIII:C levels, vWd may occasionally be difficult to differentiate from hemophilia A; however, normal bleeding times, normal vWf activity, and a sex-linked pattern of inheritance are characteristic of hemophilia A.

Factor Xa complexes, on phospholipid surfaces provided, in vivo, by platelets and/or endothelial cells (41,42), with FVa and calcium to form prothrombinase, which converts prothrombin to the active enzyme thrombin. Factor X shares all of the characteristics of the vitamin K–dependent clotting factors and serine proteases. Because FX lies at the junction of the extrinsic and intrinsic pathways of coagulation, FX deficiency is associated with abnormal prolongations of both the prothrombin time (PT) and the partial thrombo-plastin time (PTT). Factor V possesses molecular homology with FVIII:C and cerulo-plasmin, and it is synthesized in the liver and megakaryocytes and stored in the platelet alpha granule. The glycoprotein is unstable, and its activity in plasma is quite labile, with inactivation achieved through the proteolytic action of protein C and thrombin. Prothrombin is also a vitamin K–dependent clotting factor, the deficiency of which prolongs both PT and PTT assays.

Factor X can also be activated to FXa via the extrinsic pathway of coagulation, containing the FVIIa tissue factor complex. The FVIIa tissue factor complex can also "cross over" to activate FIX in the intrinsic pathway and is tightly regulated by extrinsic pathway inhibitor (EPI) or tissue factor inhibitor (TFI). Tissue factor inhibitor is thought to form a complex with FXa that subsequently inactivates FVIIa by binding to the previously formed FVIIa–tissue factor complex present on a phospholipid membrane surface, i.e., the platelet or endothelial cell. Factor VII is also a vitamin K–dependent serine protease, and its deficiency produces an isolated prolongation of the PT. Intriguingly, the Northwick Park Heart Study, examining the contributions of coagulation proteins to increased risks of cardiovascular disease and myocardial infarction, revealed a strong independent association between fibrinogen and FVII activity levels and the incidence of ischemic heart disease.

The intrinsic and extrinsic pathways culminate in the generation of fibrin monomers. The final steps after FX activation are collectively referred to as the common pathway of coagulation. The active enzyme thrombin proteolytically cleaves fibrinogen, releasing 2 moles of fibrinopeptide A and fibrinopeptide B per mole of fibrin monomer. Fibrin monomers spontaneously polymerize but are easily disrupted until FXIIIa covalently crosslinks the fibrin strands to form a stable clot. The FXIII zymogen is converted to its active form by the action of thrombin (Fig. 2). The detection and quantitation of proteolytic peptides from clotting factor proteins provide sensitive indicators of overall coagulation activity or activity of specific segments within the cascade. For example, elevated plasma levels of fibrinopeptides A and B represent thrombin effects and are directly related to the degree of thrombin generation in vivo. Thrombin generation is also corroborated by the measurement of D-dimers, the fibrinolytic by-product derived from fibrin that has been crosslinked in the presence of FXIIIa and thrombin. Factor Xa generation in vivo can be monitored in plasma by measuring proteolytic activation peptides of prothrombin, such as fragment F1.2. Elevated levels of F1.2 with normal fibrinopeptide A levels indicate the

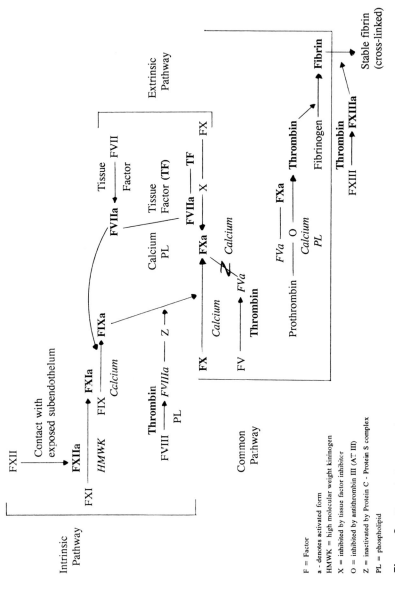

Figure 2 Coagulation cascade.

F = Factor

a - denotes activated form

HMWK = high molecular weight kininogen

X = inhibited by tissue factor inhibiter

O = inhibited by antithrombin III (AT III)

Z = inactivated by Protein C - Protein S complex

PL = phospholipid

efficiency of the circulating inhibitors of coagulation, i.e., antithrombin III (ATIII), protein S, and protein C, in controlling coagulation activity and preventing thrombin generation.

Antithrombin III is a specific inhibitor of serine proteases, and it is the primary inhibitor of thrombin, FXa, and FXIa in vivo. Antithrombin III interacts with pharmacologic heparin or with the proteoglycan heparan sulfate on endothelial cell surfaces and undergoes a conformational change induced by high negative charges. This opens the reactive center on ATIII to receive the serine proteases, which are rapidly inactivated upon complex formation. This process explains the pharmacology of heparin anticoagulation; FXa is very vulnerable to ATIII inactivation in the presence of small amounts of heparin, providing the rationale for minidose heparin regimens. Less heparin is required to inhibit FXa activity and subsequent thrombin formation than is necessary to inhibit thrombin after it is formed.

Protein C and protein S are vitamin K–dependent proteins that complex with each other to inactivate FVIIIa and FVa, and this inhibits thrombin formation. Alternatively, the protein C/protein S complex also interacts with PAI-1 and thus facilitates plasmin formation and fibrinolysis by tissue plasminogen activator and urokinase plasminogen activator. These reactions occur on platelet and endothelial cell surfaces.

Protein S circulates in the plasma free and bound to the complement pathway protein C4b binding protein. Only the free form complexes with protein C to modulate coagulation and fibrinolysis. Congenital deficiencies of ATIII, protein S, and protein C have all been associated with hypercoagulability. Interestingly, protein S deficiency produces arterial thromboembolic complications more frequently than other deficiencies of the naturally occurring inhibitors of coagulation.

IV. COAGULATION ASSAYS

The functional activity of each plasma coagulation protein may be individually evaluated in vitro in the coagulation laboratory by employing substrates deficient in the specific factor being measured. Routinely, however, coagulation is first assessed by screening assays. These include the activated partial thromboplastin time (aPTT), the prothrombin time (PT), and the thrombin time (TT). The aPTT measures the function of both the intrinsic and the common pathways of coagulation. It is performed by activating citrated plasma with a surface-activating agent such as silica or kaolin. After recalcification, the time to fibrin formation is measured. The aPTT is prolonged by a deficiency of, or inhibitor against, any of the coagulation proteins in the intrinsic and/or common pathways. A decrease of coagulation protein concentration to below 40–50% of normal activity is generally required before the aPTT will be affected. Heparin anticoagulation prolongs the aPTT to a much greater degree than it does the PT.

The PT assay measures both the extrinsic and the common pathways of coagulation and is performed by adding a source of tissue thromboplastin to plasma. The time to fibrin formation is then measured. The PT may be prolonged by a deficiency of, or inhibitor against, any of the coaglution proteins present in the intrinsic and/or common pathways. Again, a decrease in activity level below 40% of normal activity is generally required for prolongation of the PT. Because of the short circulation time of FVII, the PT is very sensitive to coumarin anticoagulation, which blocks the postribosomal carboxylation of vitamin K–dependent clotting proteins by interfering with the availability of the proper form of vitamin K to function as a coenzyme in the reaction. Vitamin K deficiency due to malabsorption, antibiotic use, or liver disease will have the same effect as coumarin on the PT.

Prolongations of the PT and/or the PTT should be approached initially by performing mixing studies with pooled normal plasma and patient plasma. Correction is indicative of a clotting factor deficiency, whereas persistent prolongation suggests the presence of a circulating inhibitor. Such inhibitors may be directed against a specific clotting factor or nonspecifically against the phospholipid template on which clotting proceeds, i.e., the lupus-like anticoagulant. Interestingly, the lupus anticoagulant has been associated with recurrent venous and arterial thromboses and multiple spontaneous abortions. Prolongations of the PT and PTT produced by coumarin anticoagulation are corrected with mixing studies; heparin behaves as a circulating anticoagulant, and prolongation of the PTT produced by heparin anticoagulation does not normalize on mixing studies. The TT specifically measures the efficiency of thrombin in converting fibrinogen to fibrin. Prolongation of the TT may be secondary to hypofibrinogenemia or dysfibrinogenemia or to the presence of fibrinogen/fibrin degradation products, heparin, or antibodies against thrombin (43).

V. PLATELETS

Platelets play a vital role in the initial hemostatic response following damage to the protective endothelial cell barrier. Formation of the platelet plug is the immediate response stimulated by exposure of circulating platelets to components of the subendothelial matrix via trauma to the naturally nonthrombogenic endothelial cell monolayer. The role of platelets in normal hemostasis may be divided into four phases: adhesion; aggregation; secretion; and the release of procoagulant activity (44).

Adhesion occurs as platelets contact the subendothelial matrix and adhere to and spread upon this surface. There are a variety of proteins located in the subendothelial matrix that function as potential adhesive sites for platelets, including fibronectin, vitronectin, and thrombospondin. Platelet attachment to these proteins occurs via glycoprotein receptors on the platelet surface (Table 2). Platelet adhesion can be supported by collagen monomers (45), but adhesion with subsequent platelet activation and aggregation requires the native triple-helical structure of collagen (46). Under conditions of flow and high shear rates such as those found in stenotic vessels, arterioles, and the microvasculature, platelet adherence to collagen in the subendothelial matrix is largely dependent on the bridging property of the highest-molecular-weight multimers of vWf protein (46,47), synthesized by endothelial cells and megakaryocytes and packaged into the alpha granules of platelets (48). There are two vWf receptor sites on the platelet membrane, glycoprotein Ib and the glycoprotein IIb-IIIa complex (49). Glycoprotein Ib is believed to be the receptor that plays the major role in platelet adhesion to collagen at high shear rates (50).

The initial layer of platelets that adheres to the subendothelium provides the framework for subsequent development of the hemostatic platelet plug. The next phase involves aggregation, platelet-platelet interactions that are irreversible and necessary for the generation of the hemostatic platelet plug. Unlike adhesion, platelet aggregation requires active platelet metabolism, which is initiated by a variety of platelet agonists.

The various agonists are divided into two categories, "strong" and "weak," according to their ability to stimulate platelet granule release in the absence (strong) or in the presence (weak) of platelet aggregation (44). Thrombin is the most potent physiologic platelet agonist identified (44), but the exact mechanism of thrombin-mediated platelet activation remains unknown. Thrombin-mediated platelet activation has been shown to be concentration-

Table 2 Platelet Membrane Glycoproteins

Complex	Function
Ia/IIa and V	Collagen receptor
Ib/IX	Von Willebrand factor receptor
Ic/IIa	Fibronectin receptor
	Laminin receptor
IIb/IIIa	Fibrinogen receptor
	Von Willebrand factor receptor
	Fibronectin receptor
	Vitronectin receptor
	Thombospondin receptor

dependent, which suggests a receptor-mediated pathway, but a definitive platelet receptor remains to be identified (44). The glycocalicin portion of the platelet surface glycoprotein Ib has been proposed as one potential thrombin receptor (51). Collagen, another strong platelet agonist, supports platelet aggregation by stimulating the generation of thromboxane A_2 (see Fig. 1) and ADP. Aspirin and nonsteroidal anti-inflammatory drugs inhibit collagen-induced aggregation by blocking the activity of cyclooxygenase in the prostaglandin pathway. These drugs do not uniformly inhibit thrombin-induced aggregation, suggesting the presence of a prostaglandin-independent pathway for activation of platelets, as well (52).

Adenosine diphosphate, which is secreted from the dense granules of activated platelets and also possibly released from hypoxic or damaged tissue (53), is a weak platelet agonist at low concentrations and is inhibited by inhibitors of prostaglandin synthesis such as aspirin (52). Epinephrine, another weak platelet agonist, also activates platelets via stimulation of prostaglandin synthesis (52). Epinephrine binds to α-adrenergic receptors on the platelet membrane but, unlike ADP, does not induce platelet shape change and exposure of membrane phospholipids (44). The physiologic importance of epinephrine acting alone in inducing platelet aggregation in vivo has been questioned (54); however, epinephrine potentiates the activity of other platelet agonists and, in conjunction with subthreshold concentrations of other agonists, can induce complete platelet aggregation in vitro (55). The mechanism of this synergistic potential and whether it occurs in vivo have not been determined.

Additional platelet agonists include platelet-activating factor (which is synthesized by endothelial cells and mast cells [16]), serotonin, and vasopressin.

Fibrinogen, an essential cofactor for platelet aggregation (56), binds to the glycoprotein IIb-IIIa complex on stimulated platelets (57) and mediates recruitment of platelets into enlarging aggregates (58,59).

Coupled with aggregation and stimulation is the secretion of the contents from the cytosolic granules of platelets, designated alpha granules, dense granules, liposomes, and microperoxisomes (44). The alpha granules contain a variety of platelet-derived proteins (platelet factor, β-thromboglobulin, and platelet-derived growth factor [PGDG]) (60), adhesive proteins (vWf protein, thrombospondin, fibronectin, and vitronectin) (44,61,62), and humoral proteins involved with coagulation and fibrinolysis (fibrinogen, FV, FXI, protein S, PAI-1, and HMWK). Platelet-derived growth factor is particularly interesting because of its mitogenic stimulation of fibroblasts and smooth muscle cells (60). This property may mediate atherogenesis and plaque formation at sites of vascular injury where platelet activation and secretion occur. This may provide a rationale for the use of small daily doses of aspirin to inhibit the platelet contribution to atherogenesis and the development of myocardial infarction. In addition, aspirin would be expected to inhibit thromboxane A_2 formation, which propagates platelet aggregation and probably mediates coronary vasospasm and anginal symptoms.

The dense granules contain ADP, adenosine triphosphate (ATP), serotonin, and calcium (63). The function of dense granule ATP, calcium, and serotonin remains unclear. Adenosine diphosphate and perhaps serotonin do function as platelet agonists and contribute to platelet recruitment into the platelet plug.

The platelet lysosomes contain an array of acid hydrolases (64) that are secreted in varying quantities after platelet stimulation. There are also a small number of microperoxisomes in platelets that possess peroxidase activity (65).

The platelet plug provides an appropriate membrane surface for the assembly of several of the coagulation protein complexes that lead to the generation of thrombin.

The prothrombinase complex, composed of FVa, FXa, and calcium, cleaves prothrombin to generate thrombin. This complex can also assemble on the phospholipid surfaces of endothelial cells, monocytes, lymphocytes, and neutrophils (44). Factor Va, a vital cofactor in the prothrombinase reaction, is found circulating in plasma and stored in platelet alpha granules (66). Although the FVa in platelet alpha granules represents only a small portion of total circulating FVa, it is believed to play a more important role than plasma FVa, since it is immediately available in high concentrations at the site of platelet activation and release to participate in the prothrombinase reaction (67). The activation of FX by the tenase complex, composed of FIXa-FVIIIa-calcium and the substrate FX, also requires a phospholipid template presumably derived from the surface of activated platelets (44). Activated platelets also help to initiate the contact phase of coagulation by enhancing the activation of FXII, FXI, and FIX (68).

Activated platelets also participate in fibrin clot retraction via interaction with fibrin within the clot (69). The cytoskeletal contraction of aggregated platelets within the clot probably contributes to clot retraction, as does the binding of FXIIIa to receptors on stimulated platelets (70).

Platelet function can be monitored in vivo indirectly with the bleeding time, and in vitro by platelet aggregation studies employing multiple agonists. The accuracy of these tests require a platelet count of at least $100,000/\mu l$ and may be affected by many medications besides aspirin and nonsteroidal anti-inflammatory drugs, such as antihistamines, beta-blockers and calcium channel antagonists, antibiotics, and thrombolytic agents. Dipyridamole does not inhibit platelet aggregation or affect the bleeding time but probably produces its antiplatelet benefits by interfering with platelet adhesion. Platelet function can also be diminished by uremia; by the presence of fibrin degradation products, dysproteinemias, or the lupus anticoagulant; and by damage induced by the cardiopulmonary bypass pump. These qualitative platelet abnormalities can frequently be reversed following infusions of desmopressin (DDAVP) at a dose of 0.3 $\mu g/kg$.

Platelet activation can be monitored in vivo by detecting elevated plasma levels of β-thromboglobulin and platelet factor 4. In addition, measurement of GMP-140 (PADGEM) is a sensitive indicator of alpha granule secretion, since it is probably derived from the alpha granule membrane. Radioimmunoassays are also available to quantitate plasma levels of generated thromboxane A_2, measured as its stable metabolite thromboxane B_2, as an indicator of cyclooxygenase pathway activity in the platelet.

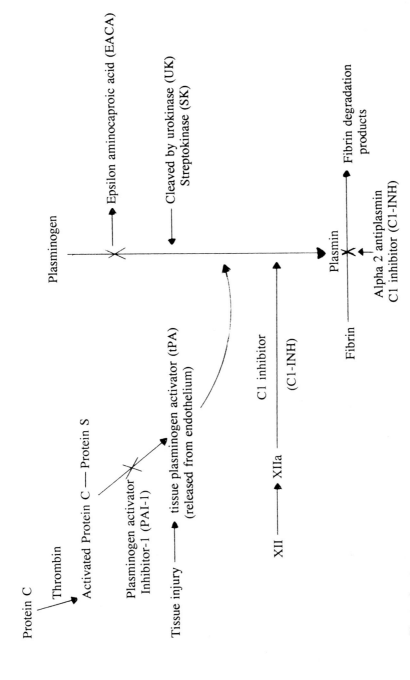

Figure 3 Fibrinolysis.

VI. FIBRINOLYSIS

Humoral coagulation and platelet aggregation are processes intended to generate fibrin clot formation. Simultaneously, fibrinolysis is initiated (Fig. 3) through the proteolytic cleavage of the zymogen plasminogen to plasmin by tissue plasminogen activator and urokinase plasminogen activator. The details of this process are provided in a later chapter.

VII. SUMMARY

In summary, the physiology of normal coagulation is extremely complex, and its orchestration is profoundly dependent on the optimal functioning of each of the separate components. Even slight alterations in the integrity of endothelial cells, in the activation of coagulation proteins and their inhibitors and modulators, and in platelet function can result in disordered coagulation producing clinical symptoms of either bleeding or thrombosis.

REFERENCES

1.   Jaffe EA. Endothelial cell structure and function. In: Hoffman R, Benz EJ, Shattil SJ, Furie B, Cohen HJ, eds. Hematology basic principles and practice. London: Churchill Livingstone, 1991:1198.
2.   Nachman RL. Thrombosis and atherogenesis: molecular connections. Blood 1992; 79:1897.
3.   Madri JA, Dryer B, Pitlick FA, Furthmayr H. The collagenous components of the subendothelium. Correlation of structure and function. Lab Invest 1980; 43:303.
4.   Terranova VP, DiFlorio R, Liyall RM, et al. Human endothelial cells are chemotactic to endothelial cell growth factor and heparin. J Cell Biol 1985; 101:2330.
5.   Albelda SM, Daise M, Levine EM, et al. Identification and characterization of cell-substratum adhesion receptors on cultured human endothelial cells. J Clin Invest 1989; 83:1992.
6.   Aihara M, Kimura A, Chiba Y, Yoshida Y. Plasma collagen cofactor correlates with von Willebrand factor antigen and ristocetin cofactor but not with bleeding time. Thromb Haemost 1988; 59:485.
7.   Aihara M, Takina H, Sawada Y, Morimoto S, et al. Effect of fibronectin and von Willebrand factor on the adhesion of human fixed washed platelets to collagen immobilized beads. Thromb Res 1986; 44:661.
8.   McCarroll DR, Levin EG, Montgomery RR. Endothelial cell synthesis of von Willebrand antigen II, von Willebrand factor, and von Willebrand factor/von Willebrand antigen II complex. J Clin Invest 1985; 75:1089.
9.   Sussman II, Rand JH. Subendothelial deposition of von Willebrand factor requires the presence of endothelial cells. J Lab Clin Med 1982; 100:526.
10. Kessler CM, Floyd CM, Frantz SC, Orthner C. Critical role of the carbohydrate moiety in human von Willebrand factor protein for interactions with type I collagen. Thromb Res 1990; 57:59.
11. Badimon L, Badimon JJ, Turitto VT, et al. Platelet thrombus formation on collagen type I. A model of deep vessel injury. Circulation 1988; 78:1431.
12. Shekhonin BV, Donogatsky SP, Idelson GL. Relative distribution of fibronectin and type I, III, IV and V collagens in normal and atherosclerotic intima of human arteries. Atherosclerosis 1987; 67:9.
13. Sakariassen KS, Baumgartner HR. Axial dependence of platelet-collagen interactions in flowing blood. Upstream thrombus growth impairs downstream platelet adhesion. Arteriosclerosis 1989; 9:33.
14. Asch E. Vitronectin binds to activated platelets and plays a role in platelet aggregation (abstr). Blood 1987; 70(suppl 1):346a.

15. Rittenhouse-Simmons S. Production of diglyceride phosphatidylinositol in activated platelets. J Clin Invest 1979; 63:580.

16. Jaffe EA. The role of blood vessels in hemostasis. In: Williams WJ, Beutler E, Erslov AJ, Lichtman MA, eds. Hematology. New York: McGraw-Hill, 1990:1322.

17. Wilcox JN, Smith KM, Schwartz SM, et al. Localization of tissue factor in the normal vessel and the atherosclerotic plaque. Proc Natl Acad Sci USA 1989; 86:2839.

18. Brox JH, Osterud B, Bjorklid E, et al. Production and availability of thromboplastin in endothelial cells: the effects of thrombin, endotoxin and platelets. Br J Haematol 1984; 57:239.

19. Broze GJ Jr, Warren LA, Novotny WF, et al. The lipoprotein-associated coagulation inhibitor that inhibits the factor VII–tissue factor complex also inhibits factor Xa: insight into its possible mechanism of action. Blood 1988; 71:335.

20. Cerveny TS, Fass DN, Mann KG. Synthesis of coagulation factor V by cultured aortic endothelium. Blood 1984; 63:1467.

21. Annamali AE, Stewart GJ, Hansel B. Expression of factor V on human umbilical vein endothelial cells is modulated by cell injury. Arteriosclerosis 1986; 6:196.

22. Dejana E, Languino LR, Polentarutti N, et al. Interaction between fibrinogen and cultured endothelial cells. Induction of migration and specific binding. J Clin Invest 1985; 75:11.

23. Van Iwaarden F, de Groot PG, Bouma BN. The binding of high molecular weight kininogen to cultured human endothelial cells. J Biol Chem 1988; 263:4698.

24. Wiggins RC, Loskutoff DJ, Cochrane CG, et al. Activation of rabbit Hageman factor by homogenates of cultured rabbit endothelial cells. J Clin Invest 1980; 65:197.

25. Best LC, Martin TS, Russell RGG, Preston FE. Prostacyclin increases cyclic AMP levels and adenylate cyclase activity in platelets. Nature 1977; 267:850.

26. Bunting S, Simmons PM, Moncada S. Inhibition of platelet activation by prostacyclin: possible consequences in coagulation and anticoagulation. Thromb Res 1981; 21:89.

27. Weiss HJ, Turitto VT. Prostacyclin (prostaglandin I_2 PGI_2) inhibits platelet adhesion and thrombus formation on subendothelium. Blood 1979; 53:244.

28. Macdonald PS, Read MA, Dusting GJ. Synergistic inhibition of platelet aggregation by endothelium derived relaxing factor and prostacyclin. Thromb Res 1988; 49:437.

29. Ignarro LJ. Biological actions and properties of endothelium derived nitric oxide formed and released from artery and vein. Circulation Res 1989; 65:1.

30. Radomski MW, Palmer RM, Moncada S. Comparative pharmacology of endothelium derived relaxing factor, nitric oxide and prostacyclin in platelets. Br J Pharmacol 1987; 92:181.

31. Buchanan MR, Butt RW, Magas Z, et al. Endothelial cells produce a lipooxygenase derived chemorepellent which influences platelet/endothelial cell interaction-effect of aspirin and salicylate. Thromb Haemost 1985; 53:306.

32. Marcum JA, Atha DH, Fritz LM, et al. Cloned bovine aortic endothelial cells synthesize anticoagulant active heparan sulfate proteoglycan. J Biol Chem 1986; 261:7507.

33. Rosenberg RD: Biochemistry of heparin antithrombin interactions, and the physiologic role of this natural anticoagulant mechanism. Am J Med 1989; 87:25.

34. Halton MW, Moar SL, Richardson M. Evidence that rabbit 1251-antithrombin III binds to protoheparan sulfate at the subendothelium of the rabbit aorta in vitro. Blood Vessels 1988; 25:12.

35. Esmon CT. The role of protein C and thrombomodulin in the regulation of blood coagulation. J Biol Chem 1989; 264:4743.

36. Maruyama I, Majerus PW. The turnover of thrombin-thrombomodulin in cultured human umbilical vein endothelial cells and A549 lung cancer cells. Endocytosis and degradation of thrombin. J Biol Chem 1985; 260:15432.

37. Stern D, Brett J, Harris K, et al. Participation of endothelial cells in the protein C–protein S anticoagulant pathway: the synthesis and release of protein S. J Cell Biol 1986; 102:1971.

38. Broekman AW, Veltkamp JJ, Bertina RM. Congenital protein C deficiency and venous thromboembolism. N Engl J Med 1983; 309:340.

39. Macfarlane RG. An enzyme cascade in the blood clotting mechanism and its function as a biochemical amplifier. Nature 1964; 202:498.

40. Furie B, Furie BC. The molecular basis of blood coagulation. In: Hoffman R, Benz EJ, Shattil SJ, Furie B, Cohen HJ, eds. London: Churchill Livingstone, 1991:1213.

41. Hultin MB. Role of human FVIII in FX activation. J Clin Invest 1982; 69:950.

42. Stern DM, Nawroth PP, Kisiell W, et al. A coagulation pathway on bovine aortic segments leading to generation of FXa and thrombin. J Clin Invest 1984; 74:1910.

43. Ockelford PA, Carter CJ. Disseminated intravascular coagulation: the application and utility of diagnostic tests. Sem Thromb Hemost 1982; 8:198.

44. Bennett JS, Shattil SJ. Platelet function. In: Williams WJ, Beutler E, Erslev AJ, Lichtman MA, eds. Hematology. New York: McGraw-Hill, 1990:1233.

45. Wilner GD, Nossel HL, LeRoy EC. Aggregation of platelets by collagen. J Clin Invest 1968; 47:2616.

46. Jaffe R, Deykin D. Evidence for a structural requirement for the aggregation of platelets by collagen. J Clin Invest 1974; 53:875.

47. Baumgartner HR, Tschopp TB, Meyer D. Shear rate dependent inhibition of platelet adhesion and aggregation on collagenous surfaces by antibodies to Factor VIII/von Willebrand factor. Br J Haematol 1980; 44:127.

48. Cramer EM, Meyer D, LeMenn R, et al. Eccentric localization of von Willebrand factor in an internal structure of platelet α-granule resembling that of Weibel-Palade bodies. Blood 1985; 66:710.

49. Ruggeri ZM, DeMarco L, Gatti L, et al.. Platelets have more than one binding site for von Willebrand factor. J Clin Invest 1983; 72:1.

50. Ruggeri ZM, Zimmerman TS. Von Willebrand factor and von Willebrand disease. Blood 1987; 70:895.

51. Jamison GA, Okumura T. Reduced thrombin binding and aggregation in Bernard-Soulier platelets. J Clin Invest 1978; 61:861.

52. Charo IF, Feinman RD, Detwiler TZ. Interrelations of platelet aggregation and secretin. J Clin Invest 1977; 60:866.

53. Holmsen H, Weiss HJ. Secretable storage pools in platelets. Annu Rev Med 1979; 30:119.

54. Peerschke EI. Induction of human platelet fibrinogen receptors by epinephrine in the absence of released ADP. Blood 1982; 60:71.

55. Huang EM, Detwiler TC. Characteristics of the synergistic actions of platelets. Blood 1981; 57:685.

56. Weiss HJ, Rogers J. Fibrinogen and platelets in the primary arrest of bleeding. N Engl J Med 1971; 285:369.

57. Mustard JF, Packham MA, Kinlough-Rathbone RL, et al. Fibrinogen and ADP induced platelet aggregation. Blood 1978; 52:453.

58. Coller BS. Activation affects access to the platelet receptor for adhesive proteins. J Cell Biol 1986; 103:451.

59. Shattil SJ, Hoxie JA, Cunningham M, et al. Changes in the platelet membrane glycoprotein IIb/IIIa complex during platelet activation. J Biol Chem 1985; 260:11107.

60. Scher CD, Shepard RC, Antoniades HN, et al. Platelet derived growth factor and the regulation of the mammalian fibroblast cell cycle. Biochem Biophys Acta 1979; 560:217.

61. Lawler J. The structural and functional properties of thrombospondin. Blood 1986; 67:1197.

62. Leung LLK. Role of thrombospondin in platelet aggregation. J Clin Invest 1984; 74:1764.

63. Plow EF, Ginsberg MH. The molecular basis of platelet function. In: Hoffman R, Benz EJ, Shattil SJ, Furie B, Cohen HJ, eds. Hematology basic principles and practice. London: Churchill Livingstone 1991:1165.

64. Bentfeld-Barker ME, Bainton DR. Identification of primary lysosomes in human megakaryocytes and platelets. Blood 1982; 59:472.

65. Breton-Soreus J, Guichard J. Ultrastructural localization of peroxidase activity in human platelets and megakaryocytes. Am J Pathol 1972; 66:277.
66. Tracy PB, Eide L, Eide E, et al. Radioimmunoassay of factor V in human plasma and platelets. Blood 1982; 60:59.
67. Tracy PB, Giles AAR, Mann KG, et al. Factor V (Quebec): a bleeding diathesis associated with a qualitative platelet factor V deficiency. J Clin Invest 1984; 74:1221.
68. Walsh PN, Griffin JH. Contributions of human platelets to the proteolytic activation of blood coagulation factor XII and XI. Blood 1981; 57:106.
69. Cohen I, Gerrard JM, White JG. Ultrastructure of clots during isometric contraction. J Cell Biol 1982; 93:775.
70. Greenberg CS, Shuman MA. Specific binding of blood coagulation factor XIIIa to thrombin stimulated platelets. J Biol Chem 1984; 259:14721.

Biochemistry of Vitamin K: Implications for Warfarin Therapy

Edwin G. Bovill and Kenneth G. Mann
University of Vermont College of Medicine, Burlington, Vermont

Jeffrey H. Lawson
Duke University Medical Center, Durham, North Carolina

James A. Sadowski
Tufts University School of Nutrition, Boston, Massachusetts

I. INTRODUCTION

Warfarin was first used clinically in 1941 (1,2) and rapidly became the standard form of outpatient anticoagulant therapy. After 50 years of clinical use, more than 1 in 200 adults (3) in the United States are taking warfarin. Over the past decade, clinical studies have demonstrated the efficacy of progressively lower doses of warfarin with fewer hemorrhagic complications. The clinical use of lower warfarin doses has challenged the traditional prothrombin time–based methods of monitoring anticoagulant therapy. For example, at the lowest doses of warfarin, little or no effect is observed on the prothrombin time, and at higher doses the prothrombin time exhibits considerable variability because of differences in the reagents used in the test systems.

The challenge to improve oral anticoagulant monitoring has been approached from two directions: (1) improvement in the conventional prothrombin time test reagents and (2) the application of novel strategies resulting from our improved understanding of the mechanisms of vitamin K metabolism and vitamin K–dependent hemostasis. This chapter will review our understanding of vitamin K metabolism and vitamin K–dependent hemostatic mechanisms. Based on the review of metabolism and hemostatic mechanisms, the final section of the chapter will cover the implications for conventional and novel monitoring strategies. Improved monitoring strategies are of particular importance in the setting of arterial thromboembolic disease, since many of these patients will be given long-term oral anticoagulant therapy.

II. VITAMIN K METABOLISM

A. Normal Vitamin K Metabolism and
Carboxylation Function

Several proteins involved in the regulation of blood clotting require vitamin K for the post-translational formation of an amino-terminal calcium-binding domain (4). The binding of calcium ions to this region of these proteins facilitates a transition to a functionally active conformation. In the absence of vitamin K or during its antagonism by coumarin anti-coagulant drugs, the biochemical maturation of the calcium-binding sites is defective, and this results in the production of clotting factors with decreased physiological activity (5). Vitamin K functions in the maturation of these proteins as a cofactor for a membrane-bound carboxylase that recognizes vitamin K–dependent proteins and converts specific glutamic acid residues in these substrates to γ-carboxyglutamic acid (Gla), producing the calcium-binding region of the molecule commonly referred to as the Gla-domain. A reduced level of carboxylation in the Gla-domain results in the production of vitamin K–dependent clotting factors with decreased abilities to generate the functionally active conformation of their Gla-domain in the presence of calcium. The biochemical basis for the anticoagulant effects of warfarin and other coumarin-based anticoagulants is attributed to their abilities to interfere with the normal metabolism of vitamin K required for the formation of the Gla-domain (6).

Evidence for the existence of a dietary factor responsible for the maintenance of hemostasis was first observed in 1929, when Heinrich Dam reported that chicks fed a diet low in fat developed hemorrhages (7). Dam named this antihemorrhagic factor vitamin K after the German word Koagulation. By 1936, Dam was able to demonstrate that a precipitate from normal plasma that contained prothrombin could restore normal coagulability when added to plasmas obtained from vitamin K–deficient chicks, and that the corresponding plasmas from vitamin K–deficient chicks were inactive (8). The concept that the bleeding associated with vitamin K deficiency was due to a simple lack of prothrombin became commonly accepted. Today, at least five other factors involved in the normal regulation of blood clotting have been shown to be vitamin K–dependent proteins that contain a Gla-domain. These five proteins are factor VII (stable factor, proconvertin), factor IX (Christmas factor, plasma thromboplastin component), factor X (Stuart-Prower factor), protein C, and protein S. Protein C and protein S are the most recent proteins to be recognized as vitamin K–dependent proteins involved in normal hemostasis (9). Activated protein C, and protein S, act as naturally occurring anticoagulants by inhibiting the procoagulant pathways through the inactivation of factors Va and VIIIa. A detailed account of this earlier history of the discovery of vitamin K and the elucidation of its function has been presented elsewhere (4).

Two major structural forms of vitamin K are present in nature (Fig. 1). Vitamin K_1 (2-methyl-3-phytyl-1,4-naphthoquinone) or phylloquinone is the major dietary source of vitamin K and is present in the highest concentrations in green and leafy vegetables and in oils extracted from soybean, rapeseed (canola), and olives. Vitamin K_2 or menaquinone(s) is a family of compounds synthesized in bacteria that contain the same aromatic nucleus as phylloquinone but a longer and more unsaturated side chain. The menaquinones of the vitamin K_2 family have been found to occur in nature with side chains ranging from 20 carbon atoms with four isoprene units to 65 carbons with 13 isoprene units. The relative contribution of menaquinones synthesized by gut flora in maintaining adequate vitamin K nutriture is not known and needs to be determined (10). Although it is a generally held belief that approximately 50% of the daily requirement for vitamin K is supplied by the gut flora, there is insufficient experimental evidence to support this conviction. Dietary vitamin K is

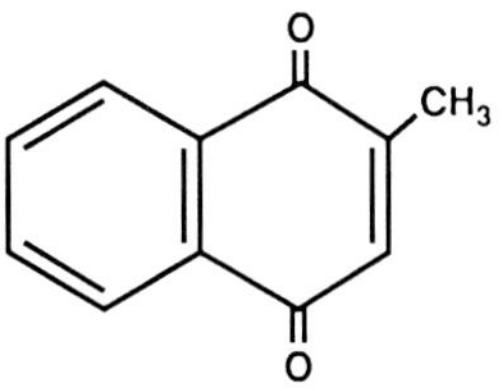

Menadione (Vitamin K₃)

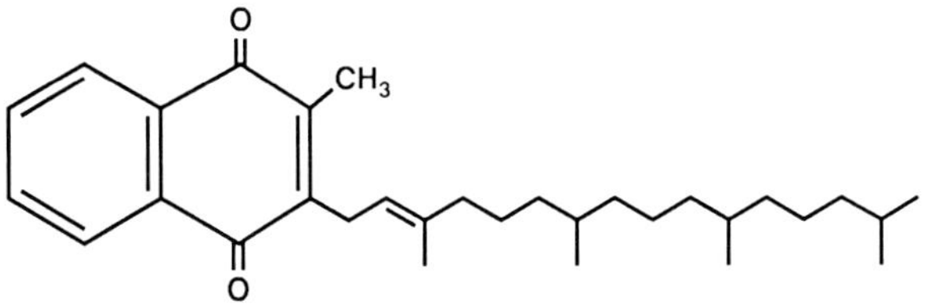

Phylloquinone (Vitamin K₁)

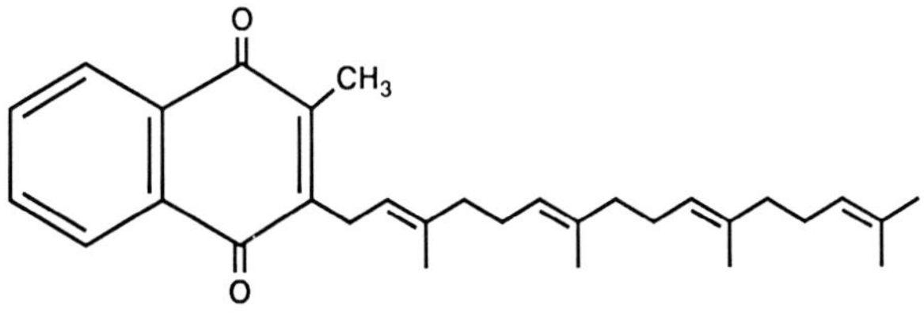

Menaquinone (Vitamin K₂, MK-4)

Figure 1 Chemical structures of compounds with vitamin K activity.

rapidly absorbed from the intestine and packaged into lipid-rich chylomicron particles that circulate in the blood and are taken up by the liver, where vitamin K is further metabolized to function as a cofactor for the vitamin K–dependent carboxylase that is involved in the synthesis of γ-carboxyglutamic acid.

B. Warfarin Disruption of Vitamin K Metabolism and Carboxylation Function

At approximately the same time that Dam observed hemorrhagic disease in chicks fed low-fat diets, which led to the discovery of vitamin K, a mysterious new hemorrhagic disease was observed in cattle feeding on spoiled sweet clover hay on the prairies of North Dakota in the United States and in Alberta, Canada. Substitution of good hay for the spoiled hay or the transfusion of blood drawn from healthy cattle demonstrated that the disease was reversible. The hemorrhagic agent was isolated and identified as 3,3′-methylenebis-(4-hydroxycoumarin), which later became known as dicumarol (11). Since the discovery of dicumarol, several hundred derivatives of coumarin have been synthesized. The most commonly used of the coumarin-based anticoagulants has been warfarin, 3-(acetonyl-benzyl)-4-hydroxycoumarin. This compound was found to be more potent than dicumarol in rats and was introduced first as a rodenticide. Application of warfarin as an anticoagulant in humans came about when it was observed through accidental poisonings and suicide attempts that, except for its depression of the clotting factors, warfarin had no other significant effects in humans. Warfarin was first introduced into human anticoagulant therapy in 1953 (12). Because of the ease with which warfarin may be administered (as a water-soluble sodium salt) and its relatively even depression of the clotting factors, it has since found wide clinical use. Research into the mode of action of vitamin K has been greatly aided through the use of warfarin to produce hypoprothrombinemia. It is tempting to suggest that γ-carboxyglutamic acid might still not have been identified as a product of vitamin K action had it not been for the discovery of coumarin anticoagulants and their use in medicine.

Coumarin anticoagulants have generally been assumed to compete directly with vitamin K for a receptor protein or proteins at the site where vitamin K normally exerts it biological activity. The overall antagonism has been presumed to result from the relative affinities of the coumarin drug and vitamin K for the active site and therefore to depend on the relative amounts of coumarin drug and vitamin K available. Many specific theories have evolved over the years, and these have been reviewed (4). Insight into the probable nature of these receptors and their function advanced with the discovery by Matschiner et al. in 1970 of a new metabolite of vitamin K (13). They found that in warfarin-treated rats, the amount of radioactivity in the liver 8 hours after an injection of radioactive vitamin K_1 was significantly higher than in controls. Chromatographic analysis of these liver extracts revealed the presence of a radioactive metabolite that was more polar than the vitamin. The metabolite was purified and characterized by mass spectroscopy as vitamin K_1-2-3-epoxide. The epoxide was further shown to be present in small amounts in the livers and hearts of normal animals fed diets containing labeled vitamin K_1 and in elevated amounts in animals that received warfarin. The identification of vitamin K_1-2-3-epoxide in normal rats and in increased levels in warfarin-treated rats suggested that the epoxide might be involved in the mechanism of action of the vitamin and warfarin.

Vitamin K epoxide was subsequently shown to possess approximately the same biological activity in vitamin K–deficient rats as in normal rats but to be totally inactive in rats that had previously been anticoagulated with warfarin (14). These results indicated that the epoxide could be rapidly converted to the vitamin in the absence of warfarin, but that in its presence the conversion was inhibited. The hypothesis was further supported by the observation that when the epoxide was administered a few minutes before the anticoagulant, protection against warfarin was as great as that obtained by administration of the vitamin before warfarin. The discovery of vitamin K epoxide and the influence of warfarin on the metabolism of vitamin K suggested that the interconversion between these two forms of the vitamin might in some way be related to the biochemical function of vitamin K (15).

In 1974, Willingham and Matschiner demonstrated the enzymatic conversion of vitamin K to its 2,3-epoxide in microsomes obtained from control and vitamin K–deficient rats (16). The epoxidation of vitamin K was shown to be dependent on molecular oxygen. Formation of vitamin K epoxide increased when precursors to prothrombin accumulated in the liver. Willingham and Matschiner hypothesized that the epoxidation of vitamin K was involved in the conversion of precursor prothrombin to biologically active prothrombin. Subsequent studies by Sadowski et al. in 1977 demonstrated a clear relationship between the in vitro formation of γ-carboxyglutamic acid in biologically active prothrombin and the epoxidation of vitamin K (17). In addition, the requirements for the in vitro synthesis of prothrombin and for the vitamin K–dependent carboxylation of glutamyl residues in microsomal prothrombin precursors were similar to the requirements for vitamin K epoxidation. Under a variety of experimental conditions, carboxylation or prothrombin synthesis was never observed without simultaneous epoxidation of vitamin K. In addition, stimulation or inhibition of the carboxylase resulted in a similar effect on epoxidation. These studies also provided another fundamental link between the two reactions when it was observed that the reduced form of vitamin K, vitamin K hydroquinone, was formed from the reduced pyridine nucleotides added to the incubation and could substitute for the vitamin in the absence of reducing equivalents for both reactions. Finally, both the epoxidation and the carboxylation were shown to be dependent on molecular oxygen. Surprisingly, both the epoxidation of vitamin K and the carboxylation of glutamyl residues in prothrombin precursors were not inhibited by the in vitro addition of warfarin, a potent in vivo antagonist of vitamin K in the synthesis of γ-carboxyglutamic acid residues in prothrombin. The in vitro refractoriness to warfarin inhibition was later understood to occur as a result of the pharmacologically high concentration of vitamin K used to study the epoxidation and carboxylation reactions. It is now generally accepted that the formation of vitamin K-2,3-epoxide from vitamin K hydroquinone provides the driving force for the glutamyl carboxylase (6,10).

A consequence of the concomitant formation of vitamin K-2,3-epoxide during the synthesis of γ-carboxyglutamic acid is that the vitamin is stoichiometrically consumed during the reaction. If the vitamin is to be used catalytically, there is a requirement for the enzymatic conversion of the epoxide back to the quinone or hydroquinone of vitamin K. Matschiner et al. first described the enzymatic conversion of vitamin K-2,3-epoxide to vitamin K in 1974 and called the enzyme vitamin K epoxide reductase (18). The epoxide reductase did not utilize reduced pyridine nucleotides as cofactors, but instead was stimulated by the addition of a nonphysiological dithiol reducing agent (dithiothreitol). Other investigators subsequently observed that the vitamin K carboxylase was also stimulated in the presence of dithiothreitol and demonstrated that much lower concentrations of vitamin K could be utilized for the carboxylation when dithiothreitol was present in the incubation mixtures (19).

Whitlon et al. were able to demonstrate that vitamin K and vitamin K-2,3-epoxide were metabolically interconverted by liver microsomes during carboxylation and proposed the metabolic pathway shown in Figure 2 (20). Based on their observations, this model proposes that the quinone form of vitamin K is converted to its active cofactor form, vitamin K hydroquinone, by two different quinone reductases. One quinone reductase requires reduced pyridine nucleotides as cofactors, while the other reductase requires some unknown reductant present in the cytosol that can be replaced by dithiothreitol in in vitro experiments. The vitamin K-2,3-epoxide formed during the carboxylation reaction is then converted back to vitamin K quinone by the vitamin K epoxide reductase in yet another reaction requiring reducing equivalents from the unknown cytosolic factor or factors but supported by dithiothreitol in vitro. Both dithiothreitol-dependent enzymatic activities (vitamin K quinone reductase and vitamin K epoxide reductase) were also shown to be strongly inhibited by warfarin, whereas the pyridine nucleotide–dependent quinone reductase was not susceptible to warfarin inhibition at the concentration of warfarin studied but required higher concentrations of the vitamin to support carboxylation.

The model proposed by Whitlon et al. provides a simplified explanation for the antagonism of clotting factor biosynthesis by warfarin and other 4-hydroxycoumarin anticoagulants. This model proposes that under normal physiological and dietary conditions, the cyclic interconversion of vitamin K to its hydroquinone and vitamin K-2,3-epoxide is

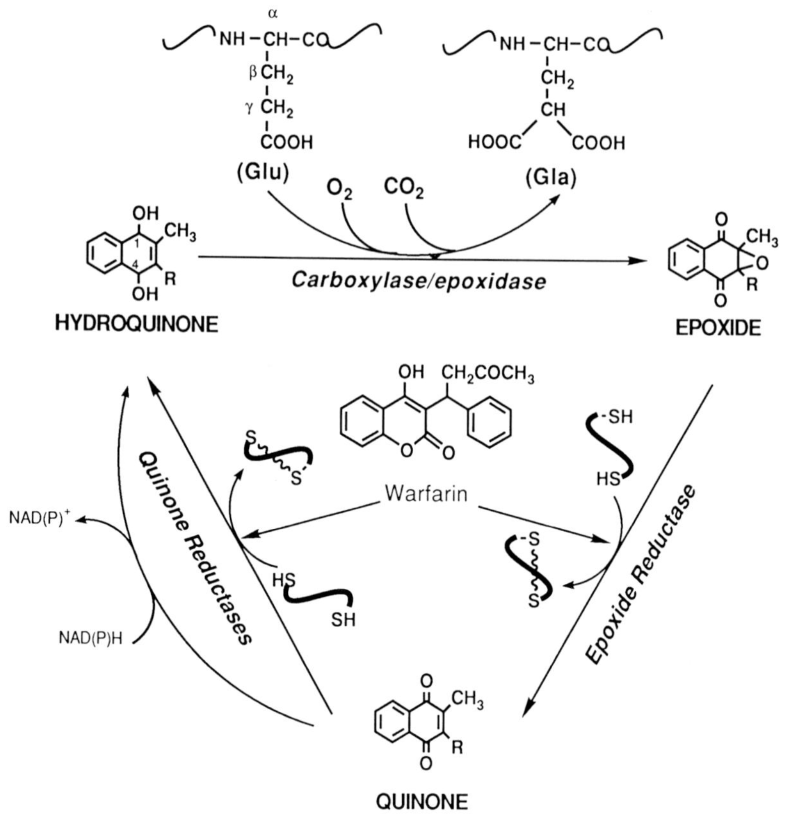

Figure 2 A schematic representation of the vitamin K cycle.

disrupted in the presence of pharmacologically effective doses of warfarin. This metabolic disruption of the cycle results in the decreased availability of the active cofactor form of vitamin K, vitamin K hydroquinone, resulting in a decreased synthesis of γ-carboxy-glutamic acid in the vitamin K–dependent blood clotting factors. It has been suggested that the daily requirement of vitamin K is approximately 1.0 μg/kg of body weight in humans. Pharmacological doses of vitamin K or dietary intake of foods containing high concentrations of the vitamin (see Table 1) can overcome this inhibition by generating the active hydroquinone cofactor through the warfarin-insensitive pyridine nucleotide–dependent pathway. However, any vitamin K epoxide formed from the hydroquinone generated by the pyridine nucleotide–dependent quinone reductase is not recycled, because of the warfarin block of the epoxide reductase. Thus, continued antagonism of warfarin by vitamin K results in a stoichiometric consumption of the vitamin, in contrast to the catalytic recycling.

Further proof for the existence of these reductase enzymes and their function in the metabolic conversion of vitamin K and its role in the carboxylation of vitamin K–dependent proteins has been provided by other investigators (6,10). However, despite extensive investigation into the nature of the vitamin K cycle, purification and characterization of the enzymes responsible for these interconversions has not been successful. Because of these shortcomings, no detailed biochemical explanation of the mechanism of warfarin at the molecular level is generally accepted. In contrast to the fragmentary nature of our understanding of hepatic vitamin K–dependent carboxylation, a comprehensive description of the

Table 1 The Vitamin K Content of Some Common Foods and Beverages

<1.0 μg/100 g	1–10 μg/100 g	10–50 μg/100 g	50–100 μg/100 g	>100 μg/100 g
Canned pears	Peanut oil	Sunflower oil	Olive oil	Soya bean oil
Banana	Corn oil	Sesame oil	Liver (beef)	Rape seed oil
Orange	Safflower oil	"Vegetable" oil	Cauliflower	Broccoli
Apple (no peel)	Apple (w/peel)	Pumpkin	Asparagus	Cabbage
Potatoes	Blueberries	Mustard	Watercress	Spinach
Onions	Cranberries	Cheese		Lettuce
Black tea	Tomatoes	Butter		Brussels sprouts
Orange juice	Sweet potatoes	Liver (pork,		Turnip greens
Apple juice	Squash	chicken)		Kale
Grapefruit juice	Whole wheat	Eggs		Chewing tobacco
Cranberry juice	flour	Green beans		
Lemonade	Milk	Peas		
Ginger ale	Corn	Oats		
Cola	Carrots			
Vinegar	Peaches			
Lemon extract	Corn flakes			
Vanilla extract	cereal			
Almond extract	Rice Krispies			
Brewed coffee	cereal			
Honey				
Salt				
Sugar				
Peanut butter				
Graham crackers				
White flour				
Egg white				
White rice				
Brown rice				
White pasta				
Chicken breast				
Lean pork				
Lean ground beef				

Source: Ref. 106.

molecular mechanisms of vitamin K–dependent hemostasis has developed over the past 10 to 15 years. The next section reviews the current state of our understanding of normal and coumarin-altered vitamin K–dependent hemostasis.

III. VITAMIN K-DEPENDENT HEMOSTATIC MECHANISMS IN THE PRESENCE OF NORMAL AND ALTERED VITAMIN K METABOLISM

A. Importance of Macromolecular Membrane-Bound Surface Complexes

The localization of blood clotting proteins to a site of vascular damage is achieved by the reversible binding of circulating coagulation proteins to specific membrane sites on the surface of damaged endothelial cells, activated platelets or monocytes, or the subendothelial matrix. The role of vitamin K–dependent proteins in hemostasis can be modeled as a series of linked, multiple-component enzyme complexes (Fig. 3) (21). A vitamin K–dependent protease is combined with a cofactor protein on a phospholipid surface in the presence of calcium ions in each successive linked reaction. The reactions are linked by the activation of a Gla-containing zymogen to its respective serine protease, ultimately leading to the conversion of fibrinogen to fibrin by α-thrombin. Once thrombin is formed, a vitamin K–dependent anticoagulant pathway is also initiated by the binding of thrombin to the cofactor protein thrombomodulin, which converts the zymogen protein C to activated protein C (22). Activated protein C inhibits the procoagulant pathways by inactivating the cofactors Va and VIIIa (23).

Blood clotting enzymes appear to be effective on a physiologic time scale only when these proteins are assembled in a "complex" where the appropriate cofactor protein is bound with the protease enzyme on an anionic phospholipid membrane in the presence of calcium ions. A schematic representation of the characterized blood clotting complexes is illustrated in Figure 3. The molecular details of complex assembly have been most rigorously described for the enzyme complex prothrombinase (24–26). The prothrombinase complex consists of activated factor V (Va), activated factor X (Xa), a charged phospholipid surface, and divalent metal ions (Ca^{2+}). Binding studies of prothrombinase assembly using synthetic phospholipid vesicles (PCPS) have demonstrated that factor Xa and factor Va bind

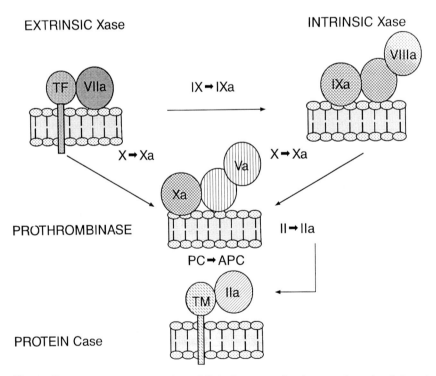

Figure 3 Schematic representation of linked macromolecular complexes involving vitamin K–dependent coagulation proteins, their cofactors, and a phospholipid membrane. TF = tissue factor; TM = thrombomodulin; Va, VIIa, VIIIa = activated factors V, VII, and VIII, respectively; II, IX, X = factor II, IX, and X; lowercase "a" represents the activated form of each factor.

independently to the membrane surface with dissociation constants of 114 nM and 3 nM respectively (27). However, when these proteins assemble together on the appropriate lipid surface, the global dissociation constant of this complex approaches 1 nM (27). In contrast, the binding constant of factors Xa and Va in solution exhibits a dissociation constant that is a 1000 times weaker, approaching 1 μM (28). From these data it has become well recognized that the assembly of factors Va and Xa occurs at a physiologic level only in the presence of the appropriate "binding site" on a charged phospholipid or platelet surface. Thus, the assembly of a functional enzymatic complex is equally dependent on both the activation of the appropriate plasma proteins and the availability of a membrane binding site.

Kinetic studies of prothrombin activation by prothrombinase have demonstrated that the complete assembled complex consisting of factor Xa, factor Va, an acidic phospholipid surface, and calcium ions activates prothrombin nearly 1×10^6 times more efficiently (k_{cat}/K_m, where k_{cat} is the turnover number and K_m is the Michaelis constant for substrate utilization) than factor Xa alone (29). The enhancement of prothrombin activation by factor Xa in the presence of factor Va, phospholipid, and calcium ions has been attributed to cocondensation of the enzyme and substrate on the same lipid surface and a 3000-fold increase in k_{cat} conferred by the interaction of factor Xa with factor Va and the phospholipid surface (27,30). Failure to assemble all of the required components of the prothrombinase complex results in the loss of biologically relevant proteolytic activity. From these observations the prothrombinase complex has served as the paradigm of vitamin K–dependent coagulation complexes.

With the prothrombinase complex as a model, the other vitamin K–dependent blood clotting complexes have been studied. It has been demonstrated that factors IXaβ and VIIIa ("intrinsic Xase") form a 1:1 stoichiometric complex on both synthetic and natural cell membranes that in many ways functions in a similar manner to prothrombinase (31). In contrast, studies of the tissue factor/factor VIIa complex ("extrinsic Xase") have suggested a slightly different model of assembly. In this case, assembly of the catalytic complex does not require acidic phospholipid, but only the presence of the membrane-bound protein tissue factor and of calcium ions (32–34). The importance of complex formation for all of the procoagulant proteins outlined above is best illustrated by comparing the catalytic efficiency (k_{cat}/K_m) of serine proteases that are either bound in an enzyme complex or free in solution. The kinetic properties of complex formation of the various blood clotting enzyme complexes are reported in Table 2. Data presented in Table 2 demonstrate that the assembled complexes are, in general, 10^6 times more efficient at performing their enzymatic functions than the uncomplexed serine proteases themselves.

B. Biochemistry of Vitamin K–Dependent Coagulation Proteins

The vitamin K–dependent plasma zymogens represent a unique class of calcium-binding proteins that can bind to membrane surfaces in the presence of divalent metal ions. The general structure of the vitamin K–dependent plasma zymogens is presented in Figure 4. It can be seen in this figure that factors II, VII, IX, and X and protein C all share considerable structural homology. The Gla-domain of these proteins consists of between 10 and 12 γ-carboxyglutamic acid residues within the first 42 amino acids at the amino-terminal end of the mature protein (35). The Gla modification of glutamic acid residues in this protein domain is essential to confer proper Ca^{2+} and lipid-binding properties on each zymogen (36). This Gla region is followed by structural protein domains that consist of epidermal

Table 2 Kinetic Properties of the Vitamin K–Dependent Enzymatic
Complexes of Blood Coagulation

Enzyme	Substrate	K_m^a (μM)	k_{cat}^b (min^{-1})	k_{cat}/K_m (M^{-1}min^{-1})
Xa	II	131	0.6	4.58×10^3
Xa/Va/PCPS/Ca^{2+}	II	1	1800.0	1.80×10^8
IXa	X	299	0.002	6.69
IXa/VIIIa/PCPS/Ca^{2+}	X	0.063	500.0	7.94×10^9
VIIa	X	4.87	0.024	4.93×10^3
VIIa/TF/PCPS/Ca^{2+}	X	0.45	69.0	1.53×10^8
VIIa	IX	NA	NA	NA
VIIa/TF/PCPS/Ca^{2+}	IX	0.243	15.6	6.42×10^7
IIa	PC	60.0	1.2	2.00×10^4
IIa/TM/PCPS/Ca^{2+}	PC	0.1	214.0	2.14×10^9

Adapted from Ref. 21.
[a]Michaelis constant for substrate utilization.
[b]Turnover number.
PCPS = phosphatidyl choline phosphatidyl serine; TF = tissue factor; TM = thrombomodulin; NA = not available; PC = protein C.

growth factor (EGF) and Kringle domains (prothrombin). The biological functions of these
protein domains are a subject of intense investigation and include calcium-binding properties and structural features that confer unique binding specificities on each of the proteins
(37–40). This structural domain is followed by a "trypsinogen-like region." Hydrolysis of a
specific Arg-X peptide bond in this region permits an alteration in the tertiary structure to
produce the catalytic domain of the protein. This structural alteration following peptide

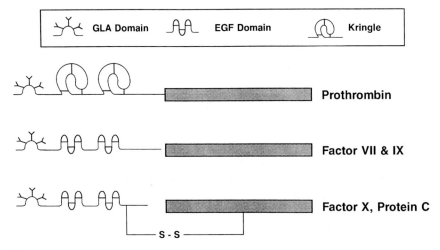

Figure 4 Domain structures of the vitamin K–dependent proteins emphasizing structural homology. (GLA = γ-carboxyglutamic acid; EGF = epidermal growth factor).

bond hydrolysis allows for proper alignment of three highly conserved amino acids, histidine, serine, and aspartic acid (HSD), that form the serine protease catalytic triad of the newly formed enzyme. Once the protein is activated, the catalytic domain shows a high degree of sequence homology and presumed three-dimensional structural homology with trypsin (41). It is the structure of this catalytic domain that confers enzymatic activity on the particular protein that is activated and very likely confers unique enzymatic specificity of the newly activated enzyme (42).

The highly conserved structural homology of these proteins can be traced to the gene level, where it has been established that each of these proteins contains a similar exon-intron structure (43). In general, each of the functional protein domains is coded for by one or two exons. The structural domain organization of these proteins suggests a common evolutionary path of new protein formation via gene duplication, gene modification, and exon shuffling (44). Thus, a functionally unique protein may arise by alteration or mutation of a specific exon, resulting in a modification of the functional domain of the newly synthesized protein.

C. Biochemistry of the Cofactor Proteins

Cofactor proteins make up a second major class of proteins involved in vitamin K–dependent complex formation. Cofactor proteins have at least three major functions in the regulation of the hemostatic process: (1) Cofactors function as regulatory molecules that enhance the enzymatic activity and specificity of the serine proteases with which they interact. (2) Cofactor proteins function by localizing coagulation reactions to a point of interaction with a damaged or activated cell membrane. (3) Cofactor proteins assist in enzymatic catalysis by modulating the binding and orientation of substrates for proteolysis by the associated serine protease.

The cofactor proteins involved in hemostasis can be separated into two major subclasses, soluble plasma cofactor proteins and cellular transmembrane cofactor proteins. The plasma cofactor proteins consist of the procoagulant cofactors factor V and factor VIII, and the anticoagulant cofactor protein S. Factors V and VIII circulate in an inactive procofactor form. Factor V circulates in plasma at a concentration of 2×10^{-8} M and has also been found in significant quantities in the alpha granules of platelets (45,46). Factor VIII circulates in plasma noncovalently associated with von Willebrand factor (vWf) at a concentration below 1×10^{-9} M (47). These procofactors require activation to their biologically active forms, factors Va and VIIIa, through limited proteolysis by thrombin (48), factor Xa (49), and plasmin (factor V) (50). Factors V and VIII are highly homologous proteins and share over 30% sequence identity (51,52). The structural features of these two cofactors is illustrated in Figure 5. Factors V and VIII share common structural features in both the "A" and "C" domains. However, the "B" domain appears to be structurally unique for either protein. Upon activation the connecting "B" domain is excised from both proteins, leaving the common structural motif for both factors Va and VIIIa consisting of three "A" domains and two "C" domains. Once activated, these proteins express their functional activity by (1) binding to the appropriate membrane or receptor site on the damaged vascular or platelet surface, (2) binding the serine protease enzyme, and (3) binding/orienting the substrate for proper proteolysis. It has been demonstrated that both proteins bind tightly to acidic phospholipid membranes, and that this lipid-binding interaction, at least in the case of factor Va, is contributed in part by the A_3 domain (53,54). In the case of factor Va, it has been shown that both the heavy chain and the light chain are required for factor Xa binding

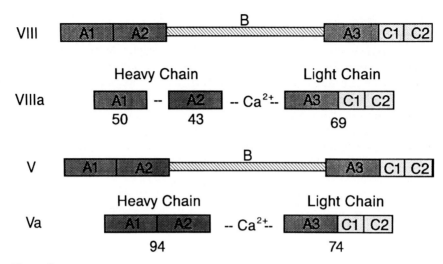

Figure 5 Schematic structure of factors V and VIII showing structural similarities of the precursor activated forms of the cofactors.

(55,56), while only the heavy chain of factor Va is responsible for prothrombin binding (55). Once activated, both proteins can be inactivated by proteolytic degradation by plasmin and activated protein C (APC) (49,57,58). This results in the formation of a number of smaller peptides that no longer possess the functional ability to serve as effective cofactor proteins. Thus, the degradation of these activated cofactor proteins by APC results in the loss of procoagulant activity from each enzyme complex.

Activated protein C must interact with membrane surfaces to exhibit maximal activity. The function of protein C is influenced by the presence of protein S (59–61). The in vivo observation that patients who are deficient in protein C or protein S have thrombotic tendencies demonstrates that degradation of these cofactor proteins by APC is an essential step in the down-regulation of hemostasis response (62). The inactivation of the activated cofactors by APC then serves as an important negative feedback control mechanism to stop a minor clotting event from becoming a major thrombotic episode.

In contrast to plasma factors V and VIII and protein S, tissue factor and thrombomodulin are integral membrane proteins. These proteins require no proteolytic processing step to become "active" cofactors. In many ways both tissue factor and thrombomodulin can be classified as cellular "receptors" that promote a cell-directed event on the surface of the cell expressing that protein. Thrombomodulin binds the protease thrombin with a dissociation constant of 1×10^{-9}M (63). Binding of thrombin to thrombomodulin alters the enzymatic specificity of thrombin, switching it from a procoagulant enzyme that converts fibrinogen to fibrin, to an anticoagulant enzyme that converts protein C to APC. Tissue factor binds both the zymogen factor VII and the protease factor VIIa with a dissociation constant for either ligand reported as being in the range of 10^{-10} to 10^{-9}M (32,34,64,65). Thrombomodulin and tissue factor do not share a high degree of structural homology and in many ways function in opposition to each other. Thrombomodulin is constitutively expressed on the cell surface of vascular endothelial cells and platelets (22). This constitutive expression of thrombomodulin results in an anticoagulant posture of presentation on the surface of normal cells in contact with blood elements. In contrast, tissue factor, under normal conditions, is not in contact with blood elements. However, tissue factor is maintained in close proximity to the vascular space and has been shown by immunohistochemical techniques to envelop the endothelial cells in the subendothelial matrix and extravascular space (66). It has been demonstrated both in vitro and in vivo that tissue factor activity can be induced on vascular endothelial cells and monocytes by a number of growth factors and mitogens. Currently, the list of agonists that stimulate tissue factor activity on endothelial cells includes fibroblast growth factor (67), platelet-derived growth factor (67), thrombin (68), interleukin-1 (69), lipopolysaccharide (70), tumor necrosis factor (71), and phorbol 12-myristate 13-acetate (72). It has also been demonstrated that when endothelial cells are stimulated to produce tissue factor, these cells down-regulate the amount of thrombomodulin on the cell surface (22). Thus, the dynamic state of procoagulant versus anticoagulant function, regulated on the surface of the vascular cells, appears to control the balance of the hemostatic response. If thrombomodulin is expressed on the cell surface, the tissue functions predominantly as an anticoagulant. If tissue factor is expressed in the cell, it rapidly becomes a procoagulant focal point for the formation of a clot or thrombus.

D. Modulation of Enzymatic Activity of Macromolecular Complexes

Although differences exist among macromolecular complexes, their similarities allow consideration of their physiological function under the following general categories: localization, amplification, and modulation of the hemostatic response. Following damage to the vascular surface, the binding of plasma coagulation proteins locally amplifies the hemostatic response by increasing the local reactant concentration and increasing the catalytic efficiency of the complex-bound proteases. The number of formed enzyme complexes then modulates the hemostatic response to the extent of the damaged cellular surface membrane that can support complex formation. Bound enzymatic complexes are, in general, protected from inactivation by protein C and antithrombin III (73,74). Dissolution of the complexes leads to both a decrease in the catalytic rate of procoagulant activity and an increase in the susceptibility of the individual components of the complex to inhibition and inactivation. Hereditary deficiency states such as the hemophilias and acquired abnormalities such as vitamin K deficiency inhibit hemostasis by decreasing the number of competent complexes formed in response to stimulation of the hemostatic system.

E. Effect of Warfarin on the Biochemistry of Vitamin K–Dependent Hemostasis

Oral anticoagulant therapy affords an opportunity to investigate vitamin K–dependent hemostatic mechanisms. Abnormal forms of the vitamin K–dependent proteins were identified as early as 1968 (75–78). These abnormal proteins were subsequently identified as the descarboxy forms of the vitamin K–dependent hemostatic proenzymes. The loss of as few as three Gla residues on prothrombin appears to severely impair lipid and calcium binding, with consequent decreased complex formation and inhibition of the hemostatic response (79–83). In contrast, prothrombin missing only one or two Gla residues retains considerable lipid- and calcium-binding properties (81,82). The enzymatic competence of minimally undercarboxylated vitamin K–dependent proteins has not been determined. It is conceivable that altered enzymatic function coupled with retention of membrane surface binding characteristics of minimally undercarboxylated proteins may play a role in the clinical response to very-low-dose (1 mg/day) warfarin therapy. There is a high degree of structural homology among the Gla-domains of the vitamin K–dependent hemostatic proteins, and they will most probably demonstrate structural and functional changes similar to those of prothrombin following oral anticoagulant therapy.

IV. CONVENTIONAL AND NOVEL STRATEGIES FOR MONITORING ORAL ANTICOAGULANT THERAPY

A. Conventional Monitoring Strategies

The mechanisms of vitamin K–dependent carboxylation and the subsequent expression of highly selective proteolytic activities reviewed in the preceding sections constitute the foundation for an expansion of the tools available for monitoring oral anticoagulant therapy. One of the primary goals of oral anticoagulation is the inhibition of thrombin generation. Figures 6 and 7 describe the metabolic and hemostatic pathways involved in thrombin generation, with identification of some of the available laboratory markers. Figure 6 outlines three potentially useful categories of assays for monitoring the anticoagulant process: vitamin K metabolites, hemostatic proenzymes, and markers of hemostatic proteolytic activity. Figure 7 amplifies the bottom portion of Figure 6 by depicting three important markers of thrombin generated during conversion of prothrombin to thrombin and by the subsequent activity and inhibition of thrombin. The proteolytic activation of prothrombin to thrombin by factor Xa releases the amino-terminal peptide fragment 1.2 (F1.2). The subsequent proteolytic cleavage of fibrinogen to fibrin by thrombin releases fibrinopeptide A (FPA). Finally, a large proportion of the thrombin generated is covalently bound by the inhibitor antithrombin III into thrombin-antithrombin (TAT) complexes. Assays have been developed for these three analytes (F1.2, FPA, and TAT).

Measurement of hemostatic proenzyme levels and specifically the prothrombin time (PT) has been almost universally the method used to monitor oral anticoagulants for the past 50 years. Although a number of investigators have evaluated the utility of measuring the plasma concentration of various hemostatic proenzymes, especially factor X (84–87), it has not been established which correlates most closely with clinical efficacy. In our experience, when the PT cannot be used because of the presence of, for example, lupus-like inhibitors, we have found the measurement of factor X by a one-stage clotting assay over a range of dilutions (1/10 to 1/80) to be the most useful monitoring tool. Recent efforts to improve the PT have focused on the production of more sensitive and standardized thromboplastins (88). Efforts to calibrate the tissue thromboplastin reagents used to initiate the PT clotting reaction, by means of the international normalized ratio (INR), have succeeded in improving inter- and intralaboratory reproducibility (88).

The INR is based on the calibration of local (usually commercial) thromboplastins used in the routine laboratory against the current World Health Organization primary international reference preparation of thromboplastin. This calibration model is based on the assumption that a linear relationship exists between the logarithm of the PT ratios of the reference and local thromboplastins. The local PT ratio may thus be converted into an INR by the following formula:

$$INR = (observed\ PT\ ratio)^{ISI}$$

where ISI is the international sensitivity index. The ISI is the experimentally determined conversion factor linking the local and international reference thromboplastins and is

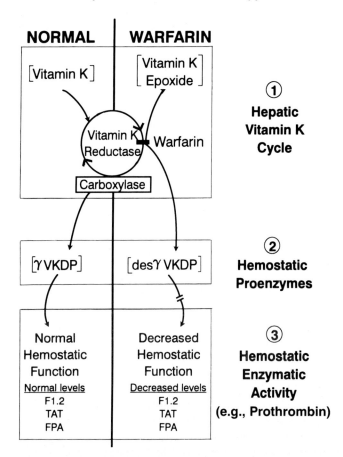

Figure 6 Assays, three categories. Diagrammatic representation of the effect of warfarin on the vitamin K–dependent hemostatic system at three levels: hepatic vitamin K cycle, hemostatic proenzyme levels, and the expression of hemostatic enzymatic activity. γVKDP = γ-carboxylated vitamin K–dependent proteins; des-γVKDP = descarboxyl vitamin K–dependent proteins; F1.2 = prothrombin activation peptide fragment 1.2; TAT = thrombin–antithrombin III complex; FPA = fibrinopeptide A.

available on most commercial thromboplastins. The INR therefore gives the PT ratio that would have been observed if the local laboratory had used the international reference thromboplastin. This form of standardization obviously benefits longitudinal reproducibility across different lost of the same thromboplastin, as one might see in a single institution. The INR also allows comparisons to be made between different manufacturers' thromboplastins, as seen in multi-institutional studies of oral anticoagulation or when a patient moves from one location to another.

An INR of 2.0 to 3.0 is recommended for most clinical indications, as reviewed in Table 3, modified from Hirsh (89). The dosing strategy for warfarin varies with the urgency of the clinical situation. Warfarin induction is smoothest if a typical maintenance dose of 4 to 5 mg/day is initiated, with the PT checked daily for 5 to 7 days until a stable prolongation of the clotting time in the target INR range is reached. The PT is then checked once or

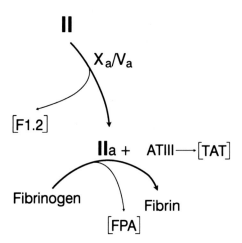

Figure 7 Schematic representation of measurable products of prothrombin activation (F1.2), thrombin activity (FPA), and thrombin inhibition (TAT). F1.2 = fragment 1.2; FPA = fibrinopeptide A; TAT = thrombin–antithrombin complex; II = prothrombin; IIa = thrombin; ATIII = antithrombin III; Xa/Va = activated forms of factors X and V.

twice a week for a month and then once or twice a month for the duration of the therapeutic course. In cases of greater therapeutic urgency, usually involving patients already receiving heparin, a warfarin dose of 10 mg/day can be used for the first couple of days, with the PT-monitoring scheme outlined above used to individualize the patient's dose in the appropriate therapeutic range. Since heparin affects the PT as well as the PTT, the INR will often decrease slightly following cessation of heparin.

The INR has found more widespread acceptance in Europe and Canada than in the United States. Recent reviews have promoted increased use of the INR in the United States (89,90), but other investigators have suggested the INR may have more limited utility with the heterogeneous groups of instruments and reagents used in the United States (91).

The most important recent contribution to the practice of oral anticoagulant therapy in North America was the demonstration by Hirsh et al. (92–94), using calibrated thromboplastins, that North American physicians used higher doses of warfarin than their European counterparts. This observation has lead to the use of lower doses of warfarin with fewer side effects and equal therapeutic efficacy (92–94). A few preliminary studies (95,96) have demonstrated the effectiveness of doses of warfarin as low as 1 mg per day. At doses this low, there is no appreciable change in the PT or traditional one-stage coagulation factor assays.

At lower doses of warfarin there are fewer hemorrhagic complications, but the effect of lower doses on the rare occurrence of warfarin-induced skin necrosis is unknown. It appears that persons heterozygous for protein C and rarely protein S deficiencies are at a higher risk for the occurrence of this latter complication. In the case of protein C deficiency this has been attributed to the relatively short half-life of protein C (6–8 h) in comparison with most of the procoagulant vitamin K–dependent proteins (e.g., prothrombin half-life = 60 h). As a result of the shorter half-life of the inhibitory proteins, patients are potentially exposed to a hemostatic imbalance favoring thrombosis during the first few days of warfarin therapy. It is possible that this potential imbalance may be less marked at lower warfarin doses, and thus the incidence of this life- and limb-threatening complication may decrease.

Table 3 Effectiveness of Oral Anticoagulant Therapy

Condition	International normalized ratio (INR)[a]		Source
	Minimal effective	Recommended	
Deep-vein thrombosis			
Prevention	1.5–2.5	2.0–3.0	Francis et al. (109)
			Powers et al. (110)
			Taberner et al. (111)
			Poller et al. (95)
Treatment	2.0–2.3	2.0–3.0	Hull et al. (92)
Acute myocardial infarction			
Prevention of stroke	2.0	2.0–3.0	Resnekov et al. (112)
			Goldberg et al. (113)
			Medical Res. Council.
			(114), VA study (115)
Prevention of mortality	2.7–4.5	3.0–4.5	Sixty Plus (116)
			Smith et al. (117)
Reduction of mortality	2.7–4.5	3.0–4.5	Sixty Plus (116)
			Smith et al. (117)
Peripheral arterial disease— prevention of death	2.6–4.5	—	Kretschmer et al. (118)
Atrial fibrillation—prevention of systemic embolism	1.5–2.5	2.0–3.0	BAATAF (94)
Cardiac-valve replacement			
Tissue valves	2.0–2.3	2.0–3.0	Turpie et al. (93)
Mechanical valves	1.9–3.6	3.0–4.5	Saour et al. (119)
Cerebral embolism	Not evaluated	—	—
Native valvular heart disease	Not evaluated	—	—

Modified, with permission, from Ref. 89.
[a]For thromboplastin with an international sensitivity index (ISI) of 2.3, the INRs and the corresponding prothrombin time ratios are as follows:

INR	1.5	2.0	2.5	3.0	3.5	4.0	4.5	5.0
Prothrombin time ratios	1.20	1.35	1.49	1.61	1.72	1.83	1.92	2.01

Recommendations are based on Hirsh et al. (107), Poller (88), and Loeliger et al. (120); a lower range might be effective. Based on an ISI of 2.3.

B. Novel Monitoring Strategies

The trend toward the lowering of warfarin doses raises two interesting questions. First, are there more direct methods for measuring the antithrombotic effect of warfarin than simple assessment of decreased proenzyme levels? This question is especially relevant to very-low-dose warfarin therapy. Second, what is the impact of dietary vitamin K on the anticoagulant effect of warfarin? Figure 6 presents a schema that suggests various alternative monitoring strategies. Selected measures of thrombin are listed in the bottom portion of Figure 6.

One of the primary goals of warfarin therapy is the inhibition of thrombin generation. Figure 7 depicts three important markers of thrombin generated during conversion of prothrombin to thrombin and by the subsequent activity and inhibition of thrombin. The proteolytic activation of prothrombin to thrombin by factor Xa releases the amino-terminal peptide fragment 1.2 (F1.2). The subsequent proteolytic cleavage of fibrinogen to fibrin by thrombin releases fibrinopeptide A (FPA). Finally, a large proportion of the thrombin generated is covalently bound by the inhibitor antithrombin III into thrombin–antithrombin III (TAT) complexes. Assays have been developed for these three analytes (F1.2, FPA, and TAT).

At the traditional level of measuring hemostatic proenzymes (Fig. 6), two novel approaches have evolved. Furie et al. (97,98) have shown that measurement of the plasma concentration of fully carboxylated "native" prothrombin correlates more closely with clinical outcome than does the PT. The Furie study was performed with somewhat higher doses of warfarin than are currently used, and further investigation using current warfarin doses is necessary to validate this approach. Blanchard et al. (99) evaluated a complementary approach using an immunoassay selective for the plasma concentration of descarboxy forms of prothrombin and observed poor correlation with clinical efficacy and complications in patients treated at relatively high warfarin doses. Others (100,101) have also begun to investigate the use of immunoassays for descarboxy vitamin K–dependent coagulation proteins in patients treated with the currently accepted lower doses of warfarin; however, demonstration of their utility must await appropriate clinical trials. The immunochemical measurement of plasma descarboxy vitamin K–dependent coagulation protein concentrations could prove particularly useful at the lower doses of warfarin as a marker of relatively low-intensity inhibition of the vitamin K cycle.

Assays available for assessment of ongoing hemostatic enzymatic activity are outlined in Figures 6 and 7. Work by a number of investigators (102) supports the hypothesis that the hemostatic system is in a state of dynamic balance between procoagulant and anticoagulant pathways, with a small amount of continuous, measurable enzymatic activity. The hemostatic markers of thrombin activity have been most thoroughly investigated (Fig. 7) and include fragment 1.2 (F1.2), fibrinopeptide A (FPA), and thrombin-antithrombin complexes (TAT). The F1.2 assay is the only one of this group that has been seriously evaluated for monitoring warfarin therapy. The plasma concentration of F1.2 is elevated in the plasma of patients at risk for thromboembolic disease with hereditary deficiencies of antithrombin III and protein C and can be suppressed in these patients and normal persons following the initiation of warfarin therapy (103). Recently, Bauer (104) and Mannucci (105) have demonstrated a dose-response relationship between the intensity of oral anticoagulant therapy assessed by INR and the degree of suppression of F1.2 plasma concentration. This dose-response relationship appears to exist across a reasonably broad range of INRs (1.3 to >4.0). However, demonstration of the practical utility of the F1.2 assay for monitoring oral anticoagulant therapy must await larger validation studies that will address the sensitivity and specificity of the assay for prediction of therapeutic effect and complications.

The measurement of vitamin K and its metabolites may prove to be a useful clinical tool especially for patients receiving lower doses of warfarin. As depicted in Figure 6, when warfarin blocks the vitamin K cycle, the epoxide form of the vitamin appears in the plasma. The measurement of vitamin K epoxide levels could prove to be useful at very low doses of warfarin when traditional assays show little or no effect. The measurement of plasma vitamin K concentration may prove effective for managing patients who appear either resistant or oversensitive to warfarin. Since vitamin K is absorbed rapidly from the gastrointestinal tract, only fasting levels reflect nutritional status (17). Preliminary data from our laboratory have demonstrated, in a limited number of patients, a relationship between ease of controlling warfarin therapy by monitoring the PT and vitamin K levels (107). Larger clinical studies are now in progress.

Finally, the role of dietary vitamin K will undoubtedly become more important at lower warfarin doses. Until recently, only limited data have been available on the vitamin K content of foods. The compilation of a comprehensive list of vitamin K content of common foods and beverages has been a long-term project of our laboratory. Table 3 presents our most recent data. The vitamin K content of different foods varies considerably, and the availability of various foods is a function of season and geographic location. Intercurrent illness may also lead to changes in intake and absorption of the vitamin, thus adding an additional element of dietary variability. Consequently, dietary counseling will probably be incorporated into future clinical practice to ensure adequate therapeutic effect at lower doses of warfarin. Careful investigation of the interactions of diet and the distributions of vitamin K metabolites at lower doses of warfarin will be necessary to fully evaluate the clinical efficacy of these regimens.

In conclusion, progress in understanding the biochemical mechanisms of vitamin K metabolism and vitamin K–dependent hemostasis has created new and promising methods for monitoring oral anticoagulant therapy. Most of these new approaches are undergoing aggressive evaluation, although none is fully validated for clinical use at the present time. In the meantime, the PT remains the mainstay of clinical monitoring. The development of more sensitive thromboplastins and their standardization by the INR should improve the therapeutic utility of this time-tested clinical tool.

REFERENCES

1. Bingham JB, Meyer OO, Pohle FJ. Studies on the hemorrhagic agent 3,3′-methylene-bis-(4-hydroxycoumarin). The effect on the prothrombin and coagulation time of dogs and humans. Am J Med Sci 1941; 202:563–78.
2. Butt HR, Allen EV, Bollman JL. Preparation from spoiled sweet clover [3,3′-methylene-bis-(4-hydroxycoumarin)] which prolongs coagulation and prothrombin time of blood, preliminary reports of experimental and clinical studies. Proc Staff Meetings Mayo Clin 1941; 16: 388–95.
3. Deykin D. Anticoagulant therapy. In: Coleman RL, et al., eds. Hemostasis and thrombosis, basic principles and clinical practice. Philadelphia: J.B. Lippincott, 1983:1003–12.
4. Sadowski JA, Bovill EG, Mann KG. Warfarin and the metabolism and function of vitamin K. In: Poller L, ed. Recent advances in blood coagulation. New York: Churchill Livingstone, 1991:93–118.
5. Bovill EG, Mann KG. Warfarin and the biochemistry of the vitamin K–dependent proteins. In: Wessler S, Becker CG, Nemerson Y, eds. New York: Plenum Press, 1987:17–46.
6. Suttie JW. The biochemical basis of warfarin therapy. In: Wessler S, Becker CG, Nemerson Y, eds. The new dimensions of warfarin prophylaxis. New York: Plenum Press, 1987:3–16.
7. Dam H. Cholesterinstoffwechsel in Huhneriern and Hunchen. Biochem Zeit 1929; 215: 475–477.
8. Dam H, Schonheyder F, Tage-Hansen E. Studies on the mode of action of vitamin K. Biochem J 1936; 30:1075.
9. Esmon CT, Vigano-D'Angelo S, D'Angelo A, Comp PC. Anticoagulation Proteins C and S. In: Wessler S, Becker CG, Nemerson Y, eds. The new dimensions of warfarin prophylaxis. New York: Plenum Press, 1987:47–54.
10. Suttie JW. Vitamin K. In: Diplock AT, ed. The fat-soluble vitamins. Lancaster, Pennsylvania: Technomic Publishing, 1985:239–245.
11. Campbell HA, Link KP. Studies on the hemorrhagic sweet clover disease. IV. The isolation and crystallization of the hemorrhagic agent. J Biol Chem 1941; 138:21.
12. Shapiro S. The purification of human prothrombin. Angiology 1953; 4:380.
13. Matschiner JT, Bell RG, Amelotti JM. Isolation and characterization of a new metabolite of phylloquinone in the rat. Biochim Biophys Acta 1970; 201:309.

14. Bell RG, Matschiner JT. Vitamin K activity of phylloquinone oxide. Arch Biochem Biophys 1969; 135:152.

15. Bell RG, Matschiner JT. Warfarin and the inhibition of vitamin K activity by an oxide metabolite. Nature 1972; 237:32.

16. Willingham AK, Matschiner JT. Changes in phylloquinone epoxidase activity related to prothrombin synthesis and microsomal clotting activity in the rat. Biochem J 1974; 140:435.

17. Sadowski JA, Schnoes HK, Suttie JW. Vitamin K epoxidase: properties and relationship to prothrombin synthesis. Biochemistry 1977; 16:3856.

18. Matschiner JT, Zimmerman A, Bell RG. Physiology and biochemistry of prothrombin conversion: the influence of warfarin on vitamin K epoxide reductase. Thromb Diathes Haemorrh 1974; (suppl 57):45.

19. Friedman PA, Shia M. Some characteristics of a vitamin K–dependent carboxylating system from rat liver microsomes. Biochem Biophys Res Commun 1976; 70:647.

20. Whitlon DS, Sadowski JA, Suttie JW. Mechanisms of coumarin action: significance of vitamin K epoxide reductase inhibition. Biochemistry 1978; 17:1371.

21. Mann KG, Nesheim ME, Church WR, Haley P, Krishnaswamy S. Surface-dependent reactions of the vitamin K–dependent enzyme complexes. Blood 1990; 76:1–16.

22. Esmon CT. The roles of protein C and thrombomodulin in the regulation of blood coagulation. J Biol Chem 1989; 264:4743–6.

23. Esmon CT. The regulation of natural anticoagulant pathways. Science 1987; 235:1348–52.

24. Krishnaswamy S, Jones KC, Mann KG. Prothrombinase complex assembly: kinetic mechanism of enzyme assembly on phospholipid vesicles. J Biol Chem 1988; 263:3823–34.

25. Nesheim ME, Kettner C, Shaw E, Mann KG. Cofactor dependence of factor Xa incorporation into the prothrombinase complex. J Biol Chem 1981; 256:6537–40.

26. Mann KG, Jenny RJ, Krishnaswamy S. Cofactor proteins in the assembly and expression of blood clotting enzymes. Annu Rev Biochem 1988; 57:915–56.

27. Krishnaswamy S. Prothrombinase complex assembly. Contributions of protein-protein and protein-membrane interactions toward complex formation. J Biol Chem 1990; 265:3708–18.

28. Pryzdial ELG, Mann KG. The association of coagulation factor Xa and factor Va. J Biol Chem 1991; 266:8969–77.

29. Nesheim ME, Taswell JB, Mann KG. The contribution of bovine factor V and factor Va to the activity of prothrombinase. J Biol Chem 1979; 254:10952–62.

30. Nesheim ME, Tracy RP, Mann KG. "Clotspeed," a mathematical simulation of the functional properties of prothrombinase. J Biol Chem 1984; 259:1447–53.

31. Van Dieijen G, Tans G, Rosing J, Hemker HC. The role of phospholipid and factor VIIIa in the activation of bovine factor X. J Biol Chem 1981; 256:3433–42.

32. Bach R, Gentry R, Nemerson Y. Factor VII binding to tissue factor in reconstituted phospholipid vesicles: induction of cooperativity by phosphatidyleserine. Biochemistry 1986; 25: 4007–20.

33. Ruf W, Rehemtulla A, Morrissey JH, Edgington TS. Phospholipid-independent and -dependent interactions required for tissue factor receptor and cofactor function. J Biol Chem 1991; 266:2158–66.

34. Lawson JH, Butenas S, Mann KG. The evaluation of complex dependent alterations in human factor VIIa. J Biol Chem 1992; 267:4834–43.

35. Stenflo J, Ohlin AK, Owen WG, Schneider WJ. β-Hydroxyaspartic acid or β-hydroxyasparagin in bovine low density lipoprotein receptor and in bovine thrombomodulin. J Biol Chem 1988; 263:21–4.

36. Nelsestuen GL. Role of gamma-carboxyglutamic acid. An unusual protein transition required for the calcium-dependent binding of prothrombin to phospholipid. J Biol Chem 1976; 251: 5648–56.

37. Toomey JR, Smith KJ, Stafford DW. Localization of the human tissue factor recognition determinant of human factor VIIa. J Biol Chem 1991; 266:19198–202.

38. Baron M, Normal DG, Harvy TS, Handford PA, Mayhew M, Tse AGD, Brownlee GG, Campbell ID. Protein Sci 1992; 1:81–90.

39. Hogg JP, Ohlin A, Stenflo J. J Biol Chem 1992; 267:703–6.

40. Berkowitz P, Huh NW, Brostrom KE, Panek MG, Weber DJ, Tulinsky A, Pedersen LG, Hiskey RG. A metal ion–binding site in the kringle region of bovine prothrombin fragment 1. J Biol Chem 1992; 267:4570–6.

41. Furie B, Bing DH, Feldmann RJ, Robison DJ, Burnier JP, Furie BC. Computer-generated models of blood coagulation factor Xa, factor IXa, and thrombin based upon structural homology with other serine proteases. J Biol Chem 1982; 257:3875–82.

42. Bajaj SP, Spitzer SG, Welsh WJ, Warn-Cramer BJ, Kasper CK, Birktoft JJ. Experimental and theoretical evidence supporting the role of Gly363 in blood coagulation factor IXa (Gly193 in chymotrypsin) for proper activation of the proenzyme. J Biol Chem 1990; 265:2956–61.

43. Furie B, Furie BC. The molecular basis of blood coagulation. Cell 1988; 53:505–18.

44. Patthy L. Evolution of the proteases of blood coagulation and fibrinolysis by assembly from modules. Cell 1986; 41:657–63.

45. Tracy PB, Eide LL, Bowie EJW, Mann KG: Radioimmunoassay of factor V in human plasma and platelets. Blood 1982; 60:59–63.

46. Viskup RW, Tracy PB, Mann KG. The isolation of human platelet factor V. Blood 1987; 69: 1188–95.

47. Sadler JE, Davie EW. The molecular basis of blood disease. Philadelphia: W.B. Saunders, 1987.

48. Nesheim ME, Mann KG. Thrombin-catalyzed activation of single chain bovine factor V. J Biol Chem 1979; 254:1326–34.

49. Foster WB, Nesheim ME, Mann KG. The factor Xa-catalyzed activation of factor V. J Biol Chem 1983; 258:13970–77.

50. Lee C, Mann KG. The activation/inactivation of human factor V by plasmin. Blood 1989; 73: 185–90.

51. Kane WH, Davie EW. Blood coagulation factors V and VIII: structural and functional similarities and their relationship to hemorrhagic and thrombotic disorders. Blood 1988; 71: 539–55.

52. Jenny RJ, Pittman DD, Toole JJ, Kriz RW, Aldape RA, Hewick RM, Kaufman RJ, Mann KG. Complete cDNA and derived amino acid sequence of human factor V. Proc Natl Acad Sci USA 1987; 84:4846–50.

53. Krishnaswamy S, Mann KG. The binding of factor Va to phospholipid vesicles. J Biol Chem 1988; 263:3823–34.

54. Kalafatis M, Jenny R, Mann KG. Identification and characterization of a phospholipid binding site of bovine factor Va. J Biol Chem 1990; 265:21580–9.

55. Guinto ER, Esmon CT. Loss of prothrombin and of factor Xa–factor Va interactions upon inactivation of factor Va by activated protein C. J Biol Chem 1984; 259:13986–92.

56. Tucker MM, Foster WB, Katzmann JA, Mann KG. A monoclonal antibody which inhibits the factor Va:factor Xa interaction. J Biol Chem 1983; 258:1210–14.

57. Vehar GA, Davie EW. Preparation and properties of bovine factor VIII (antihemophilic factor). Biochemistry 1980; 19:401–10.

58. Walker FJ, Sexton PW, Esmon CT. The inhibition of blood coagulation by activated protein C through the selective inactivation of activated factor V. Biochim Biophys Acta 1979; 571:333–42.

59. Walker FJ. Identification of a new protein involved in the regulation of the anticoagulant activity of activated protein C. Protein S–binding protein. J Biol Chem 1986; 261:10941–4.

60. Harris KW, Esmon CT. Protein S is required for bovine platelets to support activated protein C binding and activity. J Biol Chem 1985; 260:2007–10.

61. Stern DM, Nawroth PP, Karris K, Esmon CT. Cultured bovine aortic endothelial cells promote activated protein C–protein S–mediated inactivation of Factor Va. J Biol Chem 1986; 261: 713–8.

62. Griffin JH, Evatt B, Zimmerman TS, Kleiss AJ, Wideman C. Deficiency of protein C in congenital thrombotic disease. J Clin Invest 1981; 68:1370–3.

63. Galvin JB, Kurosawa S, Moore K, Esmon CT, Esmon NL. Reconstitution of rabbit thrombomodulin into phospholipid vesicles. J Biol Chem 1987; 262:2199–205.

64. Drake TA, Ruf W, Morrissey JH, Edgington TS. Functional tissue factor is entirely cell surface expressed on lipopolysaccharide-stimulated human blood monocytes and a constitutively tissue factor–producing neoplastic cell line. J Cell Biol 1989; 109:389–95.

65. Fair DS, MacDonald MJ. Cooperative interaction between factor VII and cell surface–expressed tissue factor. J Biol Chem 1987; 262:11692–8.

66. Wilcox JN, Smith KM, Schwartz SM, Gordon D. Localization of tissue factor in the normal vessel wall and in the atherosclerotic plaque. Proc Natl Acad Sci USA 1989; 86:2839–43.

67. Hartzell S, Ryder K, Lanahan A, Lau LF, Nathan D. A growth factor–responsive gene of murine BALB/c 3T3 cells encodes a protein homologous to human tissue factor. Mol Cell Biol 1989; 9:2567–73.

68. Brox JH, Osterud B, Fenton JW. Production and availability of thromboplastin in endothelial cells: the effects of thrombin, endotoxin and platelets. Br J Haematol 1984; 57:239–46.

69. Bevilacqua MP, Pober JS, Majeau GR, Cotran RS, Gimbrone MA Jr. Interleukin 1 (IL-1) induces biosynthesis and cell surface expression of procoagulant activity in human vascular endothelial cells. J Exp Med 1984; 160:618–23.

70. Crossman DC, Carr DP, Tuddenham EG, Pearson JD, McVey JH. The regulation of tissue factor mRNA in human endothelial cells in response to endotoxin or phorbol ester. J Biol Chem 1990; 265:9782–7.

71. Scarpati EM, Sadler JE. Regulation of endothelial cell coagulant properties. Modulation of tissue factor, plasminogen activator inhibitors, and thrombomodulin by phorbol 12-myristate 13-acetate and tumor necrosis factor. J Biol Chem 1989; 254:20705–13.

72. Janco RL, Morris PJ. Regulation of monocyte procoagulant by chemoattractants. Blood 1985; 65:545–52.

73. Walker FJ, Esmon CT. The effects of phospholipid and factor Va on the inhibition of factor Xa by antithrombin III. Biochem Biophys Res Commun 1979; 90:641–7.

74. Nesheim ME, Canfield WM, Kisiel W, Mann KG. Studies of the capacity of factor Xa to protect factor Va from inactivation by activated protein C. J Biol Chem 1982; 257:1443–7.

75. Hemker HC, Muller AD. Kinetic aspect of the interaction of blood clotting enzymes. V. The reaction mechanism of the extrinsic clotting system as revealed by the kinetics of one-stage estimations of coagulation enzymes. Thromb Diathes Haemorrh 1968; 19:368–82.

76. Prydz H, Gladhaug A. Factor X: immunological studies. Thromb Diathes Haemorrh 1971; 25:157–65.

77. Veltkamp JJ. Detection and clinical significance of PIVKA. Mayo Clin Proc 1971; 49:923–4.

78. Brozovic M, Howarth DJ. Demonstration of PIVKA-VII. Boerhave course on synthesis of prothrombin and related coagulation factors. Leiden, Netherlands. 1974.

79. Malhotra OP. Dicoumarol-induced prothrombins. Ann NY Acad Sci 1981; 370:426–37.

80. Malhotra OP, Nesheim ME, Mann KG. The kinetics of activation of normal and γ-carboxyglutamic acid–deficient prothrombins. J Biol Chem 1985; 260:279–87.

81. Malhotra OP. Dicoumarol-induced prothrombins containing 6, 7 and 8 γ-carboxyglutamic acid residues: isolation and characterization. Biochem Cell Biol 1989; 67:411–21.

82. Malhotra OP. Dicoumarol-induced γ-carboxyglutamic acid prothrombin: isolation and comparison with 6-, 7-, 8- and 10-γ-carboxyglutamic acid isomers. Biochem Cell Biol 1990; 68:705–15.

83. Walls JD, Berg DT, Yan B, et al. Amplification of multicistronic plasmids in the human 293 cell line and secretion of correctly processed recombinant human protein C. Gene 1989; 81:139–49.

84. Lammle B, Bounameaux H, Marbet GA, Eichlisberger R, Ducker F. Monitoring of oral anticoagulation by an amidolytic factor X assay. A long-term study in 42 patients. Thromb Haemost 1980; 46:150–3.

85. Van Wijk EM, Kahle LH, ten Cate JW. Mechanized amidolytic technique for determination of factor X and factor X antigen, and its application to patients being treated with oral anticoagulants. Clin Chem 1980; 26:885–90.

86. Erskine G, Walker ID, Davidson JF. Maintenance control of oral anticoagulant therapy by a chromogenic substrate assay for factor X. J Clin Pathol 1980; 33:445–8.

87. Fareed J, Messmore HL, Walenga JM, Bermes EW. Synthetic peptide substrates in hemostatic testing. CRC Critical Reviews in Clinical Laboratory Sciences 1983; 19:71–134.

88. Poller L, Hirsh J. Optimal therapeutic ranges for oral anticoagulation. In: Fuster V, Verstraete M, eds. Thrombosis in cardiovascular disorders. Philadelphia: W.B. Saunders, 1992:161–73.

89. Hirsh J. Oral anticoagulant drugs. N Engl J Med 1991; 324:1865–75.

90. Hirsh J. Substandard monitoring of warfarin in North America. Time for a change. Arch Intern Med 1992; 152:278–82.

91. Ng VL, Levin J, Corash L, Gottfried E. Failure of the international normalized ratio to generate constant results within a local medical community. Am J Clin Pathol 1993 (in press).

92. Hull R, Hirsh J, Jay R, Carter C, England C, Gent M, Turpie AGG, McLoughlin D, Dodd P, Thomas M, Raskob G, Ockelford P. Different intensities of anticoagulation in long-term treatment of proximal venous thrombosis. N Engl J Med 1982; 307:1676.

93. Turpie AGG, Hirsh J, Gunstensen J, Nelson H, Gent M. Randomized comparison of two intensities of oral anticoagulant therapy after tissue valve replacement. Lancet 1988; 1: 1242.

94. The Boston Area Anticoagulation Trial for Atrial Fibrillation Investigators: The effect of low dose warfarin on the risk of stroke in patients with non-rheumatic atrial fibrillation. N Engl J Med 1990; 323:1505–11.

95. Poller L, McCernan A, Thompson JM. Fixed minidose warfarin: a new approach to prophylaxis against venous thrombosis after major surgery. Br Med J 1987; 295:1309–12.

96. Bern MM, Kokich JJ, Wallach SR, et al. Very low dose warfarin can prevent thrombosis in central venous catheters. Ann Intern Med 1990; 112:234–8.

97. Furie B, Liebman HA, Blanchard RA, et al. Comparison of the native prothrombin antigen and the prothrombin time for monitoring oral anticoagulant therapy. Blood 1984; 64:445–51.

98. Furie B, Diuguid CF, Jacobs M, Diuguid DL, Furie BC. Randomized prospective trial comparing the native prothrombin antigen with prothrombin time for monitoring oral anticoagulant therapy. Blood 1990; 75:344–9.

99. Blanchard R, Furie BC, Kruger SF, et al. Immunoassays of human prothrombin species which correlate with functional coagulant activities. J Lab Clin Med 1983; 101:242–55.

100. Church WR, Bhushan FH, Mann KG, et al. Discrimination of normal and abnormal prothrombin and protein C in plasma using a calcium ion–inhibited monoclonal antibody to a common epitope on several vitamin K dependent proteins. Blood 1989; 74:2418–2425.

101. Amiral J, Grosley M, Plassart V, Mimilla F, Chambrette B. Development of a monoclonal immunoassay for the direct measurement of decarboxy prothrombin on plasma. Thromb Haemost 1991; 65(6):10.

102. Bauer KA, Rosenberg RD. The pathophysiology of the prethrombotic state in humans: insights gained from studies using markers of haemostatic system activation. Blood 1987; 70:343–50.

103. Conway EM, Bauer KA, Barzegar S, Rosenberg RD. Suppression of hemostatic system activation by oral anticoagulants in the blood of patients with thrombotic diatheses. J Clin Invest 1987; 80:1535.

104. Millenson MM, Bauer KA, Kistler JP, Barzegar S, Tulin L, Rosenberg RD. Monitoring "mini-intensity" anticoagulation with warfarin: comparison of the prothrombin time using a sensitive thromboplastin with prothrombin fragment F_{1+2} levels. Blood 79:2034–8.

105. Mannucci PW, Bottasso B, Tripodi A, Bonomi AB. Prothrombin fragment 1 + 2 and intensity of treatment with oral anticoagulants. Thromb Haemost 1991; 66:741.

106. Lynch MB, Bovill EG, Bhushan FA, Church WR, Landesman MM, Sadowski JA. The measurement of des-carboxy vitamin K dependent proteins (II, C) and vitamin K levels during

the induction of warfarin therapy. Proceedings of the Academy of Clinical Laboratory Physicians and Scientists, June 1990.

107.   Hirsh J, Poller L, Deykin D, Levine M, Dalen JE. Optimal therapeutic range for oral anticoagulants. Chest 1989; 95(Suppl 2):5S–11S (erratum, Chest 1989; 96:962).

108.   Francis CW, Marder VJ, Evarts CM, Yaukoolbodi S. Two-step warfarin therapy: prevention of postoperative venous thrombosis without excessive bleeding. JAMA 1983; 249:374–8.

109.   Powers PJ, Gent M, Jay RM, et al. A randomized trial of less intense postoperative warfarin or aspirin therapy in the prevention of venous thromboembolism after surgery for fractured hip. Arch Intern Med 1989; 149:771–4.

110.   Taberner DA, Poller L, Burslem RW, Jones JB. Oral anticoagulants controlled by the British comparative thromboplastin versus low-dose heparin in prophylaxis of deep vein thrombosis. Br Med J 1978; 1:272–4.

111.   Resnekov L, Chediak J, Hirsh J, Lewis HD Jr. Antithrombotic agents in coronary artery disease. Chest 1989; 95(suppl 2):52S–72S.

112.   Goldberg RJ, Gore JM, Dalen JE, Alpert JS. Long-term anticoagulant therapy after acute myocardial infarction. Am Heart J 1985; 109:616–22.

113.   The Working Party on Anticoagulant Therapy in Coronary Thrombosis. Assessment of short-term anticoagulant administration after cardiac infarction: report of the Working Party on Anticoagulant Therapy in Coronary Thrombosis to the Medical Research Council. Br Med J 1969; 1:335–42.

114.   Anticoagulants in acute myocardial infarction: results of cooperative clinical trial. JAMA 1973; 225:724–9.

115.   A double-blind trial to assess long-term oral anticoagulant therapy in elderly patients after myocardial infarction: report of the Sixty Plus Reinfarction Study Research Group. Lancet 1980; 2:989–94.

116.   Smith P, Arnesen H, Holme I: The effect of warfarin on mortality and reinfarction after myocardial infarction. N Engl J Med 1990; 323:147–52.

117.   Kretschmer G, Wenzl E, Schemper M, et al. Influence of postoperative anticoagulant treatment on patient survival after femoropopliteal vein by-pass surgery. Lancet 1988; 1:797–8.

118.   Saour JN, Sieck JO, Mamo LAR, Gallus AS. Trial of different intensities of anticoagulation in patients with prosthetic heart valves. N Engl J Med 1990; 322:428–32.

119.   Poller L. Therapeutic ranges in anticoagulant administration. Br Med J 1985; 290:1683–6.

120.   Loeliger EA, Poller L, Samama M, et al. Questions and answers on prothrombin time standardization in oral anticoagulant control. Thromb Haemost 1985; 54:515–7.

Mechanisms of Thrombolysis

Russell P. Tracy, Edwin G. Bovill, and Kenneth G. Mann
University of Vermont College of Medicine, Burlington, Vermont

I. INTRODUCTION

A. Thrombolysis Versus Fibrinolysis

Thrombolysis is the term that is currently used to describe the medical dissolution of blood clots through the action of drugs such as recombinant tissue-type plasminogen activator (rt-PA) and streptokinase, among others. The most widespread application of these drugs is in the treatment of acute myocardial infarction. Additional clinical applications are being explored, such as venous thrombosis and pulmonary embolism. Blood clots are composed of both platelets and fibrin (as well as of red blood cells). The term thrombolysis implies that thrombolytic agents act against all components. However, it appears that clots resulting from primary hemostatic mechanisms (so-called "platelet plugs") are relatively resistant to the action of thrombolytic agents (1). Therefore, a more accurate term to describe the effects of a drug such as rt-PA might be "fibrinolysis." Nonetheless, "thrombolysis" is the currently accepted term and will be used throughout this chapter. Successful clinical thrombolysis may also include the concept of prevention of reocclusion.

It should be emphasized that the purpose of this chapter is to provide a fundamental description of thrombolysis. Space limitations preclude a complete exposition. (For reviews see Refs. 2–4.) Furthermore, it is important to note that a complete understanding of all the mechanisms of the thrombolytic process has not yet been achieved. As this chapter is being prepared, important research is ongoing, concerning such areas as the interaction between thrombolytic and thrombogenic factors (5,6), the role of adjunctive therapy in producing effective thrombolysis (7), and the underlying biochemical factors that contribute in individual patients to the effectiveness of a fixed dose of a particular thrombolytic agent (8).

Procoagulation   Profibrinolysis

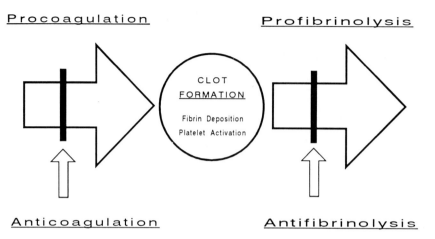

Anticoagulation   Antifibrinolysis

Figure 1 Coagulant balance. Schematic representation of the overall concept of coagulation and fibrinolysis as dynamic, linked systems, involving proactive as well as regulatory elements.

B. Coagulant Balance

We write this chapter in the context of the concept of coagulant balance, as depicted in Figure 1. Briefly stated, "coagulant balance" refers to the ongoing, linked processes of procoagulation and profibrinolysis, each held in check by appropriate inhibitory activities (anticoagulation and antifibrinolysis, respectively). Crucial to the process of procoagulation is the generation of α-thrombin, important not only for fibrin generation, but also for platelet activation. In the process of profibrinolysis, the ultimate enzyme is plasmin, which acts directly to dissolve fibrin. We believe that these processes occur normally, at low levels, in an "idling" manner, and that one or the other is accentuated under certain conditions. In the case of thrombolytic therapy, the profibrinolytic process is greatly enhanced. We believe that it is useful to keep the coagulant-balance scheme in mind as one considers the mechanisms of thrombolysis, as described below.

II. COMPONENTS OF THE FIBRINOLYTIC SYSTEM

Figure 2 illustrates the major components of the fibrinolytic system as we currently understand them. These factors are summarized in Table 1. Important factors in both the profibrinolytic and the antifibrinolytic pathway are listed.

A. Plasminogen Activators

In situ, the presence of fibrin triggers the activation of plasminogen to plasmin (9), most likely through the action of tissue plasminogen activator (t-PA). However, there are actually several activators that may play a role in either natural or pharmacological plasmin activation. The activators have been grouped into the so-called intrinsic, extrinsic, and exogenous systems, in a manner similar to that in which the procoagulant system has been grouped into intrinsic and extrinsic coagulation pathways (4,9). The intrinsic system of plasminogen activation involves the action of the contact activation components of procoagulation, namely factor XII/XIIa, high-molecular-weight kininogen, and prekallikrein/kallikrein.

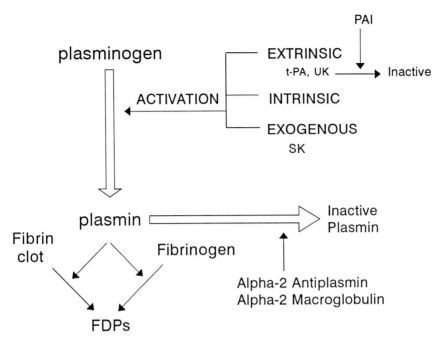

Figure 2 Components of the fibrinolytic system. Schematic representation of the major components of the fibrinolytic system. t-PA = tissue plasminogen activator; PAI1 = plasminogen activator inhibitor-1; UK = urokinase; SK = streptokinase; FDPs = fibrin(ogen) degradation products.

Table 1 Components of the Fibrinolytic System

Factor	Class	Molecular weight	Normal plasma concentration
Tissue plasminogen activator (t-PA)[a]	Activator (extrinsic)	70,000	5–20 ng/ml 0.08–0.30 nM
Urokinase (UK)[b]	Activator (extrinsic)	54,000	1–40 ng/ml 0.02–0.07 nM
Streptokinase (SK)	Activator (exogenous)	48,000	none
Plasminogen[c]	Plasmin precursor	90,000	150–200 µg/mL 1800–2200 nM
Plasminogen activator inhibitor-1 (PAI-1)[d]	t-PA inhibitor	50,000	5–30 ng/mL 0.1–0.6 nM
α_2-Antiplasmin[e]	Plasmin inhibitor	70,000	50–80 µg/mL 800–1200 nM

[a]t-PA is believed to be the most important physiological plasminogen activator, and the ratio of t-PA to active PAI-1 appears to control the rate of fibrinolysis.

[b]Although urokinase appears to be approximately as abundant as t-PA, it is not thought to play a major role in physiological fibrinolysis.

[c]Plasminogen may be considered a true zymogen (i.e., inactive enzyme precursor), much like coagulation factors such as factor X and prothrombin.

[d]Approximately 50% of the PAI-1 present in plasma is in a complex with t-PA and therefore inactive. PAI-1 is also very abundant in platelets, although primarily in a "latent," i.e., inactive, form.

[e]α_2-Antiplasmin is a very active inhibitor, but essentially inactive against plasmin already bound to fibrin.

This system differs from the other pathways of plasminogen activation in that the primary agents circulate as inactive zymogens (or proenzymes) that must be activated in order to initiate plasminogen activation. None of the other mechanisms of plasminogen activation involve zymogens per se, although plasma alterations of the other activators may be important in the regulation of activity. Little is currently known about the intrinsic activation system. It is believed that this system does not play a large role in naturally occurring plasminogen activation, although research continues in this area (4).

The extrinsic plasminogen activation system is made up of two systems, one involving t-PA and the other urokinase. Under normal conditions t-PA is supplied by the vascular endothelium, in response to a variety of stimuli such as fibrin deposition, physical trauma, etc. (9). It is believed that rt-PA serves the same function when delivered intravenously at pharmacological doses. Tissue plasminogen activator is an approximately 70,000-molecular-weight active enzyme produced by vascular endothelial cells (10). The plasma concentration of this enzyme is approximately 5 to 20 ng/ml under normal conditions. This level increases two- to threefold during the provocative venous occlusion test. This is in contrast to the levels achieved pharmacologically, which may be 1500 ng/ml or higher (11). However, there is currently little information about the systemic levels that occur during the course of natural fibrinolysis, or, probably more important, the local levels of t-PA that are achieved at the site of fibrin deposition. The peripheral-blood plasma levels are most likely a poor reflection of local concentrations, because of the ability of t-PA to bind tightly to the fibrin in a clot such as a thrombotic occlusion. As supplied by endothelial cells, t-PA is a single-chain glycoprotein that functions as a serine protease, although there is also a two-chain form with similar properties toward fibrin (12). The preferred substrate of t-PA is plasminogen, and the resulting product is the active enzyme plasmin. However, t-PA is also capable of cleaving at least one other protein substrate, fibrinogen, although this cleavage appears to be slow and probably not physiologically relevant even at pharmacological doses of t-PA (13).

Urokinase is also a serine protease with plasminogen-activation activity. This enzyme was originally described in urine (14,15). We now know urokinase circulates in plasma as a 54,000-molecular-weight single-chain enzyme (single-chain urokinase-type plasminogen activator, or scu-PA) (15). As is the case for t-PA, scu-PA is readily cleaved by plasmin into

Table 2 Comparative Properties of Thrombolytic Agents

	SK	UK	APSAC	t-PA	scu-PA
Fibrin specificity	−	−	+/−	+ +	+/+ +
Bleeding risk	+	+	+	+	+
Antigenicity	+	−	+	−	−
Circulating inhibitors	−	+	−	+	−/+
Circulating antibodies	+	−	+	−	−
Plasma half-life (min)	20	10	40	5	5
Cost	low	moderate/high	moderate/high	high	high

SK = streptokinase; UK = urokinase; APSAC = anisoylated plasminogen streptokinase complex; t-PA = tissue plasminogen activator; scu-PA = single-chain urokinase-type plasminogen activator.
Adapted from: Collen D, Stump DC, Gold HK. Thrombolytic therapy. J. Cardiovasc Pharmacol 1985; 39:405–23.

a two-chain form, which is the form that occurs in urine. The fibrinolytic role of either scu-PA or two-chain urokinase is not well defined (4). Both forms of urokinase have been used successfully as thrombolytic agents.

The exogenous system of plasminogen activation involves primarily the pharmacological use of the bacterial protein streptokinase (16). This process does not occur in natural fibrinolysis. Streptokinase is a 48,000-molecular-weight protein produced by group C β hemolytic streptococci. In plasminogen activation streptokinase, unlike the other activators, does not function as an enzyme. Rather, it forms a 1:1 stoichiometric complex with plasminogen (17). As a result of this complexation, the plasminogen protein undergoes a conformational change that exposes an active site capable of cleaving free plasminogen to plasmin and thereby acting as a plasminogen activator. The exogenous system was the first to be exploited therapeutically, and streptokinase is widely used today as a thrombolytic agent, especially in acute myocardial infarction. Both endogenous and exogenous plasminogen activators have been used for thrombolytic therapy. Table 2 summarizes the comparative characteristics of the most commonly used thrombolytic agents.

B. Plasminogen and Plasmin

Plasminogen is the target substrate of the activation systems; cleavage between amino acids Arg_{560} and Val_{561} leads to generation of the active enzyme plasmin. Plasminogen is characterized structurally by the presence of five triple-loop, disulfide-linked structures, called Kringle structures, made up of highly conserved amino acid sequences (18). Several other factors involved in coagulant balance, such as prothrombin, factor XII, t-PA, and urokinase, share the feature of Kringle structures, although the Kringle domains are not identical in these proteins. In t-PA, there is also a region homologous to a part of the protein fibronectin, the so-called finger domain, which along with one of the Kringle structures is probably responsible for the ability of t-PA to bind to fibrin (19,20). Since plasminogen also binds to fibrin, it is thought that the Kringle domains play an important role in this protein as well. Plasminogen may be cleaved by plasmin to Lys-plasminogen, a form of the molecule with a relatively small region removed from the amino-terminus; Lys-plasminogen is more readily converted to plasmin than the native form of plasminogen (Glu-plasminogen), and conversion of Glu- to Lys-plasminogen may be an important regulatory step in plasminogen activation (18).

Plasmin is derived from plasminogen and shares several structural features with it. Plasmin is a two-chain enzyme with disulfide-linked heavy and light chains. The amino-terminal heavy chain contains the five Kringle structures from the parent plasminogen molecule, which contain the lysine-binding site and appear to mediate binding to fibrin, α_2-antiplasmin, and thrombospondin.

C. Inhibitors

Plasma contains naturally occurring inhibitors of all forms of plasminogen activation, as well as inhibitors of plasmin itself. For intrinsic activation, the most potent inhibitor appears to be C1 esterase inhibitor. For the components of extrinsic activation, i.e., t-PA and urokinase, there appear to be three different inhibitors: plasminogen activator inhibitor-1 (PAI-1), PAI-2, and PAI-3 (21). At this time most investigators believe that PAI-1 is the most important of these three. A product of endothelial cells, PAI-1 is the so-called "fast-acting" inhibitor of t-PA (22), with a rate of inhibition approximately four orders of magnitude greater than that of the other inhibitors. Plasminogen activator inhibitor-1 is a 50,000-

molecular-weight protein of the serpin (*serine proteinase inhibitor*) family of inhibitors. The plasma concentration of PAI-1 is variable, probably ranging from 2 or 3 ng/ml to 50 ng/ml or higher. However, these estimates are tentative, since blood collection is extremely important in the PAI-1 assay. Platelets contain a large quantity of PAI-1, which may be elaborated during phlebotomy or sample preparation (23). Plasminogen activator inhibitor-1 exists in two forms, an active inhibitor form and an inactive latent form that may be activated in vitro by chemical methods (2). The physiological activator is unknown. Plasminogen activator inhibitor-2, from the placenta, and PAI-3, found primarily in urine, are not thought to play important roles in either naturally occurring or pharmacologic fibrinolysis under normal conditions.

Naturally occurring antistreptokinase antibodies occur in some persons who have had previous streptokinase intervention or streptococcal infections. These antibodies may inhibit the action of streptokinase and may be associated with anaphylactic reactions.

The inhibitor of plasmin of physiological relevance is α_2-antiplasmin (24), a 70,000-molecular-weight plasma glycoprotein, although α_2-macroglobulin, antithrombin III (in the presence of heparin), α_1-antitrypsin, inter-α trypsin inhibitor and, C1 esterase inhibitor are all capable of inhibiting plasmin. All of these are relatively poor inhibitors compared with α_2-antiplasmin. Until depleted, α_2-antiplasmin is the primary plasmin inhibitor. This inhibitor circulates at a concentration of approximately 1 μM and is an extremely rapid inhibitor of plasmin in solution (24). It should be noted that since the plasma concentration of plasminogen is approximately 2 μM, aggressive plasmin generation, such as is seen with thrombolytic therapy with streptokinase, is capable of generating enough plasmin to overwhelm the plasma α_2-antiplasmin, resulting in relatively unopposed plasmin activity in solution.

III. PLASMINOGEN ACTIVATION

A. Fibrin Specificity

Plasminogen is activated to the primary fibrinolytic enzyme plasmin by proteolytic cleavage. All of the activators mentioned above produce plasmin in the fluid compartment of blood. However, t-PA, in contrast to the others, is capable of performing this function on a fibrin surface, much more effectively than it does in solution. This property led to the concept of "fibrin specificity," the details of which are shown in schematic form in Figure 3. As mentioned before, t-PA and plasminogen can bind to fibrin tightly. The dissociation constant of t-PA for fibrin is approximately 0.6 μM (25). The Michaelis constant (K_m) represents the concentration of substrate, plasminogen in this case, that allows for half-maximal reaction rate, and lower values may be viewed as a measure of increased effectiveness. The K_m of t-PA for plasminogen decreases dramatically in the presence of fibrin, from 65 μM in solution to 0.16 μM on the fibrin surface (26). Since, as mentioned above, the plasma concentration of plasminogen is approximately 2 μM, which is 30 times below the solution-phase K_m, little plasmin generation by t-PA will occur in the absence of fibrin. Of course, this reaction follows the law of mass action, and if very large concentrations of t-PA are present, solution-phase plasminogen activation will occur in the absence of fibrin. In this regard, since pharmacological levels of t-PA may exceed normal circulating values by up to three orders of magnitude, the non-fibrin-dependent activation of plasminogen by t-PA cannot be disregarded.

The increase in t-PA effectiveness in the presence of fibrin may be only partly explained by changes in K_m. Changes in other parameters have been identified, and a concentration

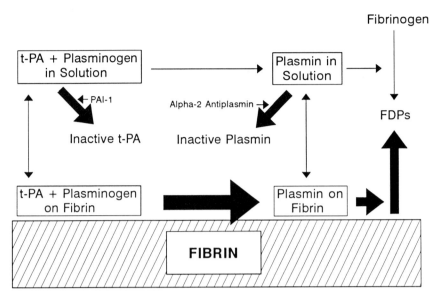

Figure 3 Fibrin specificity. Schematic representation of the increased ability of t-PA to catalyze plasmin formation on the fibrin surface, compared to solution phase. The arrows indicate relative catalytic efficiency. t-PA = tissue plasminogen activator; PAI-1 = plasminogen activator inhibitor-1; FDPs = fibrin(ogen) degradation products.

effect may also take place, since plasmin generated directly on the fibrin surface is in an ideal position to engage in fibrinolysis. Also, α_2-antiplasmin is ineffective against plasmin that is bound to a fibrin surface (25,27).

Unlike t-PA, urokinase, even though it contains a Kringle domain, does not bind to any significant degree to fibrin (14). Even so, the single-chain scu-PA, but not the two-chain form, does exhibit a measure of "fibrin specificity." The exact mechanism of this specificity is not established.

B. Plasmin as an Enzyme

Plasmin performs several functions that are of interest in fibrinolysis, which are listed in Table 3. Of course, the most prominent is the conversion of fibrin to fibrin degradation products, with the resulting decrease in clot stability. Plasmin is also able to degrade fibrinogen, which results in different, but similar, degradation products. This set of reactions is depicted in Figure 4. Before discussing these reactions in detail, we point out that plasmin is not particularly discriminatory, and plasmin free in solution, unopposed by α_2-antiplasmin, will cleave fibrinogen quite readily. In the worst case this will lead to compromised fibrin-forming ability and hemorrhagic risk. Currently, it is unclear why in certain cases α_2-antiplasmin is not able to check plasmin activity against fibrinogen. The most likely reason is that the α_2-antiplasmin levels have dropped too low during extensive plasminogen activation. However, it is also possible that occupancy of the lysine-binding sites by soluble pieces of fibrin or fibrinogen may also occur, giving rise to a highly active soluble, circulating t-PA–fibrin complexes.

Fibrinogen is a large (340,000-molecular-weight) plasma glycoprotein composed of three pairs of disulfide-linked peptide chains (28). These pairs are called A-α, B-β, and γ. Fibrinogen consists of three domains, a central E domain (comprising the disulfide-linked

Table 3 Functions of Plasmin in Blood

Substrate	Product	Action
Fibrin	FDPs	Clot dissolution, especially fibrin-rich clots
Fibrinogen	FDPs	Compromised coagulation, and loss of ability to judge coagulation status from laboratory tests, e.g., aPTT
Plasminogen	Lys-Plasminogen	Increased rate of plasmin formation
GPIb, GPIIb/IIIa	Inactive Ib, IIb/IIIa	Possible inhibition of platelet aggregation
Factor V	Factor Va	Activation of coagulation
Factor V, Va	Inactive factor V	Compromised coagulation, and loss of ability to judge coagulation status from laboratory tests, e.g., aPTT
Factor VIII, VIIIa	Inactive factor VIII	Compromised coagulation, and loss of ability to judge coagulation status from laboratory tests, e.g., aPTT

FDPs = fibrin(ogen) degradation products; aPTT = activated partial thromboplastin time; GP = glycoprotein.

amino-termini of all three pairs), and two peripheral D domains, each comprising the carboxy-terminal regions of one of the A-α, B-β, and γ chains from each pair. Thrombin cleaves the external D domain the A-α chain to release fibrinopeptide A and form fibrin I. A second thrombin cleavage releases a peptide from the B-β chain, fibrinopeptide B, and forms fibrin II. Binding sites on the fibrin II molecule are exposed and rapid polymerization

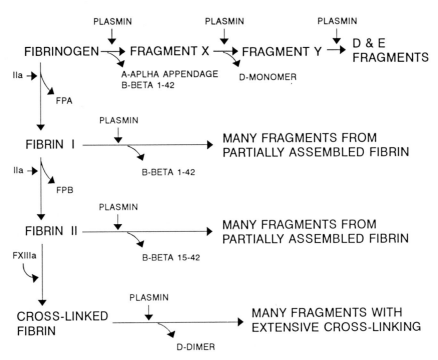

Figure 4 Cleavage of fibrinogen and fibrin by the enzymes thrombin and plasmin. Schematic representation of the cleavages catalyzed by thrombin and plasmin. IIa = thrombin; FXIIIa = factor XIIIa; X, Y, D, E = portions of the fibrinogen molecule; B-β 1–42 = the peptide from the B and β fibrinogen chains from amino acids 1 to 42; B-β 15–42 = the peptide from the B and β chains of fibrinogen from amino acid 15 to 42; FPA = fibrinopeptide A; FDB = fibrinopeptide B.

takes place. α-Thrombin also activates factor XIII to the transaminase enzyme factor XIIIa, which introduces covalent cross-links into fibrin, producing a network with long-term stability.

The plasmin cleavages of fibrinogen and fibrin proceed, much as the thrombin cleavages do, in an ordered manner (29,30). The initial cleavages of fibrinogen are in the A-α region (the "polar appendage") and the B-β region (B-β 1–42). The remaining molecule is called fragment X and is capable of forming fibrin, although in a weakened form; the pieces remaining from latter cleavages do not form fibrin and in fact most likely inhibit fibrin formation in vivo. Additional cleavages result in the release of a "D" region from fragment X, leaving fragment Y, which is then further cleaved into the remaining D and E pieces. If thrombin has acted to release fibrinopeptide B, which is actually the B-β 1–14 peptide, plasmin releases B-β 15–42, not 1–42. Finally, if thrombin and factor XIIIa have acted to produce stabilized fibrin, the plasmin cleavages release a series of cross-linked fragments, the most extensively studied of which is the D-dimer fragment. The thrombin and plasmin cleavage products are summarized in Figure 4. Immunoassays have been developed for several of the thrombin and plasmin reaction products, such as fibrinopeptide A (31) and B-β 1–42 (32). We have explored the use of commercially available assays for D-dimer, B-β 1–42, and B-β 15–42 in the context of thrombolytic therapy, and have found them to be inadequate because of cross-reactivity problems (33). Of course, they may be useful in other clinical situations characterized by less severe fibrinogenolysis.

When initiated by pharmacological intervention, plasmin generation will occur either systemically (e.g., via streptokinase) or at the site of a blood clot, whether pathological or physiological in nature (e.g., via rt-PA). Dissolution of hemostatic blood clots is most likely the leading cause of clinically significant bleeding in patients receiving thrombolytic therapy, and much research is currently under way attempting to identify more readily those persons at risk because of the presence of a preexisting physiological clot in a sensitive location such as the cerebral vasculature (34,35).

Plasmin is also capable of cleaving several other proteins (36,37), including the platelet glycoproteins Ib and IIb-IIIa (38), proteins important to platelet aggregation. The ability of plasmin to cleave factors V and VIII is possibly the most significant activity other than fibrin cleavage, since these proteins are essential to proper coagulation and the maintenance of the coagulant balance. Plasmin action on factor V has been known for many years, but the cleavage mechanism has only recently been explored (6). Plasmin initially activates factor V to factor Va, which would be a procoagulant action. However, immediately thereafter, plasmin inactivates factor Va by a second cleavage, leading to an anticoagulant effect. It appears likely that similar cleavages occur with factor VIII. The *net* result of plasmin activity on factors V and VIII is determined by which action, activation or inactivation, takes precedence; unfortunately, the factors that determine this are not yet known.

IV. REGULATION OF THROMBOLYSIS

Many of the important issues concerning the regulation of natural and pharmacological thrombolysis are discussed in this section and listed in Table 4.

A. Established Mechanisms

As mentioned in an earlier section, naturally occurring t-PA–mediated plasminogen activation is regulated by at least two mechanisms: the presence of fibrin and the action of PAI-1.

Table 4 Regulation of Thrombolysis

Regulatory action	Effector(s)
Increased plasmin formation	Increased t-PA, UK, SK level; fibrin, as a t-PA activator
Decreased plasmin formation	PAI-1 (and possibly Lp(a)) at physiological levels of t-PA
	Nothing known at pharmacological levels of t-PA; SK may be inhibited by α-SK antibodies
Decreased plasmin activity	α_2-Antiplasmin, in the fluid phase
	Nothing known to inhibit plasmin on the fibrin surface
Increased reocclusion	Thrombin activity appearing during thrombolysis, either newly generated from prothrombin or entrapped and released from lysing clot
Decreased reocclusion	Thrombin inhibition by ATIII-heparin, other inhibitors
	Platelet inhibition by aspirin, other inhibitors

t-PA = tissue plasminogen activator; UK = urokinase; SK = streptokinase; PAI-1 = plasminogen activator inhibitor-1; Lp(a) = lipoprotein (a); ATIII = antithrombin III.

Both of these mechanisms of regulation are clearly established at the molecular level (39), and for the PAI-1 mechanism there are supportive epidemiologic data as well. Elevated PAI-1 values are associated with increased risk for a second myocardial infarction, suggesting that inefficient or inadequate fibrinolysis may be responsible in part for the thrombotic component of coronary heart disease (40). Since it is also possible that prevalent coronary heart disease may have had an influence on the plasma PAI-1 levels, the ultimate significance of findings such as these will have to await incident-disease studies, several of which are ongoing. The regulation of plasminogen activation may also involve carbohydrate metabolism, since PAI-1 plasma levels are responsive to insulin levels (41). The details of the relationship of plasminogen activation and diabetes, however, have not been worked out.

Although PAI-1 is an effective regulator of plasminogen activation under normal conditions, it appears to play little role in thrombolytic therapy. The amount of circulating active PAI-1 is relatively small (1 nM or less) when compared with pharmacological concentrations of rt-PA (up to 30 nM); and in one study in which PAI-1 concentrations were examined in the context of clinical outcome, little or no effect was detected (42).

Concerning plasmin activity, the major regulatory factor, as mentioned above, is α_2-antiplasmin, although when this inhibitor is depleted, other plasma inhibitors may act to decrease plasmin activity (43). There are no other known plasmin-regulatory factors.

B. Other Potential Regulatory Mechanisms

It is possible that fibrin(ogen) degradation products (FDPs) generated by plasmin activity, either at the site of a clot (fibrin degradation products) or in solution (fibrinogen degradation products) may play a role in successful thrombolysis, especially in the setting of pharmacological thrombolysis. A possible mechanism is that FDPs, because of structural similarity to fibrinogen, may occupy platelet fibrinogen receptors and thereby inhibit platelet aggregation. Platelet aggregation proceeds by fibrinogen's acting as a bridge between platelets; the fibrinogen receptor on platelets is the membrane protein complex called glycoprotein IIb-IIIa. Inhibition of platelet aggregation by fibrin or fibrinogen fragments, while probably not important in the initial thrombolytic events, may help prevent recurrent thrombosis and reocclusion. While evidence for a relationship between FDP concentration and patency has not been forthcoming (44), this line of thinking has contributed to the development of "joint" thrombolytic regimes, characterized by the presence of rt-PA early in infusion, to effect rapid and complete thrombolysis and patency, with a secondary infusion of a non-fibrin-specific agent, such as streptokinase or urokinase. In such a regimen, the resultant increased fibrinogenolysis and FDP generation may help prevent reocclusion. Early results from such trials suggest that this may be so, although more data are needed (45).

The notion that platelet suppression is important in successful clinical thrombolysis is supported by the concept that aspirin is an important adjunct, presumably through its ability to attenuate platelet activation (46). Several laboratories are seeking both natural and synthetic platelet aggregation inhibitors, which might be used to limit reocclusion. One promising effort uses synthetic peptides that mimic the parts of fibrinogen that bind to the receptor, in a manner similar to the proposed mechanism for FDP effects (47). Another effort uses a monoclonal antibody directed at the IIb-IIIa protein to block fibrinogen binding (48). This field is advancing rapidly, and effective antiplatelet reagents, besides aspirin, should be available soon.

Other attempts at the prevention of reocclusion have centered on thrombin inibition, since some believe that effective thrombin inhibition will virtually eliminate reocclusive events. It is believed by many, but not all, investigators that heparin is an important adjunctive therapy to rt-PA for exactly this reason (49,50). There are animal-model data to support the notion that effective thrombin inhibition is important. For example, results in primates with cardiac stents reveal that inhibition of thrombin with D-Phe-Pro-Arg chloromethyl ketone, a very potent thrombin inhibitor, completely eliminates platelet aggregation, whereas aspirin is only partially effective (51). Many investigators, both in academic centers and in industry, are actively seeking the most effective thrombin inhibitor. Studies have centered on hirudin, a naturally occurring protein from leeches, which is a potent anticoagulant (52); synthetic hirudin-like peptides (53); and other synthetic thrombin inhibitors such as Argatroban (54). Over the next several years much information will be gained in this area, and, it is hoped, a consensus will be achieved concerning the importance of thrombin inhibition in maintaining patency.

The issue of thrombin inhibition has taken on added importance as researchers have come to realize that increased thrombin activity accompanies successful thrombolysis. This was demonstrated most effectively by studies revealing the presence of fibrinopeptide A during thrombolysis with rt-PA (55). While it is known that rt-PA can generate fibrinopeptide A from fibrinogen, the rate is very slow, and most likely rt-PA cannot account for all the fibrinopeptide A observed (13). However, while thrombin appears to be involved in this fibrinopeptide A generation, the origin of the thrombin remains obscure. Many believe that this thrombin originates not as newly generated thrombin from prothrombin, but from a pool of preformed thrombin that was incorporated into the blood clot during its formation, and becomes liberated during thrombolysis (56). In fact, other procoagulation factors may be incorporated as well. While the exact nature of the thrombin activity seen during thrombolysis remains unknown, it seems likely that, given the data discussed above, inhibiting thrombin activity during thrombolysis will prove to be an effective way to increase thrombolytic efficiency.

Several research groups have been seeking to regulate thrombolysis by designing and producing new plasminogen activator enzymes (for review see Ref. 47). Using recombinant DNA techniques, mutant t-PA molecules, modified for a longer plasma half-life, have been prepared and evaluated (57,58). These studies have not to date identified t-PA mutants with potentially significant clinical advantage; it remains to be seen if they will do so in the near future. In theory, an rt-PA molecule with prolonged half-life ("native" t-PA has an estimated half-life of approximately 7 min) should provide effective thrombolysis over a longer period with a lower dose.

A modified streptokinase agent has also been produced (anisoylated plasminogen-streptokinase complex [APSAC]) which has a modified rate of plasmin-generating activity. While APSAC has several theoretical advantages and has proven useful in a number of small clinical trials (59), preliminary results from the large ISIS-3 trial have not indicated that it is clinically superior to the normal streptokinase preparation (oral presentation by ISIS-3 Investigators, American College of Cardiology meeting, 1991).

There is much current interest in a newly described lipid fraction, lipoprotein (a), also called Lp(a) (60). This lipid particle is very similar to the low-density lipoprotein (LDL) particle, with the exception that the protein moiety, instead of being composed of apolipoprotein B alone, also contains the apo (a) protein structure (see Fig. 5). The apo (a) moiety bears a striking resemblance to plasminogen: it contains a large but variable number of Kringle domains, each of which is homologous to Kringle 4 from plasminogen, and it contains a sequence similar to the active site of plasmin, although the arginine residue associated with the active site–generating cleavage has been replaced with a serine residue. As a consequence of this alteration, the generation of an active enzyme cannot occur by the known serine protease activating mechanism, and enzymatic activity is not possible (60). Because of the multiple Kringle structures it has been proposed that Lp(a) may compete with plasminogen for fibrin or endothelial cell binding sites, thereby limiting plasmin generation (61). Whether this hypothesis is true remains to be proven, but this mechanism has tremendous potential as a long-term regulator of plasminogen activation, especially since

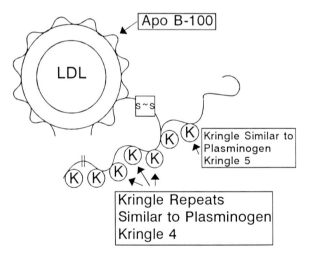

Figure 5   Structure of lipoprotein (a) [Lp(a)]. As described in the text, the Lp(a) particle is, in a general sense, a low-density lipoprotein (LDL) particle with the apo (a) moiety attached to the B-100 protein through a disulfide linkage. In the schematic, the encircled "K"s indicate Kringle structures homologous to the Kringle 4 and Kringle 5 of plasminogen. This has led to speculation, and some recent data, that Lp(a) can compete with plasminogen in certain Kringle-regulated binding events. The number of Kringle units per apo (a) is regulated genetically and is related to the plasma concentration of Lp(a). Other variations may include more than one apo (a) per Lp(a) particle, and variations in the lipid content.

plasma Lp(a) levels appear to be tightly controlled genetically (62) There is considerable epidemiologic evidence that Lp(a) is an independent risk factor for cardiovascular disease (63), and with elements of both the lipid factors (the LDL-like particle structure) and the thrombotic factors (plasminogen Kringle homology) Lp(a) has the potential to be involved with cardiovascular disease in several ways. This story should be revealed soon as research continues in this area.

ACKNOWLEDGMENTS

The authors thank Drs. Desire Collen and Dave Stump for many stimulating conversations. This work was supported in part by NHLBI HL38460, HL42940.

REFERENCES

1. Jang I, Gold H, Ziskind A, Fallon J, Holt R, Leinbach R, May J, Collen D. Differential sensitivity of erythrocyte-rich and platelet-rich arterial thrombi to lysis with recombinant tissue-type plasminogen activator. Circulation 1989; 79:920–8.
2. Loskutoff D, Curriden S. The fibrinolytic system of the vessel wall and its role in the control of thrombosis. Ann NY Acad Sci 1990; 598:238–47.
3. Robbins K. Fibrinolytic therapy: biochemical mechanisms. Semin Thromb Hemost 1991; 17:1–6.
4. Kluft C, Dooijewaard G, Emeis J. Role of the contact system in fibrinolysis. Semin Thromb Hemost 1987; 13:50–68.
5. Bajzar L, Fredenburgh J, Nesheim M. The activated protein C–mediated enhancement of tissue-type plasminogen activator–induced fibrinolysis in a cell-free system. J Biol Chem 1990; 265: 16948–54.
6. Lee C, Mann K. Activation/inactivation of human factor V by plasmin. Blood 1989; 73:185–90.
7. Willerson J, Golino P, McNatt J, Eidt J, Yao S-K, Buja L. Role of new antiplatelet agents as adjunctive therapies in thrombolysis. Am J Cardiol 1991; 67:12A–18A.
8. Tracy R, Bovill E, Terrin M, Collen D, Mann K, for the TIMI Investigators. Coagulation inhibitor values in myocardial infarction compared to those in normals. J Am Coll Cardiol 1991 (abstr.); 17:145A.
9. Stump D, Taylor F Jr, Nesheim M, Giles A, Dzik W, Bovill E. Pathologic fibrinolysis as a cause of clinical bleeding. Semin Thromb Hemost 1990; 16:260–73.
10. Collen D. Molecular mechanisms of fibrinolysis and their application to fibrin-specific thrombolytic therapy. J Cell Biochem 1987; 33:77–86.
11. Bovill E, Terrin M, Stump D, Berke A, Frederick M, Collen D, Feit F, Gore J, Hillis L, Lambrew C, Leiboff R, Mann K, Markis J, Pratt C, Sharkey S, Sopko G, Tracy R, Chesebro J, Investigators ftT. Hemorrhagic events during therapy with recombinant tissue-type plasminogen activator, heparin, and aspirin for acute myocardial infarction: results of the Thrombolysis in Myocardial Infarction (TIMI) phase II trial. Ann Intern Med 1991; 115:256–65.
12. Ranby M, Bergsdorf N, Nilsson T. Enzymatic properties of the one- and two-chain forms of tissue plasminogen activator. Thromb Res 1982; 27:175–83.
13. Weitz J, Cruickshank M, Thong B, Leslie B, Levine M, Ginsburg J, Eckhardt T. Human tissue-type plasminogen activator releases fibrinopeptides A and B from fibrinogen. J Clin Invest 1988; 82:1700–7.
14. Gurewich V. Pro-urokinase: physiochemical properties and promotion of its fibrinolytic activity by urokinase and by tissue plasminogen activator with which it has a complementary mechanism of action. Semin Thromb Hemost 1988; 14:110–5.
15. Husain S, Gurewich V, Lipinski B. Purification of a new, high molecular weight form of urokinase from urine. Thromb Haemost 1981; 46:11–17.
16. Marder V, Francis C. An assessment of regional versus systemic thrombolytic treatment of

peripheral and coronary artery thrombosis. In: Spaet T, ed. Progress in hemostasis and thrombosis. Orlando, FL: Grune & Stratton, 1984:325–56.

17. Reddy K. Streptokinase: biochemistry and clinical applications. Enzyme 1988; 40:79–89.

18. Castellino F. Biochemistry of human plasminogen. Semin Thromb Haemost 1984; 10:18–23.

19. Ichinose A, Takio K, Fujikawa K. Localization of the binding site of tissue-type plasminogen activator to fibrin. J Clin Invest 1986; 78:163–9.

20. Pannekoek H, de Vries C, van Zonneveld A-J. Mutants of human tissue-type plasminogen activator (t-PA): structural aspects and functional properties. Fibrinolysis 1988; 2:123–32.

21. Sprengers E, Kluft C. Plasminogen activator inhibitors. Blood 1987; 69:381–7.

22. Kruithof E, Tran-Thang C, Ransign A, Bachmann F. Demonstration of a fast-acting inhibitor of plasminogen activators in human plasma. Blood 1984; 64:907–13.

23. DeClerck P, Alessi M, Verstreken M, Kruithof E, Juhan-Vague I, Collen D. Measurement of plasminogen activator inhibitor 1 (PAI-1) in biological fluids with a murine monoclonal antibody based enzyme-linked immunosorbent assay. Blood 1988; 71:220–5.

24. Wiman B, Lijnen H, Collen D. On the specific interaction between the lysine-binding sites in plasmin and complementary sites in alpha-2-antiplasmin and in fibrinogen. Biochim Biophys Acta 1979; 579:142–54.

25. Collen D. Tissue-type plasminogen activator (t-PA) and single chain urokinase-type plasminogen activator (scu-PA): potential for fibrin-specific thrombolytic therapy. In: Coller B, ed. Progress in hemostasis and thrombosis. Orlando, FL: Grune & Stratton, 1986:1–18.

26. Hoylaerts M, Rijken D, Lijnen H, Collen D. Kinetics of the activation of plasminogen by human tissue plasminogen activator. Role of fibrin. J Biol Chem 1982; 257:2912–9.

27. Wiman B, Hamsten A. The fibrinolytic enzyme system and its role in the etiology of thromboembolic disease. Semin Thromb Hemost 1990; 16:207–16.

28. Doolittle R. Fibrinogen and fibrin. In: Putnam F, ed. The plasma proteins. New York: Academic Press, 1975:109–61.

29. Marder V, Shulman N, Carroll W. High molecular weight derivatives of human fibrinogen produced by plasmin. I. Physicochemical and immunological characterization. J Biol Chem 1969; 144:2111–9.

30. Sane D, Califf R, Topol E, Stump D, Mark D, Greenberg C. Bleeding during thrombolytic therapy for acute myocardial infarction: mechanisms and management. Ann Intern Med 1989; 111:1010–22.

31. Nossel H, Yudelman J, Canfield R, Butler V, Spanondis K, Wilner G, Qureshi G. Measurement of fibrinopeptide A in human blood J Clin Invest 1974; 54:43–53.

32. Weitz J, Koehn J, Canfield R, Landman S, Friedman R. Development of a radioimmunoassay for the fibrinogen-derived peptide B-beta-42. Blood 1986; 67:1014–1022.

33. Lawler C, Bovill E, Stump D, Collen D, Mann K, Tracy R. Fibrin fragment D-dimer and fibrinogen B-beta peptides in plasma as markers of clot lysis during thrombolytic therapy in acute myocardial infarction. Blood 1990; 76:1341–8.

34. Gore J, Sloan M, Price T, Young-Randall A, Bovill E, Collen D, Forman S, Knatterud G, Sopko G, Terrin M, for the TIMI Investigators. Intracerebral hemorrhage, cerebral infarction, and subdural hematoma after acute myocardial infarction and thrombolytic therapy in the Thrombolysis in Myocardial Infarction study: thrombolysis in myocardial infarction, phase II, pilot and clinical trial. Circulation 1991; 83:448–59.

35. Pendlebury W, Iole E, Tracy R, Dill B. Intracerebral hemorrhage related to cerebral amyloid angiopathy and t-PA treatment. Ann Neurol 1991; 29:210–3.

36. Gurewich V. Importance of fibrin specificity in therapeutic thrombolysis and the rationale of using sequential and synergistic combinations of tissue plasminogen activator and pro-urokinase. Semin Thromb Hemost 1989; 15:123–8.

37. Robbins K. The plasminogen-plasmin enzyme system. In: Colman R, Hirsh J, Marder V, Salzman E, eds. Hemostasis and thrombosis: basic principles and clinical practice. Philadelphia: J.B. Lippincott, 1987:318–39.

38. Adelman B, Michelson A, Loscalzo J, Greenberg J, Handin R. Plasmin effect on platelet glycoprotein Ib–von Willebrand's factor interaction. Blood 1985; 65:32–45.

39. Collen D, Juhan-Vague I. Fibrinolysis and atherosclerosis. Semin Thromb Hemost 1988; 14: 180–3.

40. Hamsten A, de Faire U, Walldius G, Dahlen G, Szamosi A, Landou C, Blomback M, Wiman B. Plasminogen activator inhibitor in plasma: risk factor for recurrent myocardial infarction. Lancet 1987; ii:3–9.

41. Vague P, Juhan-Vague I, Aillaud M, Badier C, Viard R, Alessi M, Collen D. Correlation between blood fibrinolytic activity, plasminogen activator inhibitor level, plasma insulin level, and relative body weight in normal and obese subjects. Metabolism 1986; 35:250–3.

42. Sane D, Stump D, Topol E, Sigmon K, Kereiakes D, George B, Mantell S, Macy E, Collen D, Califf R. Correlation between baseline plasminogen activator inhibitor levels and clinical outcome during therapy with tissue plasminogen activator for acute myocardial infarction. Thromb Haemost 1991; 65:275–9.

43. Tiefenbrunn A, Graor R, Robison A, Lucas F, Hotchkiss A, Sobel B. Pharmacodynamics of tissue-type plasminogen activator characterized by computer-assisted simulation. Circulation 1986; 73:1291–9.

44. Arnold A, Brower R, Collen D, van Es G, Lubsen J, Serruys P, Simoons M, Verstraete M. Increased serum levels of fibrinogen degradation products due to treatment with recombinant tissue-type plasminogen activator for acute myocardial infarction are related to bleeding complications, but not to coronary patency. J Am Coll Cardiol 1989; 14:581–8.

45. Morris J, Muller D, Topol E. Combination thrombolytic therapy: a comparison of simultaneous and sequential regimens of t-PA and urokinase. Am Heart J 1991; 122:375–80.

46. Group I-2(ISoISC. Randomised trial of intravenous streptokinase, oral aspirin, both, or neither among 17,187 cases of suspected acute myocardial infarction: ISIS-2. Lancet 1988; 2:349–60.

47. Bang N, Wilhelm O, Clayman M. After coronary thrombolysis and reperfusion, what next? J Am Coll Cardiol 1989; 14:837–49.

48. Gold H, Coller B, Yasuda T, Saito T, Fallon J, Guerrero J, Leinbach R, Ziskind A, Collen D. Rapid and sustained coronary artery recanalization with combined bolus injection of recombinant tissue-type plasminogen activator and monoclonal antiplatelet GPIIb/IIIa antibody in a canine preparation. Circulation 1988; 77:670–7.

49. Group TIS. In-hospital mortality and clinical course of 20891 patients with suspected acute myocardial infarction randomised between alteplase and streptokinase with or without heparin. Lancet 1990; 336:71–5.

50. Eisenberg P. Role of new anticoagulants as adjunctive therapy during thrombolysis. Am J Cardiol 1991; 67:19A–24A.

51. Krupski W, Bass A, Kelly A, Marzec U, Hanson S, Harker L. Heparin-resistant thrombus formation by endovascular stents in baboons: interruption by a synthetic antithrombin. Circulation 1990; 81:570–7.

52. Haskel E, Prager N, Sobel B, Abendschein D. Relative efficacy of antithrombin compared with antiplatelet agents in accelerating coronary thrombolysis and preventing early reocclusion. Circulation 1991; 83:1048–56.

53. Jakubowski J, Maraganore J. Inhibition of coagulation and thrombin-induced platelet activities by a synthetic dodecapeptide modeled on the carboxy-terminus of hirudin. Blood 1990; 75:399–406.

54. Jang I, Gold H, Ziskind A, Leinbach R, Fallon J, Collen D. Prevention of platelet-rich arterial thrombosis by selective thrombin inhibition. Circulation 1990; 81:219–25.

55. Eisenberg P, Sherman L, Rich M, Schwartz D, Schechtman K, Geltman E, Sobel B, Jaffe A. Importance of continued activation of thrombin reflected by fibrinopeptide A to the efficacy of thrombolysis. J Am Coll Cardiol 1986; 7:1253–62.

56. Francis C, Markham R, Barlow G, Florack T, Dobrzynski D, Marder V. Thrombin activity of fibrin thrombi and soluble plasmic derivatives. J Lab Clin Med 1983; 102:220–30.

57. Collen D, Stassen J, Larsen G. Pharmacokinetics and thrombolytic properties of deletion mutants of human tissue-type plasminogen activator in rabbits. Blood 1988; 71:216–9.

58. Cambier P, van de Werf F, Larsen G, Collen D. Pharmacokinetics and thrombolytic properties of a non-glycosylated mutant of human tissue-type plasminogen activator, lacking the finger growth factor domains, in dogs with copper coil–induced coronary artery thrombosis. J Cardiovasc Pharmacol 1988; 11:468–72.

59. Fears R. Development of anisoylated plasminogen-streptokinase activator complex from the acyl enzyme concept. Semin Thromb Hemost 1989; 15:129–39.

60. Scanu A, Fless G. Lipoprotein (a): heterogeneity and biological relevance. J Clin Invest 1990; 85:1709–15.

61. Miles L, Fless G, Levin E, Scanu A, Plow E. A potential basis for the thrombotic risks associated with lipoprotein(a). Nature 1989; 339:301–3.

62. Boerwinkle E, Menzel H, Kraft H, Utermann G. Genetics of the quantitative Lp(a) lipoprotein trait. III. Contribution of Lp(a) glycoprotein phenotypes to normal lipid variation. Hum Genet 1989; 82:73–8.

63. Uterman G. The mysteries of lipoprotein(a). Science 1989; 246:904–10.

5

Heparin: Biochemistry, Pharmacology, Pharmacokinetics, and Dose-Response Relationships

Clive Kearon
McMaster University, Hamilton, Ontario, Canada

Jack Hirsh
Hamilton Civic Hospitals Research Centre, Henderson General Hospital, and McMaster University, Hamilton, Ontario, Canada

I. INTRODUCTION

The anticoagulant effects of heparin were first identified in 1916 by McLean, a medical student, who incidentally discovered that an extract of liver, "heparphosphatid," was a potent inhibitor of coagulation, while he was studying the thromboplastic action of different tissues (1,2). McLean's supervisor, Howell, and his colleagues subsequently performed studies purifying and elucidating the properties of this substance, which was renamed heparin (2,3). In the early 1930s, Charles and Scott developed methods of isolating heparin in a highly purified state and in substantial quantities, paving the way for clinical studies (3). By the late 1930s purified preparation of heparin had been used successfully in the prophylaxis and treatment of various thrombotic disorders (3,4).

In 1939, Brinkhous and associates demonstrated that heparin required a plasma cofactor, which they termed heparin cofactor, for its anticoagulant activity (5). It had been noted from the end of the 19th century that the procoagulant thrombin gradually lost activity after being added to defibrinated plasma; a specific thrombin inhibitor, termed antithrombin, was thought to be responsible (6). In 1968, Abildgaard isolated small amounts of α_2-globulin from human plasma and showed that it had both antithrombin and heparin cofactor activity (7). These observations supported earlier suspicions (8,9) that the antithrombin constituent of blood and heparin cofactor were the same substance, which Abildgaard renamed antithrombin III (ATIII). In the 1970s, studies by Rosenberg's and Lindahl's groups established that binding of heparin to ATIII converts it from a progressive slow inhibitor to a very rapid inhibitor of coagulation (6,10–12). Heparin then dissociates from the complex and can be reutilized (6).

The first randomized, controlled trial of intravenous heparin therapy was performed in 1960 by Barrett and Jordan, who showed unequivocally that anticoagulant therapy was effective in preventing recurrence of pulmonary embolism (13). Subsequent randomized, controlled trials have expanded the therapeutic role of heparin so that it is now indicated for prophylaxis (14,15) and treatment (13,16,17) of venous thrombosis and pulmonary embolism; unstable angina (18,19); and acute myocardial infarction with or without thrombolytic therapy (20–27). Heparin is also used as an adjunct to percutaneous transluminal angioplasty; to prevent thrombosis on artificial surfaces during cardiac bypass surgery and hemodialysis; during and after peripheral vascular surgery; and in selected patients with disseminated intravascular thrombosis.

In this chapter, the biochemistry of heparin and its interaction with ATIII, the physiological role of heparin and related compounds, therapeutic actions, pharmacokinetics and dose-response relationships, and side effects will be reviewed. In addition, the potential of a new class of heparins, the low-molecular-weight heparins (LMWHs), will be discussed, and their biophysical, pharmacokinetic, antithrombotic, and hemorrhagic properties will be compared with those of standard heparin.

II. BIOCHEMISTRY

A. Structure of Heparin

Heparin is made up of a heterogeneous group of highly sulfated glycosaminoglycan molecules of different sizes and structures (6,28–30). Glycosaminoglycans (also called mucopolysaccharides) are large-molecular-weight linear carbohydrates composed of repeating disaccharide units, of which one is an *N*-acetyl-hexosamine and the other a hexose or hexuronic acid. The repeating disaccharide units of heparin are composed of D-glycosamine and a uronic acid (either glucuronic or iduronic) that are sulfated to a variable degree, resulting in a highly negatively charged molecule. Heparin molecules vary according to (1) size or length, depending on the number of disaccharide residues; (2) constituents, depending on whether glycuronic or iduronic acid is present; and (3) sulfation and charge, depending on the extent and positioning of sulfate residues. All of these factors contribute to functional heterogeneity between heparin molecules.

B. Interaction of Heparin with Antithrombin III

The molecular weight and net charge (degree of sulfation) of heparin molecules are the factors that largely determine protein binding and heparin pharmacokinetics (30,31). The anticoagulant effect of heparin is mediated largely through its ability to bind to ATIII and catalyze its anticoagulant effect. Binding of heparin to ATIII requires the presence of a specific pentasaccharide sequence containing a 3-0-sulfated glycosamine unit as its third residue (6,10–12,30,32–35). This pentasaccharide sequence combines with lysine sites on the ATIII molecule and produces a conformational change that exposes an arginine reactive site on the heparin-ATIII complex. In turn, the arginine center inhibits the active center serine of thrombin and other coagulation enzymes, thereby inducing an anticoagulant effect. After this sequence has been completed, heparin dissociates from antithrombin III and is available to activate further antithrombin III molecules.

C. Interaction of Heparin–Antithrombin III Complex with Coagulation Factors

The anticoagulant effect of heparin is not mediated exclusively by ATIII and is not confined to inhibition of thrombin (IIa) (6,30). At high concentrations, heparin also catalyzes the inhibition of IIa by a second plasma protease inhibitor, heparin cofactor II, but at the concentrations at which heparin is utilized clinically, this interaction is thought to be of little importance (36). More important, the heparin-ATIII complex inhibits the activated coagulation enzymes X, XI, XII, and IX (X_a, XI_a, XII_a, and IX_a). Thrombin and Xa are the coagulation factors that are most sensitive to inactivation; on average, inhibition of thrombin is about 10 times greater than the inhibition of Xa, but relative sensitivities vary with the length of heparin molecules (6,30).

The inhibition of thrombin requires that heparin bind to both ATIII and thrombin (ternary complex formation), whereas the inhibition of factor Xa requires that heparin bind to ATIII alone (6,34). Heparin molecules with fewer than 18 saccharide residues are unable to bind to thrombin and ATIII simultaneously and thus cannot catalyze the inhibition of thrombin (Fig. 1). In contrast, even smaller heparin fragments that contain the high-affinity pentasaccharide sequence are able to catalyze the inhibition of factor Xa by ATIII. There is increasing evidence that heparins principal inhibitory effect on coagulation is the inhibition of thrombin-induced activation of factor V and factor VIII (37–39).

D. Preparations of Standard Heparin

Commercial preparations of heparin are heterogeneous, their components having molecular weights ranging from 3000 to 30,000 (mean 15,000). Only about one-third of the heparin has the specific pentasaccharide sequence required for binding with ATIII, and this fraction is responsible for most of its anticoagulant effect (40,41). Heparin is common to all higher animal species, in which it appears to be synthesized by mast cells (6). Commercially, heparin is most commonly obtained from the lungs or intestinal mucosa of cows or pigs, from which it is extracted as either the sodium or the calcium salt.

III. PHYSIOLOGICAL FUNCTION AND THERAPEUTIC EFFECTS OF HEPARIN

A. Anticoagulant Actions

The physiological role of heparin is uncertain. Its synthesis by mast cells, which are present in the perivascular tissues, suggests that heparin is not involved in maintaining blood fluidity. However, vascular endothelial cells synthesize heparin-like heparan sulfate molecules independently of mast cells (42), and pretreatment of vascular surfaces with heparinase (which destroys heparin) greatly reduced the normal inhibition of thrombin by ATIII in animal preparations (43,44). These two observations suggest that the heparin-antithrombin system plays an important physiological role in the prevention of intravascular thrombosis.

Congenital deficiency states for heparin have not been described, but congenital deficiency of ATIII does occur and is associated with a hypercoagulability state (45). Antithrombin III deficiency is inherited as an autosomal dominant disorder, and carriers have ATIII levels that are between 40% and 60% of normal. Affected persons have a high prevalence (30–80%) of thrombosis, which often occurs before the fifth decade, is idiopathic and recurrent, may occur in unusual locations, and is associated with a positive family history of thrombosis (45). The serious consequences of this condition attest to the physiological importance of the ATIII system as an antithrombotic regulatory mechanism.

Although heparin has been shown to interact with the fibrinolytic system, it does not appear to have a direct thrombolytic effect (29,46–51), but favors clot removal by preventing extension or recurrence of thrombosis (23,26,52,53).

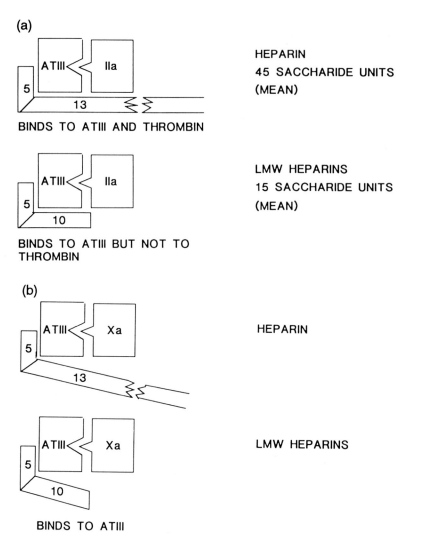

Figure 1 (a) Inactivation of thrombin. To inactivate thrombin, heparins must bind antithrombin III (ATIII) through the high-affinity pentasaccharide and to thrombin through an additional 13 saccharide units. Low-molecular-weight (LMW) heparins that contain less than 18 saccharide units cannot bind to thrombin and therefore are unable to inactivate thrombin. (b) Inactivation of factor Xa. To inactivate factor Xa, heparins must bind to ATIII through the high-affinity pentasaccharide but do not need to bind to factor Xa. Therefore, both standard heparin and LMW heparins are able to inactivate factor Xa. (From Ref. 172.)

B. Nonanticoagulant Actions

The function of heparin is not confined to its anticoagulant effects. In addition it may increase physiological functions such as vessel wall permeability (54) and activation of lipoprotein lipase (44), or decrease them, as with inhibition of platelet function (55), reduced proliferation of vascular smooth muscle cells (56), inhibition of delayed hypersensitivity reactions (57), suppression of aldosterone secretion (58), and regulation of angiogenesis (59). While this review focuses on the effects heparin has on hemostasis, it will also consider actions of heparin that may contribute to side effects when it is used therapeutically, particularly interference with platelet function.

1. Heparin-Platelet Interactions

The relationship between heparin and platelet function is complex; heparin has been shown both to increase and to decrease platelet aggregation under different circumstances (60,61). The importance of these interactions lies mainly in the contribution to bleeding of heparin-induced platelet inhibition. Whereas the anticoagulant effect of heparin is confined to 30% of standard heparin molecules, all heparin fractions can interfere with platelet function, and there is evidence that large heparin molecules having absent or low affinity for ATIII are particularly potent inhibitors of platelets (62). Platelet inhibition, coupled with heparin's ability to increase vascular permeability, probably accounts for dissociations between the antithrombotic and hemorrhagic effects of heparin (54,55,63,64).

It has been proposed that heparin molecules contain two types of binding site (6). One of these sites has the capacity to bind to either platelets or ATIII but has greater affinity for the inhibitor. When bound to ATIII, this site would not be available to interfere with platelet function; such a binding site predominates on the lower-molecular-weight fractions. The second site binds to platelets and impairs their function independently of ATIII binding; this site predominates on larger-molecular-weight heparins, particularly those with no affinity for ATIII, which would lack the first site. Such differences in platelet binding sites could account for the differences in physiological (platelet aggregation) and hemorrhagic (blood loss assay) effects that have been observed between low-molecular-weight heparins and standard heparin under experimental conditions (65–70) and clinically (71–73).

In addition to the inhibitory effect that heparin may have on platelets, platelets can also inhibit the anticoagulant effect of heparin, by binding and protecting factor Xa from inactivation by heparin-ATIII complex (74,75), and by secreting the heparin-neutralizing protein platelet factor 4 (76). The anticoagulant effect of heparin may also be diminished by a number of other endogenous proteins and endothelial constituents, as discussed in the following section.

Thrombocytopenia can also occur as a side effect of heparin therapy (see below), a phenomenon that is unrelated to the usual inhibitory effect of heparin on platelet function.

IV. PHARMACOKINETICS

A. Administration

Heparin is not absorbed after oral administration and therefore must be given by injection, the preferred routes of administration being the intravenous and subcutaneous (29). Intramuscular injection may produce large hematomas by accidental puncture of an intramuscular vein and therefore should be avoided. There is evidence that heparin administration by intermittent intravenous injection is associated with more bleeding than administration by continuous intravenous infusion (77–79); the latter method is therefore preferred for intravenous therapy.

The efficacy and safety of heparin administered by either continuous infusions or subcutaneously are comparable provided that the dosages used are adequate (80–84). However, if the subcutaneous route is selected, the initial dose must be sufficiently high to counteract the reduced bioavailability that is associated with this method of administration. If an immediate anticoagulant effect is required, the initial subcutaneous dose should be accompanied by an intravenous bolus injection to avoid the 1 to 2 h delay in anticoagulant effect that occurs with subcutaneous heparin alone.

B. Distribution

Following its injection and passage into the blood stream, heparin binds to a number of plasma proteins (76,85–91) that can reversibly neutralize its anticoagulant activity and so reduce its bioavailability. Heparin also binds to endothelial cells (92–94) and macrophages (93,95), further complicating its pharmacokinetics. Interindividual differences in protein and cell binding capacity for heparin contributes to variability of the anticoagulant response to administered heparin, which is commonly seen in patients with thromboembolic disorders (96), and to the laboratory phenomenon of heparin resistance (91) (see below).

C. Interactions

In addition to loss of heparin effect as a result of competitive binding and neutralization, the ability of heparin-ATIII to inactivate thrombin and factor Xa is reduced when these coagulation enzymes are bound to fibrin and platelets, respectively. Fibrin binds thrombin and protects it from inactivation by structurally obstructing binding of heparin-ATIII (97,98). In plasma, approximately 20 times more heparin is needed to inactivate fibrin-bound thrombin than to inactivate free thrombin (98). This resistance of fibrin-bound thrombin to inhibition by heparin may also explain why preventing the extension of venous thrombosis requires higher concentrations of heparin than preventing its formation (99), as well as why heparin fails to inhibit thrombin activity in some patients after successful coronary thrombolysis (100–102). Thrombin also binds to subendothelial matrix proteins, where it is again protected from inhibition by heparin (103). As previously noted, binding of factor Xa to platelet surfaces has a similar effect (74,75).

There is little information on the influence of specific diseases, or of the concurrent use of other medications, on the pharmacokinetics of heparin (104,105). Liver or renal disease does not appear to influence heparin pharmacokinetics at standard therapeutic concentrations. Similarly, there is no convincing evidence that heparin pharmacokinetics is influenced by concomitant use of other medications. Heparin elimination is, however, increased in patients with acute pulmonary embolism by a mechanism that is poorly understood (96,106). It has been suggested that intravenous nitroglycerin may increase the required dose of heparin (107), but this was not confirmed in a recent randomized crossover study (108).

However, pharmacodynamic interactions between therapeutic heparin and either disease states or other medications are not uncommon and may contribute to side effects, particularly bleeding, or, to a lesser extent, to loss of anticoagulant effects. Bleeding in patients receiving heparin therapy is increased by any process that additionally impairs hemostatic mechanisms (109,110). Such processes include reduction in platelet numbers (e.g., lymphoproliferative disorders, therapeutic agents) or function (e.g., polycythemia rubra vera, aspirin) or reduction in the concentration of coagulation proteins (e.g., hepatic disease, oral anticoagulants). Medications may also contribute to bleeding in heparinized patients by disrupting gastrointestinal mucosal integrity (e.g., aspirin [111]). Pregnancy, malignancy, acute thrombosis, and major surgery may be associated with heparin resistance as a result of an increase in procoagulant activity (91,96) (see below).

There appears to be no clinically important difference in the bioavailability of sodium and calcium heparin; antithrombotic efficacy and hemorrhagic side effects have been

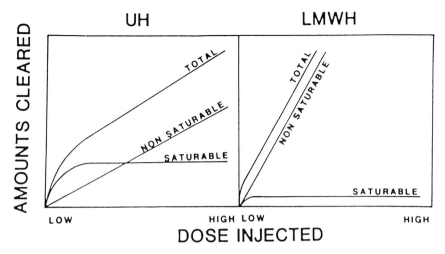

Figure 2 Schematic representation of the pharmacokinetic model of heparins. After parenteral injection, heparin disappearance results from the activity of a saturable and of a linear nonsaturable mechanism that operate simultaneously. UH = unfractionated heparin; LMWH = low-molecular-weight heparin. (From Ref. 31.)

similar when the two salts have been directly compared in clinical trials assessing subcutaneous heparin prophylaxis for deep venous thrombosis (112,113).

D. Clearance

After administration of an intravenous bolus of heparin, activity falls rapidly as equilibration occurs with binding to plasma proteins and cellular constituents, particularly endothelial cells. This is followed by a more gradual clearance that can best be explained by a combination of a saturable and a nonsaturable mechanism (31,114,115). The saturable phase of heparin clearance appears to be due to uptake by endothelial cells and macrophages, with depolymerization and metabolism to smaller, less sulfated derivatives (92,94,95,116). The nonsaturable mechanism obeys first-order kinetics, the rate of clearance being linearly related to dose, and can be accounted for by renal elimination (31,117). The relative contribution of each of these mechanisms to clearance of heparin depends on the dose and the size of the heparin fractions administered (Fig. 2) (31,118,119). Low doses of standard heparin are predominantly eliminated by the highly efficient but low-capacity saturable mechanism (31,94). With larger doses of heparin, capacity of the saturable mechanism is exceeded, so that at high doses, renal clearance predominates. Larger heparin molecules are preferentially cleared by the saturable mechanism (31,94); this has important implications for dose-response relationships and for differences between the pharmacokinetic properties of standard and low-molecular-weight heparins (see below).

V. DOSE-RESPONSE RELATIONSHIPS

A. Monitoring Heparin Therapy

Since there is no suitable chemical assay for heparin, the investigation of its kinetics has depended on measurements of its biologic activity (114,120). There are a number of ways to measure this, of which some focus on specific coagulation factor activities and others assess a more global effect on coagulation. As with many other properties of heparin, its influence on these assays also varies according to molecular weight (6,30,41,121). The most widely available specific heparin assays measure the level of anti-X_a or antithrombin (anti-IIa) activity.

1. Heparin Assays

Heparin can be assayed by measuring its ability to inactivate factor Xa activity or factor IIa (thrombin) activity. These assays are performed by adding factor Xa or thrombin to the test (heparin-containing) plasma and then measuring the residual activity of the coagulation enzyme after a short period of incubation. Residual activity can be measured with a clotting assay or a chromogenic assay. The assays can be performed either with or without added ATIII. The therapeutic range for the anti-Xa assay is 0.3 to 0.7 U/ml.

2. Protamine Titration of Thrombin Time

In protamine titration of thrombin time, thrombin is added to the test plasma and thrombin clotting time is measured. Protamine is then added to the plasma, and the concentration of protamine required to normalize the clotting time is calculated. Protamine is a highly basic naturally occurring protein that combines with and neutralizes heparin on a one-to-one basis (122,123). As the antithrombin effects of heparin are predominantly due to the larger-molecular-weight molecules, this test is more sensitive to this fraction. The therapeutic range of this assay is 0.2 to 0.4 U/ml.

3. Activated Partial Thromboplastin Time

In clinical practice, the anticoagulant effects of heparin are usually monitored by the activated partial thromboplastin time (APTT), a test that provides a global assessment of the intrinsic and common coagulation pathways and is sensitive in particular to the inhibitory effects of heparin on thrombin, Xa, and IXa. In this test, plasma that has been decalcified is preincubated with an activating surface (usually kaolin) and cephalin (a source of phospholipid), and time to clotting is then determined after recalcification. Unfortunately, the ability of heparin to prolong the APTT depends on the responsiveness of the different commercial APTT reagents, which may vary with the type of clot detection mechanism, the contact activator, and the phospholipid composition of the reagent (124–126). For many APTT reagents, the therapeutic effect is achieved with an APTT ratio of 1.5 to 2.5 (measured by dividing the observed APTT by the mean of the laboratory control values of APTT), corresponding to an anti-Xa heparin level of 0.3 to 0.7 U/ml or a protamine-titration heparin level of 0.2 to 0.4 U/ml. The response of the APTT ratio to heparin may also be reduced in the presence of elevated levels of procoagulants (91). Efforts are being made to develop a reliable international standard for the APTT system, but until this is available, therapeutic ranges need to be established in local laboratories, corresponding to the therapeutic range of the specific heparin assays.

B. Why Monitor Heparin Therapy?

The recommended therapeutic range for the treatment of venous thrombosis was originally based on a study performed on rabbits demonstrating that thrombus extension was prevented by a heparin dose that prolonged the APTT ratio to 1.5–2.5 (127). The results of subsequent randomized, controlled trials confirm that a relationship exists between the clinical effectiveness of heparin and its ex vivo effect on the APTT for the following conditions: prevention of recurrent thrombosis in patients with proximal vein thrombosis (80,128);

prevention of mural thrombus in patients with acute myocardial infarction (21); prevention of recurrent ischemia following streptokinase therapy for acute myocardial infarction (129, 130); and prevention of coronary artery reocclusion following t-PA therapy (131) (Table 1).

Maintaining the APTT ratio above 1.5 is associated with protection against thrombosis, but, unfortunately, bleeding complications may occur within the therapeutic range. The risk of bleeding is increased by a number of factors (see below) that include both the heparin dose and the degree of prolongation of the APTT (109,110,132).

C. Achieving a Therapeutic Effect with Heparin

The anticoagulant effect of standard heparin is heterogeneous because (1) only one-third of the heparin molecules administered have anticoagulant activity (40,41); (2) the anticoagulant profile of heparin is influenced by the chain length of the molecules (6,30,41,121); (3) clearance of heparin is influenced by chain length (30,31,94,118,119); and (4) bioavailability is inversely proportional to the capacity of plasma proteins (76,85–91), endothelial cells (92–94), and macrophages to bind heparin (93,95). In addition, because there are two mechanisms responsible for heparin clearance, one of which is effective only at clearing low doses, the half-life of heparin is highly dose-dependent; the apparent biological half-life of heparin increases from approximately 30 min with an intravenous bolus of 25 U/kg to 60 min with an intravenous bolus of 100 U/kg and to 150 min with a bolus of 400 U/kg (120,133,134).

The saturable nature of the binding sites that (1) reduce heparin bioavailability and (2) accelerate its clearance results in a within-subject nonlinear relationship of heparin effect to dose administered. Large increments in heparin dose are required to increase heparin effects at lower dosages, but at higher dosages, further small increments in dose achieve large increases in both the intensity and the duration of heparin activity (133). The form of this dose-response relationship translates into a narrow therapeutic window for heparin administration and calls for close monitoring.

The therapeutic effects that are achieved with a given dose of heparin also depend on the route of administration; the mean maintenance dosage in 11 studies using continuous

Table 1 Relationship Between Failure to Reach Lower Limit of Therapeutic Range and Thromboembolic Events from Subgroup Analysis of Prospective Studies

Study	Type of patients	Outcome	N	Relative risk
Hull et al. (80)	DVT	Recurrent VTE	115	15.0
Basu et al. (128)	DVT	Recurrent VTE	157	10.7
Turpie et al. (21)	AMI	LVMT	112	22.2[a]
Kaplan et al. (129)	AMI	Recurrent MI/AP	75	6.0[b]
Camilleri et al. (130)	AMI	Recurrent MI/AP	70	13.3

[a]Estimated by assuming a normal distribution of the reported heparin levels.
[b]Kaplan used a partial thromboplastin time (PTT) measurement and reported the relative risk associated with PTT values less than 50 compared with PTT values of more than 100.
DVT = deep vein thrombosis; AMI = acute myocardial infarction; VTE = venous thromboembolism; LVMT = left ventricular mural thrombosis; AP = angina pectoris.

intravenous heparin was 30,516 U/24 h, in 5 studies using subcutaneous heparin it was 33,459 U/24 h, and in 6 studies using intermittent intravenous heparin it was 36,062 U/24 h (29). For the two preferred routes of administration, continuous intravenous and twice-daily subcutaneous injection, additional insights relating to the dose of heparin required to maintain therapeutic APTTs over a 24-h period can be obtained from a recent prospective study that compared the two routes. The mean daily dose was 7% higher in the subcutaneous-injection group than in the continuous-intravenous-infusion group (33,800 vs. 31,700 U, $p = 0.01$) (84).

When heparin is given by either intravenous infusion or subcutaneous injection, an initial intravenous loading dose is required if a rapid onset of effect is desired. This bolus occupies a large proportion of the plasma protein heparin-binding sites, allowing the subsequent infusion or subcutaneous injection to maintain heparin levels in the desired range.

A logical approach to selecting the size of this bolus and an initial infusion rate (or subcutaneous dose) would be to vary them according to the patient's size. However, because of the many factors that influence heparin dose-response relationships, indexing heparin dosage to actual or ideal body weight has not proved valuable. A satisfactory approach is to give an initial bolus of 5000 units intravenously (unless this is contraindicated, e.g., within 24 h of surgery) followed by an infusion of 32,000 units over 24 h. This is the average infusion rate that is required to achieve optimal anticoagulation. Because of the short half-life of heparin at therapeutic doses, infusion rates should be adjusted on the basis of APTT measurements as little as 6 h apart, with the first being performed 6 h after initiating heparin. A heparin dose adjustment nomogram has been developed for APTT reagents for which the therapeutic range is 1.9 to 2.7 times control (based on a protamine titration heparin level of 0.2 to 0.4 U) (Table 2) (135). With this protocol, an APTT above the lower limit of the therapeutic range was reached in 82% of patients after 24 h and in 91% after 48 h; those proportions were significantly better than in a historical control group. This nomogram is not applicable to all APTT reagents and should be adapted to the heparin responsiveness of the thromboplastin in local use.

In post–myocardial infarction patients who have received thrombolytic therapy, particularly with streptokinase, a systemic lytic state may be observed, with prolongation of clotting parameters (136,137). When intravenous heparin is given in this situation, the same 5000-unit intravenous bolus may be given, followed by 24,000 units over a 24-h period. During the first 24 h of heparin therapy, upward adjustments of heparin dose are made in response to a low APTT, but downward adjustments are not made if the APTT is above the therapeutic range, as this may be due to a systemic lytic state rather than excessive heparin effect. The benefits of adding therapeutic doses of heparin to thrombolytic agents and adequate doses of aspirin in patients with acute myocardial infarction is uncertain (24,25,27) and is being investigated in the Global Utilization of Streptokinase and Tissue Plasminogen Activator for Occluded Coronary Arteries (GUSTO) study. It is hoped that optimal route and timing of heparin administration with different thrombolytic agents will also be clarified by the GUSTO study.

When the subcutaneous route is used for therapeutic anticoagulation, a suitable initial heparin dosage is 17,500 units every 12 h (12,500 units after thrombolytic therapy). Dosage is adjusted according to APTT measurements performed 6 h after the last dose.

D. Heparin Resistance

Approximately 20% of patients require doses of heparin of more than 35,000 U/24 h to achieve therapeutic APTT ratios. These patients, whose response to heparin as measured by

Table 2 Heparin Dose Adjustment Protocol[a]

Patient's APTT[b]	Dosing instructions			Timing of next APTT
	Repeat bolus dose	Stop infusion (min)	Change rate (dose) of infusion ML/H[c] (U/24 h)	
<50	5000 U	0	+3 (+2880)	6 h
50–59	0	0	+3 (+2880)	6 h
60–85[d]	0	0	0	Next morning
86–95	0	0	−2 (−1920)	Next morning
96–120	0	30	−2 (−1920)	6 h
>120	0	60	−4 (−3840)	6 h

[a]Starting dose of 5,000 U I/V bolus followed by 31,000 U/24 h as a continuous infusion. First APTT performed 6 h after the bolus injection, dosage adjustments made according to protocol and the APTT repeated as indicated in the right hand column.
[b]Normal range for APTT with Dade Actin FS reagent is 27–35 s.
[c]40 U/ml.
[d]Therapeutic range of 60–85 s equivalent to a heparin level of 0.2–0.4 U/ml by protamine titration or 0.35–0.7 U/ml as an anti-factor Xa level. The therapeutic range will vary with the responsiveness of the APTT reagent to heparin.
APTT = activated partial thromboplastin time.

laboratory test results is atypically poor, are often considered to be heparin-resistant. The mechanism of heparin resistance has been clarified by the results of two recent studies (91; Levine et al., 1992, in preparation). The great majority of heparin-resistant patients have increased levels of heparin-binding proteins that compete with ATIII for heparin binding. As a result, for any given dosage of heparin they have lower levels of heparin activity, measured by anti-factor Xa heparin assay, than non-heparin-resistant patients. Thus their mean heparin requirement was found to be 36,000 U/24 h, in comparison with 32,000 U/24 h for non-heparin-resistant patients. Many heparin-resistant patients also have elevated levels of factor VIII and possibly of other procoagulants, which produce a dissociation between the APPT and the heparin level, the APPT being proportionately low relative to the heparin level. Therefore, if the anticoagulant effect of heparin in these heparin-resistant patients is monitored by the APPT, even higher doses of heparin are required (mean dose of 44,000 U/24 h). The results of a recent randomized trial indicate that these heparin-resistant patients can be safely monitored by the anti-factor Xa assay (Levine et al., 1992).

Antithrombin III deficiency is a very uncommon cause of heparin resistance and was not encountered in any of 120 consecutive heparin-resistant patients (Levine et al., 1992).

E. Low-Dose Heparin Prophylaxis of Thromboembolism

In addition to the use of heparin for the treatment of acute thrombotic episodes, low-dose subcutaneous heparin provides an effective and safe form of prophylaxis in medical and surgical patients who are at risk for thromboembolism (14,15). It is usually administered in a fixed dose of 5000 units every 8 or 12 h. With these regimens, the APTT rarely rises beyond the normal range and heparin levels do not exceed 0.1 anti-Xa U/ml, so that monitoring of coagulation parameters is not necessary. For patients at particularly high risk, three studies have demonstrated that the efficacy of low-dose heparin is improved without compromising safety by adjusting the dose to achieve a minimal heparin effect (138–140). One of these studies, which aimed for an APTT at the upper limit of normal, used a mean daily dose of 15,000 units of heparin (138), while the other two prolonged the APTT ratio to 1.1–1.2 with a mean daily dose in excess of 18,000 units (139,140). The adjusted dose regimen has limitations for routine use, since it requires careful monitoring and the use of a responsive APTT system.

VI. SIDE EFFECTS

A. Bleeding

Four variables have been reported to influence bleeding during heparin treatment: the dose of heparin, the patient's anticoagulant response, the method of heparin administration, and patient factors (109–111,132,141,142). There is indirect evidence that the frequency of bleeding is increased by heparin dose and anticoagulant effect (109,110,132). Pooled analysis of randomized trials comparing different methods of heparin administration yields an average incidence of major bleeding of 6.8% in the continuous-infusion group and 14.2% in the intermittent-intravenous group (odds ratio 0.42; $p = 0.01$). However, the comparison is confounded by the difference in the 24-h heparin dose, which was greater in the intermittent-intravenous group in five of the six studies. Thus, the observed increase in bleeding could be contributed to by the higher dose of heparin in the intermittent-intravenous group.

For studies comparing continuous intravenous heparin with subcutaneous heparin, there was a similar bleeding incidence of 5.2% and 4.1% respectively (odds ratio 1.1) (109). Other factors that predispose to anticoagulant-induced bleeding are a serious concurrent illness (109,141), chronic heavy alcohol consumption (142), and a reduced functional capacity (110).

The concomitant use of aspirin has long been identified as a risk factor for heparin-induced bleeding (109,111,142). This observation bears close examination because heparin and aspirin in combination are used frequently in the initial treatment of acute coronary artery syndromes. Aspirin increases operative and postoperative bleeding in patients who receive the very high doses of heparin required during open heart surgery (143). However, the risk of adding aspirin to a short course of regular therapeutic doses of heparin does not appear to be excessive. In the ISIS-3 study, subcutaneous heparin 12,500 units twice a day started 4 h after initiating a thrombolytic regimen with aspirin 162 mg/day was associated with an increase in major noncerebral bleeds of 0.26% (1.02% vs. 0.76%; $p < 0.01$) and an increase in cerebral bleeds of 0.16% (0.56% vs. 0.40%; $p < 0.05$) (27). In GISSI-2, the same heparin regimen was started 12 h after initiating thrombolytic therapy with aspirin 300–325 mg and was associated with an increase in major noncerebral bleeds of 0.45% (0.99% vs. 0.55%; $p < 0.001$) but no difference in cerebral bleeds (0.35% vs. 0.37%) (24,25).

Renal failure and patient age and sex have also been implicated as risk factors for heparin-induced bleeding (109,144). The reported association with female sex has not been consistent among studies and remains in question. The influence of patient-related factors on heparin-associated bleeding is illustrated by a recent study of patients with proximal vein thrombosis (84). Patients received an initial intravenous bolus of 5000 units of heparin followed by a continuous infusion of 30,000 U/24 h for patients with clinical risk factors for bleeding and of 40,000 U/24 h in patients free of risk factors for bleeding. The incidence of major bleeding was 11% in the high-risk group (who received the lower starting dose) and 1% in the low-risk group (who received the higher starting dose) ($p = 0.007$).

1. *Management of Bleeding on Heparin*

Management of bleeding associated with heparin therapy depends on the site and severity of the bleed, the route of heparin administration, and the associated anticoagulant effect at the time of bleeding. Bleeding during an intravenous infusion can usually be managed with supportive measures and by stopping the infusion, as the half-life for heparin at therapeutic levels is approximately 60 min, and heparin effect is rapidly lost. It may be necessary to reverse heparin effect more rapidly if bleeding is life-threatening (e.g., massive gastrointestinal bleeding, or intracranial bleeding) or if a heparin overdose has occurred when heparin elimination will be markedly delayed. The anticoagulant effects of heparin can be reversed with protamine sulfate, which binds firmly with heparin (122,123). The dose of protamine sulfate is determined by the amount of circulating heparin, which in turn depends on the amount of heparin that was administered and the time interval since the last heparin dose. The full neutralizing dose is 1 mg of protamine sulfate for 100 units of heparin; it needs to be reduced by half this at 1 h and by three-quarters at 2 h. Protamine should be infused over 10 min to avoid hypotension and may need to be repeated because of its rapid clearance. Smaller repeated doses of protamine will be required to reverse therapeutic doses of heparin that have been given subcutaneously.

B. Thrombocytopenia

The prime significance of heparin-induced thrombocytopenia is the risk of associated arterial thrombosis (cerebrovascular, coronary, peripheral), and consequently it is important to monitor for its occurrence with regular platelet counts (145). The reported incidence of heparin-associated thrombocytopenia varies widely. Thrombocytopenia is more common with heparin derived from bovine lung than with heparin from porcine gut. Pooled analysis of recent prospective studies of full-dose intravenous heparin yielded a frequency of thrombocytopenia (defined as a platelet count less than 100×10^9 per liter) of 5.4% (16/294) for bovine and 1.3% (6/463) for porcine heparin (145). The frequency of thrombocytopenia in association with low-dose subcutaneous heparin appears to be lower than with full-dose intravenous therapy; no cases were detected among 214 prospectively studied patients who were receiving a porcine preparation (145). Arterial thrombosis as a complication of heparin-induced thrombocytopenia is also rare; only three cases were found among 1629 prospectively studied patients, yielding a frequency of 0.18% (145). Arterial thrombosis occurs as a consequence of platelet aggregation in vivo, but venous thrombosis could result from heparin resistance caused by the neutralizing effect of heparin-induced release of platelet factor 4.

Thrombocytopenia usually begins between 3 and 15 days after commencing heparin therapy (median 10 days), but it has been reported within hours of commencing heparin in patients who have been exposed to heparin previously. The platelet count usually returns to baseline levels within 4 days of stopping heparin. Heparin-associated thrombocytopenia is thought to be caused by an immunoglobulin G (IgG)-heparin immune complex involving both the Fab and the Fc portion of the IgG molecule (145) If the platelet count falls progressively or precipitously to less than 100,000/ml, heparin should be stopped and an alternative management strategy instituted. If warfarin treatment has already been started and the international normalized ratio (INR) is approaching or in the therapeutic range, warfarin can be continued without the addition of alternative treatment. If warfarin has not been started, and heparin is being used to treat venous thromboembolism, a caval filter can be inserted or an alternative antithrombotic agent used. Two alternative antithrombotic agents have been evaluated in descriptive studies. These are the snake venom Ancrod and the heparinoid Lomoparin. A dosage regime for Ancrod (which is still experimental in the United States but can be obtained from Knoll Pharmaceutical and stored in the pharmacy for compassionate use) is shown in Table 3 (146).

The diagnosis of suspected heparin-induced thrombocytopenia can be confirmed by laboratory tests, but these are rarely useful in making clinical decisions at the time a patient presents. A test based on ^{14}C-serotonin release of washed donor platelets plus heat-treated patient serum in the presence of therapeutic (0.1 U/ml) and high (100 U/ml) heparin concentrations (147) has been shown to be both sensitive and specific (148).

C. Osteoporosis

Prolonged administration of therapeutic doses of heparin is required in a small number of patients, usually because oral anticoagulants (vitamin K antagonists) are contraindicated (e.g., in pregnancy) or have been ineffective at preventing thrombosis (e.g., in association with adenocarcinomas). Under these circumstances, heparin therapy may be associated with osteoporosis. The frequency of this complication has been difficult to determine, as the need for long-term heparin treatment is rare, and when it occurs, randomization to heparin or alternative therapy is usually not clinically justifiable. In the one randomized trial that did address this question (149), one of the 20 women allocated to long-term antenatal heparin prophylaxis (10,000 units twice daily) developed clinical osteoporosis, whereas no control patient did. A number of other descriptive series and case-control studies have also evaluated clinical or radiological endpoints (150–163), and taken in combination these studies suggest that heparin-induced osteoporosis is largely confined to patients who receive moderately high doses (i.e., $\geq$20,000 U/24 h) for more than 5 months.

D. Other Side Effects

Heparin has been reported to produce two distinct types of skin lesions, urticarial lesions and skin necrosis. Urticarial lesions occur at the site of subcutaneous injection and may be caused by a contaminant of heparin. Changing to a different preparation (i.e., a different

Table 3 Dosage Regimen for Ancrod

Initial dose: 2 U/kg IV over 6 h
Maintenance: by either subcutaneous injection or intravenous infusion.

A. Subcutaneous injection: subsequent dose based on the fibrinogen level 12 h after IV infusion.

Fibrinogen level	Daily SC dose of Ancrod
<0.5 gm/l	0
0.5 to 1.0 gm/l	1 U/kg
>1.0 gm/l	2 U/kg

B. Continuous intravenous infusion: subsequent doses by IV infusion based on a fibrinogen level.

Fibrinogen	Daily IV dose of Ancrod
<0.5 g/L	0
0.5 to 1 g/L	1 U/kg over 24 h
1.0 to 1.5 g/L	1 U/kg over 18 h
1.5 to 2.0 g/L	1 U/kg over 12 h
>2.0 g/L	1 U/kg over 8 h

salt or different animal origin) may resolve this problem. Skin necrosis usually occurs as a complication of subcutaneous heparin administration but has also been observed in association with intravenous administration (164). The mechanism of skin necrosis is uncertain; it is inconsistently associated with thrombocytopenia but may be caused by a heparin-associated immune reaction. Histological studies have found hemorrhagic infarction of skin and subcutaneous fat with acute necrotizing angiitis, in keeping with a hypersensitivity reaction. Since skin necrosis seems to be unrelated to the source of the heparin, a different preparation of standard heparin is unlikely to be tolerated. The heparinoid Lomoparin, which has minimal cross-reactivity with standard heparin, may be a safe alternative for these patients, but this has yet to be demonstrated unequivocally.

Generalized hypersensitivity reactions may also occur secondary to heparin administration (165). Symptoms include urticaria, conjunctivitis, rhinitis, bronchospasm, angioneurotic edema, and anaphylactic shock.

Selective hypoaldosteronism is a rare but probably real side effect of heparin administration (166) and appears to be due to inhibition of 18-hydroxycorticosterone synthesis from corticosterone (167,168). It is usually of no clinical importance, although significant metabolic derangements and death have been reported (169–171).

VII. LOW-MOLECULAR-WEIGHT HEPARINS

The earlier part of this chapter has focused on standard heparin, which is currently in widespread use throughout North America. It has been noted that standard heparin is heterogeneous with respect to molecular weights (length) and that pharmacokinetic and pharmacodynamic properties vary between heparin fractions of different sizes. In particular, smaller heparin molecules bind less to plasma proteins and endothelial cells; are cleared predominantly by nonsaturable renal mechanisms rather than by the rapid, saturable cellular route; inhibit platelet function to a lesser extent; have little effect on vascular permeability; and have a higher anti-X_a to anti-II_a ratio than larger heparin molecules. These observations provided the stimulus to develop low-molecular-weight heparins (LMWHs) for clinical use, and these new compounds, which are currently in widespread use in Europe, are likely to be approved for use in North America in the next few years (172). In anticipation of their more widespread use, the differences between LMWHs and standard heparin will be briefly outlined.

A. Biochemistry and Anticoagulant Effects of Low-Molecular-Weight Heparins

Low-molecular-weight heparins are fragments of heparin produced by either chemical or enzymic depolymerization (173). Low-molecular-weight heparins are approximately one-third the size of heparin; like standard heparin, they are heterogeneous with respect to molecular size, with a molecular weight distribution of 1000 to 10,000 and a mean molecular weight of 4000 to 5000. Depolymerization of heparin results in a change in the anticoagulant profile of the resulting low-molecular-weight fractions, with a progressive loss of their ability to catalyze thrombin inhibition (174,175). In addition to LMWHs produced by depolymerization, two other glycosaminoglycans have been developed for clinical use. These are dermatan sulfate and the heparinoid Lomoparin (Organon), which is a mixture of heparan sulfate (80% of the mixture), dermatan sulfate, and chondroitin sulfate.

Low-molecular-weight heparins produce their anticoagulant effect by binding to ATIII through the same unique pentasaccharide sequence as standard heparin (32,34,35), a sequence present on fewer than one-third of LMWH molecules. Since a minimum chain length of 18 saccharides (including the pentasaccharide sequence) is required for ternary complex formation (heparin-ATIII-thrombin), only the larger molecules in each preparation are able to inactivate thrombin (Fig. 1). In contrast, all LMWH fragments that contain the high-affinity pentasaccharide sequence catalyze the inactivation of factor Xa. Virtually all standard heparin molecules contain at least 18 saccharide units, while only 25–50% of different LMWHs contain fragments of this or greater length (33,176–179). Therefore, in contrast to standard heparin, which has a ratio of anti-factor Xa to anti-IIa activity of approximately 1:1, the various commercial LMWHs have anti-factor Xa to anti-IIa ratios that vary between 4:1 and 2:1, depending on their molecular size distribution (172).

B. Pharmacokinetics of Low-Molecular-Weight Heparins

The pharmacokinetics of LMWHs differ from those of standard heparin largely as a result of their reduced binding and clearance by plasma proteins (28,85,88,89), macrophages, and endothelial cells (31,93,180,181). These differences probably account for their longer plasma half-life, which is approximately two to four times longer than that of standard heparin (115,182–186). Minimal protein binding contributes to excellent bioavailability of LMWHs at low doses and a predictable anticoagulant dose response (187). Since they are cleared principally by the kidneys, the half-life of LMWHs is largely independent of the dose administered, and, unlike that of standard heparin, it is prolonged with renal failure (115,188,189).

C. Antithrombotic and Hemorrhagic Effects of Low-Molecular-Weight Heparins

When compared with standard heparin in experimental models of thrombosis and hemorrhage, LMWHs are slightly less effective as antithrombotic agents but produce much less bleeding (65–70,190–195). These experimental observations have not been evaluated properly in humans, but there is suggestive evidence that less bleeding occurred with LMWHs than with standard heparin when both were given for prophylaxis with matching of ex vivo anticoagulant effect (71), and when both were given in high doses for the treatment of venous thrombosis (72,73). The improved antithrombotic-to-bleeding ratio with LMWHs is thought to be due to less impairment of platelet function (55,89,196), reduced binding of von Willebrand factor (89), and reduced effects on vascular permeability (54). Low-molecular-weight heparins have been compared with standard heparin and have been shown to be more effective than standard heparin for the prevention of venous thrombosis in high-risk patients, and to be more effective and safe than standard heparin for the treatment of venous thrombosis (172). Coupled with more uniform bioavailability and predictable dose-response relationships, these properties open the way for therapeutic anticoagulation with LMWHs without the need for frequent monitoring. This could make it feasible to treat some acute thrombotic disorders on an outpatient basis, an advance that would reduce cost and improve patient convenience.

D. Unresolved Issues with Low-Molecular-Weight Heparins

Like standard heparin (197), LMWHs do not cross the placental barrier (198–200), and descriptive studies suggest they are safe and effective (201) in pregnancy, but experience is limited. As previously noted, the long-term use of standard heparin may be complicated with osteoporosis. Although there is a case report of successful use of a LMWH in a patient whose treatment with standard heparin was complicated with symptomatic osteoporosis (201), it is not known if the risk of osteoporosis is reduced or eliminated by LMWHs.

There is an impression that the incidence of thrombocytopenia is lower with LMWHs than with standard heparin, but this has never been confirmed in a properly designed clinical study. There are reports that LMWHs can be associated with thrombocytopenia, both in previously unexposed persons (202) and in those with a history of heparin-induced thrombocytopenia (HIT) (203), and that LMWH preparations cross-react with plasma from patients with recent HIT (204). In contrast to the LMWHs, the heparinoid lomoparin, which is essentially free of contaminating heparin, has minimal cross-reactivity in in vitro assays for HIT (205), and it has been used successfully in patients with a history of HIT (205) Prospective studies of large numbers of patients treated with LMWHs will be required to resolve these issues.

REFERENCES

1. McLean J. The thromboplastic action of cephalin. Am J Physiol 1976; 41:250–7.
2. McLean J. The discovery of heparin. Circulation 1959; 19:75–8.
3. Best CH. Preparation of heparin and its use in the first clinical cases. Circulation 1959; 19:79–86.
4. Jorpes JE. Heparin: a mucopolysaccharide and an active antithrombotic drug. Circulation 1959; 19:87–91.
5. Brinkhous KM, Smith HP, Warner ED, Seegers WH. The inhibition of blood clotting: an unidentified substance which acts in conjunction with heparin to prevent the conversion of prothrombin into thrombin. Am J Physiol 1939; 125:683–7.
6. Rosenberg RD. The heparin-antithrombin system: a natural anticoagulant mechanism. In: Colman RW, Hirsh J, Marder VJ, Salzman EW, eds. Hemostasis and thrombosis: basic principles and clinical practice. Philadelphia: J.B. Lippincott 1987; 1373–92.
7. Abildgaard U. Highly purified antithrombin III with heparin cofactor activity prepared by disc electrophoresis. Scand J Clin Lab Invest 1968; 21:89–91.
8. Waugh DF, Fitzgerald MA. Quantitative aspects of antithrombin and heparin in plasma. Am J Physiol 1956; 184:627–639.
9. Monkhouse FC, France ES, Seegers WH. Studies on the antithrombin and heparin cofactor activities of a fraction absorbed from plasma by aluminum hydroxide. Circ Res 1955; 3: 397–402.
10. Rosenberg RD, Lam L. Correlation between structure and function of heparin. Proc Natl Acad Sci USA 1979; 76:1218–22.
11. Lindahl U, Backstrom G, Hook M, Thunberg L, Fransson L-A, Linker A. Structure of the antithrombin-binding site of heparin. Proc Natl Acad Sci USA 1979; 76:3198–202.
12. Hook M, Bjork I, Hopwood J, Lindahl U. Anticoagulant activity of heparin: separation of high-activity and low-activity heparin species by affinity chromatography on immobilized antithrombin. FEBS Lett 1976; 66:90–3.
13. Barritt DW, Jordan SC. Anticoagulant drugs in the treatment of pulmonary embolism: a controlled trial. Lancet 1960; 1:1309–12.
14. Clagett GP, Reisch JS. Prevention of venous thromboembolism in general surgical patients. Results of meta-analysis. Ann Surg 1988; 208:227–40.
15. Collins R, Scrimgeour A, Yusuf S, Phil D, Peto R. Reduction in fatal pulmonary embolism and venous thrombosis by perioperative administration of subcutaneous heparin. N Engl J Med 1988; 318:1162–73.
16. Hull RD, Delmore TJ, Genton E, Hirsh J, Gent M, Sackett D, McLoughlin D, Armstrong P.

Warfarin sodium versus low dose heparin in the long-term treatment of venous thrombosis. N Engl J Med 1979; 301:855–8.

17. Lagerstedt CJ, Olsson CG, Fagher BO, Oqvist BO, Albrechtsson U. Need for long term anticoagulant treatment in symptomatic calf-vein thrombosis. Lancet 1985; 2:515–8.

18. Theroux P, Ouimet N, McCans J, Latour J-G, Joly P, Levy G, Pelletier E, Juneau M, Stasiak J, DeGuise P, Pelletier GB, Rinzler D, Waters DD. Aspirin, heparin or both to treat unstable angina. N Engl J Med 1988; 319:1105–11.

19. Serneri GGN, Gensini GF, Poggesi L, Trotta F, Modesti PA, Boddi M, Ieri A, Margheri M, Casolo GC, Bini M, Rostagno C, Carnovali M, Abbate R. Effect of heparin, aspirin, or alteplase in reduction of myocardial ischaemia in refractory unstable angina. Lancet 1990; 335:615–8.

20. SCATI Group. Randomised controlled trial of subcutaneous calcium-heparin in acute myocardial infarction. Lancet 1989; 2:182–6.

21. Turpie AGG, Robinson JG, Doyle DJ, Kulji AS, Mishkel GJ, Sealey BJ, Cairns JA, Skingley L, Hirsh J, Gent M. Comparison of high dose with low dose subcutaneous heparin to prevent left ventricular mural thrombosis in patients with acute transmural anterior myocardial infarction. N Engl J Med 1989; 320:352–94.

22. ISIS (International Studies of Infarct Survival) Pilot Study Investigators. Randomized factorial trial of high-dose intravenous streptokinase, or oral aspirin and of intravenous heparin in acute myocardial infarction. Eur Heart J 1987; 8:634–42.

23. Bleich SD, Nichols T, Schumacher R, Cooke D, Tate D, Steiner C, Brinkman D. The role of heparin following coronary thrombolysis with tissue plasminogen activator (t-PA) (abstr). Circulation 1989; 80(suppl 2):II–13.

24. Gruppo Italiano per lo Studio della Sopravvivenza nell'Infarto Miocardico. Gissi-2: a factorial randomised trial of alteplase versus streptokinase and heparin versus no heparin among 12,490 patients with acute myocardial infarction. Lancet 1990; 336:65–71.

25. The International Study Group. In-hospital mortality and clinical course of 20,891 patients with suspected acute myocardial infarction randomised between alteplase and streptokinase with or without heparin. Lancet 1992; 336:71–5.

26. Hsia J, Hamilton WP, Kleiman N, Roberts R, Chaitman BR, Ross AM, HART Investigators. A comparison between heparin and low-dose aspirin as adjunctive therapy with tissue plasminogen activator for acute mycardial infarction. N Engl J Med 1990; 323:1433–7.

27. ISIS-3 (Third International Study of Infarct Survival) Collaborative Group. ISIS-3: a randomised comparison of streptokinase vs tissue plasminogen activator vs anistreplase and of aspirin plus heparin vs aspirin alone among 41,299 cases of suspected acute myocardial infarction. Lancet 1992; 339:753–70.

28. Andersson LO, Barrowcliffe TW, Holmer E, Johnson EA, Soderstrom G. Molecular weight dependency of the heparin potentiated inhibition of thrombin and activated Factor X. Effect of heparin neutralization in plasma. Thromb Res 1979; 15:531–41.

29. Hirsh J. Heparin. N Engl J Med 1991; 324:1565–74.

30. Jackson CM. Mechanism of heparin action. In: Hirsh J, ed. Clinical haematology. London: Balliere Tindall, 1990;483–504.

31. Boneu B, Caranobe C, Sie P. Pharmacokinetics of heparin and low molecular weight heparin. In: Hirsh J, ed. Clinical haematology. London: Bailliere Tindall, 1990:531–44.

32. Choay J, Lormeau JC, Petitou M, Sinay P, Fareed J. Structural studies on a biologically active hexasaccharide obtained from heparin. Ann NY Acad Sci 1981; 370:644–9.

33. Lindahl U, Thunberg L, Backstrom G, Riesenfel J, Nordling K, Bjork I. Extension and structural variability of the antithrombin binding sequence in heparin. J Biol Chem 1984; 259:12368–76.

34. Casu B, Oreste P, Torri G, Zoppetti G, Choay J, Lormeau JC, Petitou M, Sinay P. The structure of heparin oligosaccharide fragments with high anti-(factor Xa) activity containing the minimal antithrombin III binding sequence. Biochem J 1981; 197:599–609.

35. Choay J, Petitou M, Lormeau JC, Sinay P, Casu BJ, Gatti G. Structure-activity of relationship in

heparin: a synthetic pentasaccharide with high affinity for antithrombin III and eliciting high antifactor Xa activity. Biochem Biophys Res Commun 1983; 116:492–9.

36. Ofosu FA, Modi GJ, Hirsh J, Buchanan M, Blajchman MA. Mechanisms for inhibition of the generation of thrombin activity by sulfated polysaccharides. Ann NY Acad Sci 1986; 485:41–55.

37. Ofosu FA, Sie P, Modi GJ, Fernandez FA, Buchanan MR, Blajchman MA, Boneu B, Hirsh J. The inhibition of thrombin-dependent feedback reactions is critical to the expression of anticoagulant effects of heparin. Biochem J 1987; 243:579–88.

38. Ofosu FA, Esmond CT, Blajchman MA, Modi GJ, Smith LA, Anuari N, Buchanan MR, Fenton II JW, Hirsh J. Unfractionated heparin inhibits thrombin-catalyzed amplification reactions of coagulation more efficiently than those catalyzed by factor Xa. Biochem J 1989; 257:143–50.

39. Beguin S, Lindhout T, Hemker HC. The mode of action of heparin in plasma. Thromb Haemost 1988; 60:457–62.

40. Lam LH, Silbert JE, Rosenberg RD. The separation of active and inactive forms of heparin. Biochem Biophys Res Commun 1976; 69:570–7.

41. Andersson LO, Barrowcliffe TW, Holmer E, Johnson EA, Sims GEC. Anticoagulant properties of heparin fractionated by affinity chromatography on matrix-bound antithrombin III and by gel filtration. Thromb Res 1976; 9:575–83.

42. Marcum JA, Fritze L, Galli SJ, Karp G, Rosenberg RD. Microvascular heparinlike species with anticoagulant activity. Am J Physiol 1983; 245:H725–33.

43. Marcum JA, Rosenberg RD. Heparinlike molecules with anticoagulant activity are synthesized by cultured endothelial cells. Biochem Biophys Res Commun 1985; 126:365–72.

44. Bengtsson-Olivecrona G, Olivecrona T. Binding of active and inactive forms of lipoprotein lipase to heparin: effects of pH. Biochem J 1985; 226:409–13.

45. Hirsh J, Piovella F. Congenital antithrombin III deficiency. Am J Med 1989; 87(suppl 3B): 34–8.

46. Highsmith RF, Rosenberg RD. The inhibition of human plasmin by human antithrombin-heparin cofactor. J Biol Chem 1974; 249:4335–8.

47. Edelberg JM, Pizzo SV. Kinetic analysis of the effects of heparin and lipoproteins on tissue plasminogen activator mediated plasminogen activation. Biochemistry 1990; 29:5906–11.

48. Andrade-Gordon P, Strickland S. Interaction of heparin with plasminogen activators and plasminogen: effects on the activation of plasminogen. Biochemistry 1986; 25:4033–40.

49. Paques EP, Stohr HA, Heimburger N. Study on the mechanism of action of heparin and related substances on the fibrinolytic system: relationship between plasminogen activators and heparin. Thromb Res 1986; 42:797–807.

50. Agnelli G, Borm J, Cosmi B, Levi M, ten Cate JW. Effects of standard heparin and a low molecular weight heparin (Kabi 2165) on fibrinolysis. Thromb Haemost 1988; 60:311–3.

51. Fry ETA, Sobel BE. Lack of interference by heparin with thrombolysis or binding of tissue-type plasminogen activator to thrombi. Blood 1988; 71:1347–52.

52. Agnelli G, Pascucci C, Cosmi B, Nenci GG. Effects of therapeutic doses of heparin on thrombolysis with tissue-plasminogen activator in rabbits. Blood 1990; 76:2030–6.

53. Cercek B, Lew AS, Hod H, Yano J, Reddy NKN, Ganz W. Enhancement of thrombolysis with tissue-ready plasminogen activator by pretreatment with heparin. Circulation 1986; 74:583–7.

54. Blajchman MA, Young E, Ofosu FA. Effects of unfractionated heparin, dermatan sulfate and low molecular weight heparin on vessel wall permeability in rabbits. Ann NY Acad Sci 1989; 556:245–54.

55. Fernandez FA, Nguyen P, Van Ryn J, Ofosu FA, Hirsh J, Buchanan MR. Hemorrhagic doses of heparin and other glycosaminoglycans induce a platelet defect. Thromb Res 1986; 43:491–5.

56. Clowes AW, Karnovsky MJ. Suppression by heparin of smooth muscle cell proliferation in injured arteries. Nature 1977; 365:625–6.

57. Sy M, Schneeberger E, McCluskey R, Greene M, Rosenberg R, Venacerraf B. Inhibition of delayed-type hypersensitivity by heparin depleted of anticoagulant activity. Cell Immun 1983; 82:23–32.

58. O'Kelly R, Magee F, McKenna TJ. Routine heparin therapy inhibits adrenal aldosterone production. J Clin Endocrinol Metab 1983; 56:108–12.

59. Folkman J. Regulation of angiogenesis: a new function of heparin. In: Folkman J, ed. Biochemical pharmacology. New York: Pergamon Press, 1985;905–9.

60. Eika C. Inhibition of thrombin-induced aggregation of human platelets in heparin. Scand J Haematol 1971; 8:216–22.

61. Kelton JG, Hirsh J. Bleeding associated with antithrombotic therapy. Semin Hematol 1980; 17:259–91.

62. Salzman EW, Rosenberg RD, Smith MH, Lindon JN, Favreau L. Effect of heparin and heparin fractions on platelet aggregation. J Clin Invest 1980; 65:64–73.

63. Ockelford PA, Carter CJ, Cerskus A, Smith CA, Hirsh J. Comparison of the in vivo hemorrhagic and antithrombotic effect of a low antithrombin III affinity heparin fraction. Thromb Res 1982; 27:679–90.

64. Heiden D, Mielke CH Jr, Rodvien R. Impairment by heparin of primary haemostasis and platelet (14-C)5-hydroxytryptamine release. Br J Haematol 1977; 36:427–36.

65. Andriuolli G, Mastucchi R, Barnti M, Sarret M. Comparison of the antithrombotic and hemorrhagic effects of heparin and a new low molecular weight heparin in rats. Haemostasis 1985; 15:324–330.

66. Bergqvist D, Nilsson B, Hedner U, Pederson PChr, Ostergaard PB. The effect of heparin fragments of different molecular weights on experimental thrombosis and haemostasis. Thromb Res 1985; 38:589–601.

67. Cade JF, Buchanan MR, Boneu B, Ockelford P, Carter CJ, Cerskus AL, Hirsh J. A comparison of the antithrombotic and hemorrhagic effects of low molecular weight heparin fractions. Thromb Res 1984; 35:613–25.

68. Carter CJ, Kelton JG, Hirsh J, Cerskus A, Santos AV, Gent M. The relationship between the hemorrhagic antithrombotic properties of low molecular weight heparin in rabbits. Blood 1982; 59:1239–45.

69. Esquivel CO, Bergqvist D, Bjork CG, Nilsson B. Comparison between commercial heparin, low molecular weight heparin and pentosan polysulfate on hemostasis and platelets in vivo. Thromb Res 1982; 28:389–99.

70. Holmer E, Matsson C, Nilsson S. Anticoagulant and antithrombotic effects of low molecular weight heparin fragments in rabbits. Thromb Res 1982; 25:475–85.

71. Levine MN, Hirsh J, Gent M. Prevention of deep vein thrombosis after elective hip surgery: a randomized trial comparing low molecular weight heparin with standard unfractionated heparin. Ann Intern Med 1991; 114:545–51.

72. Hull RD, Raskob GE, Pineo GF, Green D, Trowbridge AA, Eliott CG, Lerner RG, Hall J, Sparling T, Brettell HR, Norton J, Carter CJ, George R, Merli G, Ward J, Mayo W, Rosenbloom D, Brant R. Subcutaneous low-molecular-weight heparin compared with continuous intravenous heparin in the treatment of proximal-vein thrombosis. N Engl J Med 1992; 326:975–82.

73. Prandoni P, Lensing AWA, Buller HR, Carta M, Cogo A, Vigo M, Casara D, Ruol A, ten Cate JW. Comparison of subcutaneous low-molecular-weight heparin with intravenous standard heparin in proximal deep-vein thrombosis. Lancet 1992; 339:441–5.

74. Marciniak E. Factor Xa inactivation by antithrombin III: evidence for biological stabilization of factor Xa by factor V–phospholipid complex. Br J Haematol 1973; 24:391–400.

75. Walker FJ, Esmon CT. The effects of phospholipid and factor Va on the inhibition of factor Xa by antithrombin III. Biochem Biophys Res Commun 1979; 90:641–7.

76. Holt JC, Niewiarowski S. Biochemistry of α-granule proteins. Semin Hematol 1985; 22: 151–63.

77. Salzman E, Deykin D, Shapiro ERM, Rosenberg R. Management of heparin therapy. N Engl J Med 1975; 292:1046–50.

78. Glazier RL, Crowell EB. Randomized prospective trial of continuous vs intermittent heparin therapy. JAMA 1976; 236:1365–7.

79. Wilson JR, Lampman J. Heparin therapy: a randomized prospective study. Am Heart J 1979; 97:155–8.
80. Hull RD, Raskob GE, Hirsh J, Jay RM, Leclerc JR, Geerts WH, Rosenbloom D, Sackett DL, Anderson C, Harrison L, Gent M. Continuous intravenous heparin compared with intermittent subcutaneous heparin in the initial treatment of proximal-vein thrombosis. N Engl J Med 1986; 315:1109–14.
81. Doyle DJ, Turpie AGG, Hirsh J, Best C, Kinch D, Levine MN, Gent M. Adjusted subcutaneous heparin or continuous intravenous heparin in patients with acute deep vein thrombosis. Ann Intern Med 1987; 107:441–5.
82. Bentley PG, Kakkar VV, Scully MF, McGregor IR, Webb P, Chan P, Jones N. An objective study of alternative methods of heparin administration. Thromb Res 1980; 18:177–188.
83. Walker MG, Shaw JW, Thompson GJL, Cumming JGR, Lea Thomas M. Subcutaneous calcium heparin versus intravenous sodium heparin in treatment of established acute deep vein thrombosis of the legs: a multicentre prospective randomised trial. Br Med J 1987; 294: 1189–92.
84. Pini M, Pattacini C, Quintavalla R, Poli T, Megha A, Tagliaferri A, Manotti C, Dettori AG. Subcutaneous vs intravenous heparin in the treatment of deep venous thrombosis—a randomized clinical trial. Thromb Haemost 1990; 64:222–6.
85. Lane DA, Pejler G, Flynn AM, Thompson EA, Lindahl U. Neutralization of heparin-related saccharides by histidine-rich glycoprotein and platelet factor 4. J Biol Chem 1986; 261:3980–6.
86. Lijnen HR, Hoylaerts M, Collen D. Heparin binding properties of human histidine-rich glycoprotein. Mechanism and role in the neutralization of heparin in plasma. J Biol Chem 1983; 258:3803–8.
87. Peterson CB, Morgan WT, Blackburn MN. Histidine-rich glycoprotein modulation of the anticoagulant activity of heparin. J Biol Chem 1987; 262:7567–74.
88. Preissner KT, Muller-Berghaus G. Neutralization and binding of heparin by S-protein/ vitronectin in the inhibition of Factor Xa by antithrombin III. J Biol Chem 1987; 262: 12247–53.
89. Sobel M, McNeill PM, Carlson PL, Kermode JC, Adelman B, Conroy R, Marques D. Heparin inhibition of von Willebrand factor–dependent platelet function in vitro and in vivo. J Clin Invest 1991; 87:1787–93.
90. Dawes J, Pavuk N. Sequestration of therapeutic glycosaminoglycans by plasma fibronectin. Thromb Haemost 1991; 65:829.
91. Young E, Prins MH, Levine MN, Hirsh J. Heparin binding to plasma proteins, an important mechanism for heparin resistance. Thromb Haemost 1992; 67:639–643.
92. Mahadoo J, Hiebert L, Jaques LB. Vascular sequestration of heparin. Thromb Res 1977; 12: 79–90.
93. Barzu T, Molho P, Tobelem G, Petitou M, Caen J. Binding and endocytosis of heparin by human endothelial cells in culture. Biochim Biophys Acta 1985; 845:196–203.
94. Glimelius B, Busch C, Hook M. Binding of heparin on the surface of cultured human endothelial cells. Thromb Res 1978; 12:773–82.
95. Friedman Y, Arsenis C. Studies on the heparin sulphamidase activity from rat spleen. Intracellular distribution and characterization of the enzyme. Biochem J 1974; 139:699–708.
96. Hirsh J, Van Aken WG, Gallus AS, Dollery CT, Cade JF, Yung WL. Heparin kinetics in venous thrombosis and pulmonary embolism. Circulation 1976; 53:691–5.
97. Hogg PJ, Jackson CM. Fibrin monomer protects thrombin from inactivation by heparin–antithrombin III: implications for heparin efficacy Proc Natl Acad Sci USA 1989; 86:3619–23.
98. Weitz JI, Hudoba M, Massel D, Maraganore J, Hirsh J. Clot-bound thrombin is protected from inhibition by heparin-antithrombin III but is susceptible to inactivation by antithrombin III– independent inhibitors. J Clin Invest 1990; 86:385–91.
99. Hirsh J. From unfractionated heparins to low molecular weight heparins. Acta Chir Scand (Suppl) 1990; 556:42–50.

100. Eisenberg PR, Sherman L, Rich M, Schwartz D, Schechtman K, Geltman EM, Sobel BE, Jaffe AS. Importance of continued activation of thrombin reflected by fibrinopeptide A to the efficacy of thrombolysis. J Am Coll Cardiol 1986; 7:1255–62.
101. Owen J, Friedman KD, Grossman BA, Wilkins C, Berke AD, Powers ER. Thrombolytic therapy with tissue plasminogen activator or streptokinase induces transient thrombin activity. Blood 1988; 72:616–20.
102. Rapold JH, Kuemmerli H, Weiss M, Baur H, Haeberli A. Monitoring of fibrin generation during thrombolytic therapy of acute myocardial infarction with recombinant tissue-type plasminogen activator. Circulation 1989; 79:980–9.
103. Bar-Shavit R, Eldor A, Vlodavsky I. Binding of thrombin to subendothelial extracellular matrix. Protection and expression of functional properties. J Clin Invest 1989; 84:1096–1104.
104. Colburn WA. Pharmacologic implications of heparin interactions with other drugs. Drug Metabol Rev 1976; 5:281.
105. Hodby ED, Hirsh J, Adeniyi-Jones C. The influence of drugs upon the anticoagulant activity of heparin. Can Med Assoc J 1972; 106:562–64.
106. Chui HM, Van Aken WG, Hirsh J, Regoeczi E, Horner AA. Increased heparin clearance in experimental pulmonary embolism. J Lab Clin Med 1977; 90:204–15.
107. Habbab MA, Haft JI. Heparin resistance induced by intravenous nitroglycerin (abstr). Circulation 1986; 74(suppl 2):321.
108. Bode V, Welzel D, Franz G, Polensky U. Absence of drug interaction between heparin and nitroglycerin. Randomized placebo-controlled crossover study. Arch Intern Med 1990; 150:2117–9.
109. Levine MN, Hirsh J, Kelton JG. Heparin-induced bleeding. In: Lane DA, Lindahl U, eds. Heparin. Chemical and biological properties. Clinical applications. London: Edward Arnold, 1989:517–32.
110. Nieuwenhuis HK, Albada J, Banga JD, Sixma JJ. Identification of risk factors for bleeding during treatment of acute venous thromboembolism with heparin or low molecular weight heparin. Blood 1991; 78:2337–43.
111. Yett HS, Skillman JJ, Salzman EW. The hazards of heparin plus aspirin. N Engl J Med 1978; 244:1209–12.
112. Bergqvist D, Hallbrook T. A comparison between subcutaneous low-dose sodium and calcium heparin. Acta Chir Scand 1978; 144:339–342.
113. Allen JG, Arendrup H, Toftgaard C, Madsen EM, Sorensen S, Lindegaard P. Calcium-heparin or sodium-heparin in low-dose heparin prophylaxis. Thromb Haemost 1979; 42:1064.
114. De Swart CA, Sixma JJ, Andersson LO, Holmer E, Versschoor L, Nijmeyer B. Kinetics in normal humans of anticoagulant activity, radioactivity and lipolytic activity after intravenous administration of (S) heparin and (S) heparin fractions. Scand J Haematol 1985; 25:50–63.
115. Boneu B, Caranobe C, Cadroy Y, Dol F, Gabaig AM, Dupouy D, Sie P. Pharmacokinetic studies of standard unfractionated heparin, and low molecular weight heparins in the rabbit. Semin Thromb Hemost 1988; 14:18–27.
116. Dawes J, Pepper DS. Catabolism of low-dose heparin in man. Thromb Res 1979; 14:845–60.
117. Pipper J. The fate of heparin in rabbits after intravenous injection. Filtration and tubular secretion in the kidneys. Acta Pharmacol 1947; 3:373–84.
118. Boneu B, Caranobe C, Gabaig AM. Evidence for a saturable mechanism of disappearance of standard heparin in rabbits. Thromb Res 1987; 28:343–50.
119. Boneu B, Buchanan MR, Caranobe C. The disappearance of a low molecular weight heparin fraction (CY 216) differs from standard heparin in rabbits. Thromb Res 1987; 46:845–53.
120. Olsson P, Lagergren H, Ek S. The elimination from plasma of intrvenous heparin. Acta Med Scand 1963; 173:619–30.
121. Johnson EA, Kirkwood TBL, Stirling Y, Perez-Requejo JL, Ingram GIC, Bangham DR, Brozovic M. Four heparin preparations: anti-Xa potentiating effect of heparin after subcutaneous injection. Thromb Haemost 1976; 35:586–591.

122. Graham DT, Pomeroy AR, Smythe DB. Measurement of the heparin neutralizing capacity of protamine. Thromb Haemost 1979; 41:583–589.

123. Douglas AS (ed.). Therapeutic use of heparin. In: Douglas AS, ed. Anticoagulant therapy. Oxford: Blackwell Scientific Publications, 1962:120–5.

124. Shojania AM, Tetreault J, Turnbull G. The variations between heparin sensitivity of different lots of activated partial thromboplastin time reagent produced by the same manufacturer. Am J Clin Pathol 1988; 89:19–23.

125. D'Angelo A, Seveso MP, D'Angelo SV, Gilardoni F, Dettori AG, Bonini P. Effect of clot-detection methods and reagents on activated partial thromboplastin time (APTT). Implications in heparin monitoring by APTT. Am J Clin Pathol 1990; 94:297–306.

126. Stevenson KJ, Easton AC, Curry A, Thomason JM, Poller L. The reliability of activated partial thromboplastin time methods and the relationship to lipid composition and ultrastructure. Thromb Haemost 1986; 55:250–8.

127. Chui HM, Hirsh J, Yung WL, Regoeczi E, Gent M. Relationship between the anticoagulant and antithrombotic effects of heparin in experimental venous thrombosis. Blood 1977; 49:171–84.

128. Basu D, Gallus AS, Hirsh J, Cade J. A prospective study of the value of monitoring heparin treatment with the activated partial thromboplastin time. N Engl J Med 1972; 287:324–7.

129. Kaplan K, Davison R, Parker M, Mayberry B, Feiereisel P, Salinger M. Role of heparin after intravenous thrombolytic therapy for acute myocardial infarction. Am J Cardiol 1987; 59:241–4.

130. Camilleri JF, Bonnet JL, Bouvier JL. Thrombolyse intraveineuse dans l'infarctus du myocarde: influence de la qualité de l'anticoagulation sur le taux de récidives précoces d'angor ou d'infarctus. Arch Mal Coeur 1988; 81:1037–41.

131. De Bono DP, Simoons ML, Tijssen J. Effect of early intravenous heparin on coronary patency, infarct size, and bleeding complications after alteplase thrombolysis: results of a randomised double blind European Cooperative Study Group Trial. Br Heart J 1992; 67:122–8.

132. Morabia A. Heparin doses and major bleeding. Lancet 1986; 1:1278–9.

133. De Swart CAM, Nijmeyer B, Roelofs JMM, Sixma JJ. Kinetics of intravenously administered heparin in normal humans. Blood 1982; 60:1251–8.

134. Bjornsson TD, Wolfram KM, Kitchell BB. Heparin kinetics determined by three assay methods. Clin Pharmacol Ther 1982; 31:104–13.

135. Cruickshank MK, Levine MN, Hirsh J, Roberts RS, Siguenza M. A standard heparin nomogram for the management of heparin therapy. Arch Intern Med 1991; 151:333–7.

136. Fennerty AG, Levine MN, Hirsh J. Hemorrhagic complications of thrombolytic therapy in the treatment of myocardial infarction and venous thromboembolism. Chest 1989; 95:885–975.

137. Hirsch DR, Goldhaber SZ. Laboratory parameters to monitor safety and efficacy during thrombolytic therapy. Chest 1991; 99:113–20.

138. Leyvraz PF, Richard J, Bachmann F. Adjusted versus fixed dose subcutaneous heparin in the prevention of deep vein thrombosis after total hip replacement. N Engl J Med 1983; 309:954–958.

139. Poller L, Taberner DA, Sandilands DG, Galasko CSB. An evaluation of APTT monitoring of low-dose heparin dosage in hip surgery. Thromb Haemost 1982; 47:50–3.

140. Taberner DA, Poller L, Thomson JM, Lemon G, Weighill FJ. Randomized study of adjusted versus fixed low dose heparin prophylaxis of deep vein thrombosis in hip surgery. Br J Surg 1989; 76:933–5.

141. Landefeld CS, Cook EF, Flatley M, Weisberg M, Goldman L. Identification and preliminary validation of predictors of major bleeding in hospitalized patients starting anticoagulant therapy. Am J Med 1987; 82:703–13.

142. Walker AM, Jick H. Predicators of bleeding during heparin therapy. JAMA 1980; 244:1209–12.

143. Sethi GK, Copeland JG, Goldman S, Moritz T, Zadina K, Henderson WG. Implications of preoperative administration of aspirin in patients undergoing coronary artery bypass grafting. J Am Coll Cardiol 1990; 15:15–20.

144. Jick H, Sloan D, Borda IT, Chapiro S. Efficacy and toxicity of heparin in relation to age and sex. N Engl J Med 1968; 279:284–6.

145. Warkentin TE, Kelton JG. Heparin-induced thrombocytopenia. Annu Rev Med 1989; 40: 31–44.

146. Demers C, Ginsberg JS, Brill-Edwards P, Panju A, Warkentin TE, Anderson DR, Turner C, Kelton JG. Rapid anticoagulation using ancrod for heparin-induced thrombocytopenia. Blood 1991; 78:2194–7.

147. Sheridan D, Carter C, Kelton JG. A diagnostic test for heparin-induced thrombocytopenia. Blood 1986; 67:27–30.

148. Chong BH, Berndt MC. Heparin-induced thrombocytopenia. Blut 1988; 58:53–7.

149. Howell R, Fidler J, Letsky E, DeSwiet M. The risks of antenatal subcutaneous heparin prophylaxis: a controlled trial. Br J Obstet Gynecol 1983; 90:1124–8.

150. Griffith CC, Nichols G, Asher JD, Flanagan B. Heparin osteoporosis. JAMA 1965; 193:85–8.

151. Jaffe MD, Willis PW. Multiple fractures associated with long term sodium heparin therapy. JAMA 1965; 193:152–4.

152. Buchwald H, Rhode TD, Schneider PD, Varco RL, Blackshear PJ. Long-term, continuous intravenous heparin administration by an implantable infusion pump in ambulatory patients with recurrent venous thrombosis. Surgery 1980; 88:507–16.

153. Rupp WM, McCarthy HB, Rohde TD. Risk of osteoporosis in patients treated with long-term intravenous heparin. Curr Surg 1982; 39:419–22.

154. Sackler JP, Liu L. Heparin-induced osteoporosis. Br J Radiol 1973; 46:548–50.

155. Miller WE, DeWolfe VG. Osteoporosis resulting from heparin therapy. Cleve Clin Q 1966; 33:31–4.

156. Aarskog D, Aksnes L, Lehmann L. Low 1,23-dihydroxyvitamin D in heparin-induced osteopenia. Lancet 1980; 2:650–1.

157. Griffiths HT, Liu DTY. Severe heparin osteoporosis in pregnancy. Postgrad Med 1984; 60: 424–5.

158. Hellgren M, Nygards E-B. Long-term therapy with subcutaneous heparin during pregnancy. Gynecol Obstet Invest 1982; 13:76–89.

159. Megard M, Cuche M, Grapeloux A, Bojoly C, Meunier PJ. Ostéoporose de l'héparinothérapie: analyse histonophométrique de la biopsie osseuse. Nouv Presse Med 1982; 11:261–4.

160. Squires JW, Pinch LWC. Heparin-induced spinal fractures. JAMA 1979; 241:2417–8.

161. Wise PH, Hall AJ. Heparin-induced osteopenia in pregnancy. Br Med J 1980; 1:110–1.

162. Dahlman T, Lindvall N, Hellgren M. Osteopenia in pregnancy during long term heparin treatment: a radiological study post-partum. Br J Obstet Gyn 1990; 97:221–8.

163. Ginsberg JS, Kowalchuk G, Hirsh J. Heparin effect on bone density. Thromb Haemost 1990; 64:286–9.

164. White PW, Sadd JR, Nensel RE. Thrombotic complications of heparin therapy: including six cases of heparin-induced necrosis. Ann Surg 1979; 190:595–608.

165. Curry N, Bandana EJ, Pirofsky B. Heparin sensitivity: report of a case. Arch Intern Med 1973; 132:744–5.

166. O'Kelly R, Magee F, McKenna J. Routine heparin therapy inhibits adrenal aldosterone production. J Clin Endocrinol Metab 1983; 56:108–12.

167. Abbott EC, Gornal AC, Sutherland DJA, Stiefel M, Laidlaw JC. The influence of a heparin-like compound on hypertension electrolytes and aldosterone in man. CMAJ 1966; 94:1155–64.

168. Conn JW, Rovner DR, Cohen EL, Anderson JE. Inhibition of heparinoid on aldosterone biosynthesis in man. J Clin Endocrinol Metab 1966; 26:527–32.

169. Phelps KR, Oh MS, Carroll HJ. Heparin-induced hyperkalaemia. Report of a case. Nephron 1980; 25:254–8.

170. Leehey D, Ganti C, Lim V. Heparin-induced hypoaldosteronism. JAMA 1981; 246:2189–90.

171. Wilson ID, Goetz FC. Selective hypoaldosteronism after prolonged heparin administration. Am J Med 1964; 36:635–40.

172. Hirsh J, Levine MN. Review: low molecular weight heparin. Blood 1992; 79:1–17.
173. Ofosu FA, Barrowcliffe TW. Mechanisms of action of low molecular weight heparins and heparinoids. In: Hirsh J, ed. Clinical haematology. London: Bailliere Tindall 1990: 505–25.
174. Danielsson A, Raub E, Lindahl U, Bjork I. Role of ternary complexes in which heparin binds both antithrombin and proteinase, in the acceleration of the reactions between antithrombin and thrombin or factor Xa. J Biol Chem 1986; 261:15467–73.
175. Jordan R, Favreau L, Braswell E, Rosenberg RD. Heparin with two binding sites for antithrombin or platelet factor 4. J Biol Chem 1982; 257:400–6.
176. Jordan RE, Oosta GM, Gardner WT, Rosenberg RD. The kinetics of hemostatic enzyme-antithrombin interactions in the presence of low molecular weight heparin. J Biol Chem 1980; 255:10081–90.
177. Lane A, Denton J, Flynn AM, Thunberg L, Lindahl U. Anticoagulant activities of heparin oligosaccharides and their neutralization by platelet factor 4. Biochem J 1984; 218:725–32.
178. Holmer E, Kurachi K, Soderstrom G. The molecular-weight heparin dependence of the rate-enhancing effect of heparin on the inhibition of thrombin, factor Xa, factor IXa, factor XIa, factor XIIa and kallikrein by antithrombin. Biochem J 1981; 193:395–400.
179. Holmer E, Soderberg K, Bergqvist D, Lindahl V. Heparin and its low molecular weight derivatives: anticoagulant and antithrombotic properties. Haemostasis 1986; 16:1–7.
180. Barzu T, Molho P, Tobelem G, Petitou M, Caen JP. Binding of heparin and low molecular weight heparin fragments to human vascular endothelial cells in culture. Nouv Rev Fr Haematol 1984; 26:243–7.
181. Barzu T, Van Rijn JLMC, Petitou M, Tobelem G, Caen JP. Heparin degradation in the endothelial cells. Thromb Res 1987; 47:601–9.
182. Bradbrook ID, Magnani HN, Moelker HC, Morrison PG, Robinson J, Rogers HJ, Spector RG, Vandinther T, Wijnand H. ORG 10172: a low molecular weight heparinoid anticoagulant with a long half life in man. Br J Clin Pharmacol 1987; 23:667–75.
183. Bratt G, Tornebohm E, Widlund L, Lockner D. Low molecular weight heparin (Kabi 2165, Fragmin): pharmacokinetics after intravenous and subcutaneous administration in human volunteers. Thromb Res 1986; 42:613–20.
184. Briant L, Caranobe C, Saivin S, Byrou B, Houin G, Boneu B. Unfractionated heparin and CY 216: pharmacokinetics and bioavailabilities of the antifactor Xa and IIa effects after intravenous and subcutaneous injection in the rabbit. Thromb Haemost 1989; 61:348–53.
185. Zimmerman LH, Levine RA, Farber HW. Hypoxia induces a specific set of stress proteins in cultured endothelial cells. J Clin Invest 1991; 87:908–14.
186. Stiekema JCJ, Wijnand HP, Van Dinther ThG, Moelker HCT, Dawes J, Vinchenzo A, Toeberich H. Safety and pharmacokinetics of the low molecular weight heparinoid Org 10172 administered to healthy elderly volunteers. Br J Clin Pharmacol 1989; 27:39–48.
187. Handeland GF, Abildgaard U, Holm HA, Arnesen K-E. Dose adjusted heparin treatment of deep venous thrombosis: a comparison of unfractionated and low molecular weight heparin. Eur J Clin Pharmacol 1990; 39:107–12.
188. Caranobe C, Barret A, Gabaig AM, Dupouy D, Sie P, Boneu B. Disappearance of circulating anti-Xa activity after intravenous injection of standard heparin and of low molecular weight heparin (CY216) in normal and nephrectomized rabbits. Thromb Res 1985; 40:129–33.
189. Palm M, Mattsson C. Pharmacokinetics of heparin and low molecular weight heparin fragment (Fragmin) in rabbits with impaired renal or metabolic clearance. Thromb Haemost 1987; 58:932–5.
190. Ockelford PA, Carter CJ, Mitchell L, Hirsh J. Discordance between the anti-Xa activity and antithrombotic activities of an ultra-low molecular weight heparin fraction. Thromb Res 1982; 28:401–9.
191. Van Ryn-McKenna J, Gray E, Weber E, Ofosu FA, Buchanan MR. Effects of sulphated polysaccharides in inhibition of thrombus formation initiated by different stimuli. Thromb Haemost 1989; 61:7–9.

192. Van Ryn-McKenna J, Ofosu FA, Hirsh J, Buchanan M. Antithrombotic and bleeding effects of glycosaminoglycans with different degrees of sulfation. Br J Haematol 1989; 71:265–9.

193. Boneu B, Buchanan MR, Cade JR, Van Ryn J, Fernandez F, Ofosu FA, Hirsh J. Effects of heparin, its low molecular weight fractions and other glycosaminoglycans on thrombus growth in vivo. Thromb Res 1985; 40:81–9.

194. Henny CP, ten Cate H, ten Cate JW, Moulijn AC, Sie TH, Warren P, Buller HR. A randomized blind study comparing standard heparin and a new low molecular weight heparinoid in cardiopulmonary bypass surgery in dogs. J Lab Clin Med 1985; 106:187–96.

195. Hobbelen PMJ, Vogel GMT, Meuleman DG. Time courses of the antithromboitc effects, bleeding enhancing effects, and interations with factors Xa and thrombin after administration of low molecular weight heaprinoid ORG 10172 or heparin to rats. Thromb Res 1987; 48:549–58.

196. Fabris F, Fussi F, Casonato A, Visentin L, Randi M, Smith MR, Girolami A. Normal and low molecular weight heparins: interaction with human platelets. Europ J Clin Invest 1983; 13: 135–9.

197. Ginsberg JS, Hirsh J, Levine MN, Burrows R. Risks to the fetus of anticoagulant therapy during pregnancy. Thromb Haemost 1989; 61:197–203.

198. Forestier F, Daffos F, Capella-Pavlovsky M. Low molecular weight heparin (PK 10169) does not cross the placenta during the second trimester of pregnancy: study by direct fetal blood sampling under ultrasound. Thromb Res 1984; 34:557–60.

199. Forestier F, Daffos F, Rainaut M, Toulemonde F. Low molecular weight heparin (CY216) does not cross the placenta during the third trimester of pregnancy. Thromb Haemost 1987; 57:234 (letter).

200. Omri A, Delaloye JF, Andersen H, Bachmann F. Low molecular weight heparin Novo (LHN-1) does not cross the placenta during the second trimester of pregnancy. Thromb Haemost 1989; 61:55–6.

201. Melissari E, Das S, Kanthou DC, Pemberton KD, Kakkar VV. The use of LMW heparin in treating thromboembolism during pregnancy and prevention of osteoporosis (abstr). Thromb Haemost 1991; 65:926.

202. Vitoux JF, Mathieu JF, Roncato M, Fiessinger JN, Aiach M. Heparin-associated thrombocytopenia. Treatment with low molecular weight heparin. Thromb Haemost 1986; 55:37–46.

203. Horellou MH, Conard J, Lecrubier C, Samana M, Roque-D'Orbcatel O, de Fenoyl O, Di Maria G, Bernadou A. Persistent heparin induced thrombocytopenia despite therapy with low molecular weight heparin. Thromb Haemost 1987; 13:126–30.

204. Leroy J, Leclerc MH, Delahousse B. Treatment of heparin-associated thrombocytopenia and thrombosis with low molecular weight heparin (CY 216). Semin Thromb Haemost 1984; 11: 326–9.

205. Chong BH, Ismail F, Cade J, Gallus AS, Gordon S, Chesterman CN. Heparin-induced thrombocytopenia: studies with a new low molecular weight heparinoid, Org 10172. Blood 1989; 73:1592–6.

Pharmacological Strategies for Antithrombotic Therapy

Thomas H. Müller and Brian D. Guth

Dr. Karl Thomae GmbH, Biberach, Germany

I. PATHOPHYSIOLOGY OF THROMBUS FORMATION

The inner surface of the blood vessels in adults has been estimated to cover an area of at least 500 m^2. Reliable repair mechanisms are therefore required to prevent leakage of this highly branched blood container when it is subjected to injury. If this life-saving repair system reacts overaggressively, however, either excessive thrombus formation at the site of injury or an embolized thrombus at a distant site can completely occlude a blood vessel, causing ischemic damage of the supplied tissue. Such processes manifest clinically as life-threatening thromboembolic disease, e.g., stroke, or pulmonary or myocardial infarction.

In a healthy blood vessel, platelets are separated from the highly thrombogenic elements of the vessel wall by a monolayer of intact endothelial cells. Disruption of this layer through injury or endothelial cell dysfunction triggers the adhesion of single platelets at the site of injury. Platelets thus activated will stimulate additional resting platelets in the immediate vicinity, causing their aggregation. Thus, more and more platelets are recruited into a platelet thrombus. This platelet–vessel wall interaction, in response to the exposure of thrombogenic structures, provides a very effective mechanism to promptly stop leakage of the blood vessel.

In parallel, an intriguing sequence of finely tuned proteolytic activities of coagulation proteins is able to polymerize soluble fibrinogen circulating in the blood into an insoluble fibrin clot. This rapid-phase transition of the soluble plasma protein to the solid blood clot is localized primarily to the site of injury and represents another pivotal system for maintaining vascular integrity. The extent of fibrin clot formation at the vessel wall–blood interface reflects the balance between procoagulant activities and local fibrinolysis. Intimate cooperation between the coagulation system and both activated blood cells (especially platelets) and the cells of the vessel wall (endothelial and smooth muscle cells) ensures an adequate response to vascular injury.

Because of the complicated regulation of hemostasis and thrombosis, an almost unlimited diversity of pharmacological approaches to antithrombotic therapy exists. The objective of such antithrombotic therapy is to prevent excessive pathological thrombus formation without impairing the essential physiological mechanisms of hemostasis. Therefore, we prefer here to examine the various pharmacological strategies in terms of the blood–vessel wall interaction, despite the incomplete understanding of this interaction. We start by reviewing the mechanisms of action of the clinically established drugs for antithrombotic therapy. Thereafter, we will present some of the innovative pharmacological strategies attempting to improve the efficacy or reduce the side effects of antithrombotic therapy.

II. PLATELET INHIBITORS

A. Acetylsalicylic Acid

In comparison with its long-established use as an antiinflammatory, antipyretic, and analgesic agent, acetylsalicylic acid (aspirin) has only recently been accepted as an antithrombotic drug, even though its inhibition of human platelet aggregation was identified more than 20 years ago (1,2). This platelet-inhibitory function is mainly attributed to irreversible inhibition of cyclooxygenase activity by acetylation of the serine hydroxyl group (position 529) of the enzyme prostaglandin G/H synthase (3).

Cyclooxygenase activity, which generates biological mediators from arachidonic acid, is present in almost every cell type. Platelets respond to receptor-mediated activation with an increased liberation of arachidonic acid from phospholipids in the cell membrane (Fig. 1). The arachidonic acid molecules are then rapidly converted to prostaglandin endoperoxides by prostaglandin G/H synthase. The platelet-specific enzyme thromboxane synthase can further oxygenate these endoperoxides to form thromboxane A_2. Thromboxane A_2 can easily pass through the platelet membrane and bind to thromboxane A_2/prostaglandin

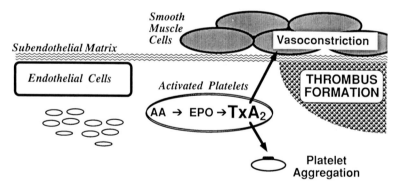

Figure 1 Platelets synthesize thromboxane A_2 in response to activation. Arachidonic acid (AA) released by platelets in response to activation at the site of vascular injury is rapidly converted by cyclooxygenase to prostaglandin endoperoxides (EPO) and then by thromboxane synthetase to thromboxane A_2 (TxA_2). Thromboxane A_2 is a potent prothrombotic agent that acts locally to stimulate platelets to aggregate and vascular smooth muscle cells to contract. Both activities enhance local thrombus formation.

endoperoxide receptors on the surface of platelets and vascular smooth muscle cells. The binding of thromboxane A_2 to these platelet receptors triggers the activation and aggregation of additional platelets, whereas the receptor on vascular smooth muscle cells mediates vasoconstriction (4). Both the potent proaggregatory activity and the vasoconstriction of thromboxane A_2 help to further recruit resting platelets for additional thromboxane generation and platelet aggregation. This positive feedback mechanism results in an explosive local burst of thromboxane A_2. The rapid inactivation of thromboxane A_2 in blood by hydrolysis to thromboxane B_2, however, may limit the propagation of this thromboxane A_2 burst to the microenvironment of the vascular injury.

Repeated treatment with aspirin in an oral dosage as low as 1 mg/kg/day is sufficient to eliminate thromboxane A_2 synthesis by activated platelets. Indeed, recent clinical trials of low-dose aspirin regimens have demonstrated an antithrombotic efficacy that appears to be comparable to that observed with higher aspirin doses of up to 1 g/day.

Cyclooxygenase activity is also required for the generation of antithrombotic prostaglandins by cells of the vessel wall (Fig. 2). Endothelial cells, for example, respond to stimulation by adenosine diphosphate (ADP), thrombin, or bradykinin with the synthesis of prostacyclin. Prostacyclin is a very potent endogenous inhibitor of platelet activation and aggregation and also a potent vasodilator. Its physiological importance as a negative feedback mechanism for thrombus formation is emphasized by its short plasma half-life as well as by its unique ability to suppress platelet activation and aggregation not only mediated by thromboxane A_2, but also if induced by ADP or even high concentrations of collagen or thrombin. Cyclooxygenase inhibition in response to conventional doses of aspirin not only suppresses the generation of thromboxane A_2 by activated platelets but also impairs the generation of prostacyclin by vascular cells (Fig. 3).

Since vascular cells, in contrast to platelets, can recover from aspirin-induced cyclooxygenase inhibition by de novo synthesis of the enzyme, it has been hypothesized that a very-low-dose aspirin regimen might spare vascular prostacyclin synthesis. In a recent study (5), healthy volunteers were treated with 75 mg of an aspirin formulation that releases only 10 mg of aspirin per hour. A 4-day treatment with this controlled-release preparation did not reduce the five- to sixfold increase in vascular prostacyclin synthesis in response to a systemic infusion of bradykinin, which directly stimulates endothelial cells. This finding seems to support the feasibility of an aspirin regimen able to confine its effects to the

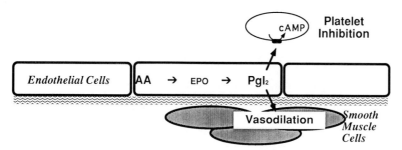

Figure 2 Endothelial cells release prostacyclin. Arachidonic acid (AA) is metabolized in endothelial cells via prostaglandin endoperoxides (EPO) to prostacyclin (PGI_2). Cyclooxygenase and prostacyclin synthetase activity are required for these two consecutive steps. Prostacyclin is a potent antithrombotic acting locally to inhibit platelets and to produce vasodilation.

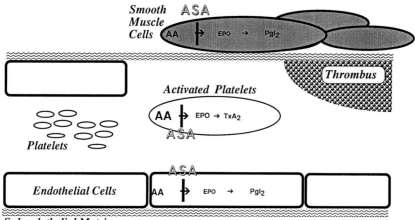

Figure 3 Aspirin inhibits cyclooxygenase in platelets and cells of the vessel wall. Aspirin (ASA) suppresses not only the generation of prothrombotic thromboxane A_2 (TxA_2) by activated platelets, but also the synthesis of antithrombotic prostacyclin (PGI_2).

presystemic circulation and thereby preserve vascular prostacyclin generation. However, both in vitro and ex vivo studies of the platelet–vessel wall interaction suggest that the endoperoxides released by activated platelets are the major source ($>80\%$) of vascular prostacyclin synthesis in response to local thrombus formation (Fig. 4). This local "cross-talk" between activated platelets and vascular cells, with its importance for prostacyclin

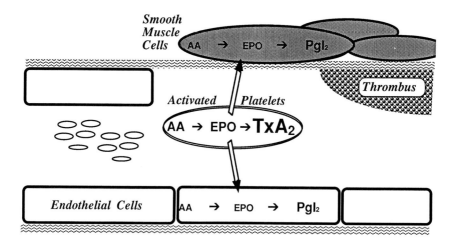

Figure 4 Endoperoxide shift: the local transfer of endoperoxides from activated platelets to adjacent cells of the vessel wall. Prostaglandin endoperoxides (EPO) released by activated platelets are converted by endothelial and vascular smooth muscle cells to antithrombotic prostacyclin (PGI_2). This local "cross-talk" between activated platelets and vascular cells represents an antithrombotic feedback mechanism to prevent further platelet activation and generation of prothrombotic thromboxane A_2 (TxA_2).

formation, will still be impaired by a platelet-inhibitory dose of aspirin. Thus, even very-low-dose aspirin regimens cannot avoid the undesired suppression of the major source of precursor for prostacyclin synthesis, which is dependent on functional platelets (Fig. 5). Whether such low-dose aspirin therapy achieves adequate antithrombotic protection in vivo remains unclear.

Additional antithrombotic mechanisms have been attributed to aspirin. On the basis of bleeding-time measurements it has been postulated that aspirin competitively inhibits the enzyme acetylcholinesterase (6). This inhibition should result in a local increase of the acetylcholine concentration, thereby inducing the release of endothelium-derived relaxing factor (EDRF), which induces relaxation of vascular smooth muscle cells and thus is a potent vasodilator.

Salicylate, the first-pass metabolite of aspirin, dose-dependently impairs the γ-carboxylation of coagulation factors II, VII, IX, and X (7–9). Post-translational modification by a vitamin K–dependent carboxylase is required for the functional activity of these coagulation factors. It appears, however, that only high-dose aspirin regimens are associated with this modest warfarin-like activity. The role of aspirin in fibrinolysis has also been investigated. From ex vivo measurements in whole blood it has been concluded that the fibrinolytic activity of the blood is increased for up to 4 h after aspirin ingestion (10). This observation could merely reflect the effect of aspirin on platelets present in the blood, an effect indirectly modulating the overall fibrinolytic response. Thus, a platelet-independent effect of aspirin on fibrinolytic activity remains to be demonstrated by more specific experiments as suggested by recent data (11). There are independent observations, however, indicating that in subjects at rest, aspirin reduces the increase in tissue plasminogen activator (tissue-type plasminogen activator) activity induced by venous occlusion by more than 50% (12).

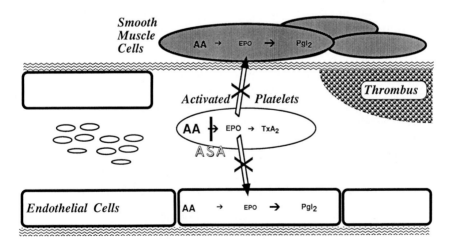

Figure 5 A platelet-selective dose of aspirin eliminates the endoperoxide shift. Ultra-low doses of aspirin (ASA) are expected to block thromboxane A$_2$ (TxA$_2$) synthesis by activated platelets without inhibiting the cyclooxygenase activity of vascular cells. However, by eliminating endoperoxide generation in activated platelets, they automatically suppress the shift of prostaglandin endoperoxides (EPO), which is the major source for prostacyclin (PGI$_2$) generation by the cells of the adjacent vessel wall.

Comparing the dose-response relationship for the different biochemical mechanisms of action for aspirin and a dose-dependence of the antithrombotic efficacy of aspirin in patients could help both to identify the clinically relevant mechanism(s) of action and to optimize the dosage. In 54 patients with peripheral vascular disease (Fontaine stage II), seven different oral aspirin doses ranging from 1 mg to 1000 mg/day have been evaluated in a placebo-controlled, double-blind study (13). The deposition of radioactively labeled platelets on the diseased femoral artery was measured before and at the end of a 3-month course of aspirin treatment. Despite the small number of patients in this study, a significant reduction of platelet deposition was observed for those patients treated with a daily dose of either 20 mg or 1000 mg, but not in patients receiving 1 mg or 50 to 500 mg aspirin daily.

Only in recent clinical trials has the antithrombotic efficacy of low-dose aspirin regimens for secondary prevention of cardiovascular events been directly compared with that of higher doses. The antithrombotic efficacy of aspirin is similar for a daily dose of 30 mg and for one of 283 mg (14). These results are consistent with the hypothesis that aspirin's primary antithrombotic mechanism of action is the inhibition of cyclooxygenase activity.

The substantial gastrointestinal side effects associated with high-dose aspirin regimens (15) are also reduced by the low-dose regimen (14,16). With the exception of these dose-related gastrointestinal side effects, a slightly increased risk of bleeding complications (17), and the problem of aspirin-induced bronchoconstriction in patients with asthma (18), aspirin is well tolerated. Conflicting findings have been reported in large prospective studies concerning the incidence of cancer among daily aspirin users (19,20).

B. Dipyridamole

The disappointing results of the initial clinical trials of aspirin for the prevention of thrombosis have stimulated the search for agents to be combined with aspirin for improved antithrombotic therapy. On the basis of the pharmacological profile observed for dipyridamole in vitro and in vivo in animal models of thrombosis (21), it appeared that dipyridamole could substantially improve the aspirin-induced inhibition of thromboxane A_2 generation.

The dipyridamole-induced inhibition of thrombus formation has been attributed to inhibition of cyclic adenosine monophosphate (cAMP)–specific phosphodiesterase activity in platelets (22). But such inhibition requires dipyridamole concentrations of at least 10 μM which are much higher than the therapeutic dipyridamole plasma levels of 1 to 6 μM used in humans. However, dipyridamole at these therapeutic levels inhibits the reuptake of adenosine into blood cells (23) and cells of the vascular wall (24).

A significant elevation of the plasma adenosine level has been demonstrated in patients treated with dipyridamole and accounts for the vasodilation induced by dipyridamole (25). The additional inhibitory effect of adenosine on platelet activation and aggregation is difficult to demonstrate ex vivo. In vivo, however, adenosine may substantially suppress thrombus formation by modulating the blood–vessel wall interaction.

Platelets activated at the site of vascular injury not only start to generate thromboxane A_2, but also secrete ADP and adenosine triphosphate (ATP) stored in their dense granules. Adenosine diphosphate activates adjacent unstimulated platelets by binding to a specific receptor on the platelet surface, analogous to thromboxane A_2–induced platelet aggregation. This proaggregatory feedback mechanism may result in a transient large increase in the ATP and ADP concentration in the microenvironment of the forming thrombus. Diffusion of ADP and ATP to adjacent endothelial cells exposes the adenosine nucleotides to the ectonucleotidase activity on the cell surface, causing rapid degradation to adenosine (Fig. 6). As mentioned above, adenosine is a very potent inhibitor of platelet activation and aggregation because of its stimulation of a receptor-linked adenylcyclase and a subsequent increase in intraplatelet cAMP (26,27). This is similar to the mechanism of action of prostacyclin.

The conversion of prothrombotic ADP released by activated platelets to antithrombotic adenosine exemplifies another local feedback mechanism for an efficient regulation of thrombus formation. The potent vasodilation and platelet inhibition produced by adenosine is terminated by the rapid uptake of adenosine into red blood cells, endothelial cells, and other vascular cells. Dipyridamole efficiently blocks this adenosine uptake. Thus, dipyridamole should enhance this local antithrombotic feedback mechanism in the proximity of a growing thrombus, as demonstrated in an in vitro model of blood–vessel wall interaction using human whole blood and human endothelial cells (28). In patients with artificial heart valves, the red blood cells are exposed to high mechanical shear forces and probably release adenine nucleotides. Dipyridamole alone significantly inhibits thrombosis in these patients (29).

Recently, several groups have independently demonstrated the potentiation of the antiplatelet and vasodilator activity of EDRF by dipyridamole (30,31). Endothelium-derived relaxing factor is released from endothelial cells in response to various prothrombotic stimuli and increases the guanylate cyclase activity of platelets. By inhibiting the cyclic guanosine monophosphate (cGMP)–specific phosphodiesterase that degrades cGMP, dipyridamole in combination with EDRF substantially increases intraplatelet cGMP (Fig. 7). This mechanism of dipyridamole is supported not only by direct measurements of cGMP, but also by dipyridamole's strong suppression of platelet aggregation even in response to ADP in concert with EDRF (31). However, an ex vivo demonstration of this EDRF-dependent effect is complicated by the extremely rapid inactivation of EDRF.

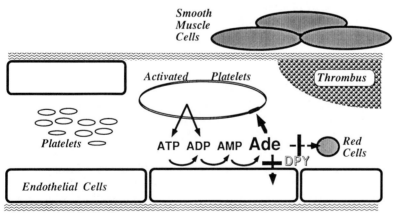

Figure 6 Dipyridamole increases the local adenosine concentration. Ectonucleotidases on the surface of endothelial cells rapidly degrade the adenosine triphosphate (ATP) and prothrombotic adenosine diphosphate (ADP) released from activated platelets to adenosine. Dipyridamole (DPY) amplifies this local increase of adenosine by blocking its uptake into endothelial cells and blood cells. Adenosine binds to platelets, increases the intraplatelet cyclic AMP level, and thus prevents further platelet activation and aggregation. Additionally, an enhanced adenosine concentration provides substantial local vasodilation.

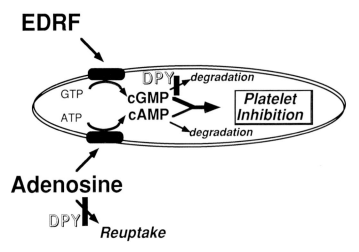

Figure 7 Dipyridamole enhances the platelet inhibition by endothelium-derived relaxing factor (EDRF). Therapeutic levels of dipyridamole (DPY) effectively inhibit the degradation of intraplatelet cGMP by blocking the cGMP-dependent phosphodiesterase. Endothelium-derived relaxing factor released from endothelial cells in response to prothrombotic stimuli triggers the formation of cGMP in platelets. In combination with the concomitant increase of the intraplatelet cAMP resulting from the increase of adenosine (see Fig. 6), platelets are effectively inhibited at the site of vascular injury.

An attractive approach to antithrombotic therapy is the reduction of the thrombogenicity of the damaged vessel wall exposed to the circulating blood after an injury. Selective removal of the endothelial cell layer of the carotid artery in rabbits by air injury increases the deposition of radioactively labeled platelets relative to the noninjured opposite artery. Long-term oral pretreatment of the rabbits with doses of dipyridamole, resulting in plasma levels similar to those used therapeutically in humans, significantly reduced platelet deposition in the injured artery in a plasma level–dependent manner (32). Measurements of the 13-hydroxyoctadecadienoic acid (13-HODE) content of the aorta demonstrated that dipyridamole treatment was associated with a significant increase in the content of this lipoxygenase product of linoleic acid. In contrast, treatment with salicylate for 7 days increased platelet adhesion to the injured carotid arteries twofold and reduced the 13-HODE content of the vessel wall by 67%. Such changes in the thromboresistance of an injured vessel wall must still be analyzed in patients with vascular disease.

The deposition of radioactively labeled platelets on active atherosclerotic lesions was measured by gamma-camera imaging in patients with symptomatic ischemic peripheral vascular disease before and 5 weeks after the start of treatment with either oral aspirin 20 mg/day, dipyridamole 75 mg t.i.d., or both (33). Only combined treatment with aspirin and dipyridamole significantly reduced platelet accumulation in the atherosclerotic arteries of these patients.

Although further evidence from recently completed clinical trials (34–36) suggests an additional benefit for the combination of aspirin and dipyridamole in comparison with aspirin alone in the secondary prevention of thromboembolic events, dipyridamole's role in antithrombotic therapy has been controversial (37). Long-term experience with dipyridamole confirms that side effects such as headache, nausea, and gastric discomfort observed at the beginning of treatment usually disappear with prolonged treatment. In contrast to aspirin, dipyridamole does not induce gastrointestinal ulcers or hemorrhagic tendencies.

C. Ticlopidine

Ticlopidine is an example of a drug with a remarkable delay between its discovery and its approval and clinical acceptance for prevention of thromboembolic disease. Ticlopidine has only recently been approved for sale in several European countries and in the United States despite its having been evaluated in humans as early as in 1975 (38). The exact mechanism of the antithrombotic action of ticlopidine remains unknown.

This uncertainty concerning ticlopidine's mechanism of action may be due in part to the complication that ticlopidine shows very limited activity in vitro. Therefore, ticlopidine's antithrombotic effect, which may be mediated by a metabolite, must be investigated either ex vivo (39) or in vivo. The main antithrombotic activity is thought to be the specific inhibition of ADP-mediated platelet activation and aggregation (40). This effect may result from the inhibition of a step yet to be precisely characterized in the signal transduction sequence initiated by the binding of ADP to specific receptors on the platelet membrane (41) (Fig. 8). Similar to the generation of thromboxane A_2, the release of ADP from activated platelets is an important amplification mechanism for platelet aggregation. Therefore, it is not surprising that the ticlopidine-induced inhibition of ADP-mediated platelet activation translates into an inhibition of ex vivo platelet aggregation induced not only by ADP but also by low concentrations of collagen, thrombin, and other stimuli (42). This proposed mechanism of action is consistent with the ex vivo demonstration that ticlopidine can prevent the transformation of the glycoprotein IIb-IIIa complex on the platelet surface to a fibrinogen receptor (42). These findings do not, however, support the conclusion that ticlopidine directly interacts with the glycoprotein IIIb-IIIa complex (43), as a direct modification of the human glycoprotein IIb-IIIa complex in response to ticlopidine treatment is very unlikely (44).

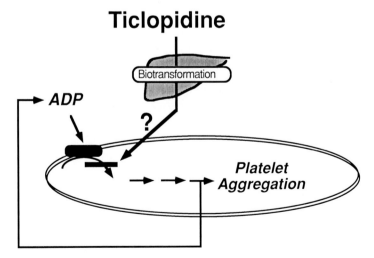

Figure 8   Ticlopidine blocks the adenosine diphosphate (ADP) pathway of platelet activation. The transmembrane signaling for ADP-mediated platelet activation and aggregation is impaired by an unidentified metabolite of ticlopidine.

The active metabolite responsible for this effect of ticlopidine on platelets has not yet been determined, despite the identification of 13 different metabolites. It is suspected that a highly reactive metabolite generated in the liver binds irreversibly to platelets or mega-karyocytes, as indicated by a delayed onset and offset of platelet inhibition. Up to 5 days of ticlopidine treatment with an oral dose of 500 mg/day were required in volunteers to inhibit ADP-induced platelet aggregation ex vivo by more than 90% (42). The duration of action corresponds to the platelet life span.

Large clinical trials have evaluated the effect of ticlopidine on cardiovascular morbidity and mortality (45,46). They reveal that approximately 1% of ticlopidine-treated patients develop a severe neutropenia, which is reversible after withdrawing ticlopidine. Up to 20% of patients develop diarrhea, as well as other symptoms of gastrointestinal intolerance, and skin rashes. Moreover, ticlopidine apparently increased the serum cholesterol level by approximately 10% (45), with potential implications for the long-term progression of vascular disease.

D. Prostaglandins

Prostacyclin and prostaglandin E_1 are very potent inhibitors of platelet aggregation and effective vasodilators. Both bind to specific receptors on the platelet surface, thereby activating membrane-bound platelet adenylcyclase (Fig. 9). The resulting increase in the intraplatelet cAMP concentration suppresses the Ca^{2+}-dependent mechanisms of platelet activation, i.e., not only aggregation but also the activation-induced release reaction and perhaps even platelet adhesion. Based on this mechanism, treatment with prostaglandins would be expected to inhibit platelets in a way distinctly superior to that achieved with selective inhibition either of thromboxane (via aspirin) or of ADP-mediated platelet activa-tion (via ticlopidine) (47). These high expectations based on in vitro studies are further supported by promising in vivo findings in animals (48) and even clinical data (49). However, an adequate exploitation of these natural antithrombotic compounds for the treatment of patients appears to be limited by several severe problems.

The rapid hydrolysis of prostacyclin in blood (half-life <3 min) apparently limits its antithrombotic activity to the site and the duration of local synthesis by the cells of the ves-sel wall. Therefore, a continuous infusion and high doses of the chemically labile prosta-cyclin are required to inhibit platelet activation and aggregation in patients. More stable analogues of prostacyclin such as iloprost, cicaprost, and taprosten have been designed to overcome this limitation. In addition to the very short half-life, desensitization of the platelet

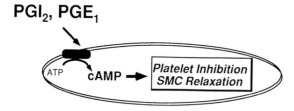

Figure 9   Prostaglandins prevent platelet activation. Binding of prostacyclin (PGI_2) or prostaglandin E_1 (PGE_1) to specific receptors on the surface of platelets and vascular smooth muscle cells (SMCs) increases the intracellular cAMP level. Thus, platelet activation and aggregation are inhibited and relaxation of vascular smooth muscle cells is induced.

prostacyclin receptors appears to limit the effect of continued exposure of platelets to prostacyclin and its analogues (50,51). Moreover, it has been demonstrated that the density of prostacyclin receptors is already reduced in patients with acute coronary artery disease (52,53).

Additionally, relatively small doses (5 ng/kg/min) suffice to dilate the peripheral vasculature, resulting in flushes, decreased diastolic blood pressure, and increased heart rate (54). These cardiovascular side effects significantly limit the doses tolerated by patients. It seems that the benefit of treatment with prostacyclin, prostaglandin E_1, and their analogues is at present best established in patients with ischemic peripheral vascular disease, in whom profound vasodilation and suppression of ischemic pain might be advantageous.

III. FUTURE APPROACHES TO ANTITHROMBOTIC THERAPY

A. Platelet Inhibitors

1. Phosphodiesterase Inhibitors

Prostaglandins are very potent endogenous inhibitors of platelet activation and aggregation and perhaps even of platelet adhesion and thus actively participate in the local regulation of thrombus formation. Their mechanism of action is to increase intraplatelet cAMP or cGMP levels (see Fig. 7 and 9). The major problem complicating clinical use of these agents appears to be rapid down-regulation of prostaglandin receptors on the platelet surface in response to prolonged exposure to agonists, as would be required for the long-term prevention of thromboembolic events. This problem may be circumvented by indirectly elevating intraplatelet cAMP or cGMP levels with phosphodiesterase inhibitors, which suppress the degradation of intraplatelet cAMP or cGMP. However, the problem of achieving platelet selectivity with phosphodiesterase inhibitors remains to be solved. Such selectivity is desirable in order to avoid the profound cardiovascular effects observed with platelet-inhibitory prostaglandins as well as phosphodiesterase inhibitors. So far, no phosphodiesterase inhibitor has been identified that can effectively inhibit platelet aggregation ex vivo without also causing significant cardiovascular side effects, including headache. Despite these disappointing results, it is possible that lower, better-tolerated doses of such phosphodiesterase inhibitors are sufficient to suppress thrombus formation in vivo. This effect may be due to a local amplification of labile endogenous antithrombotic substances (e.g., prostacyclin) that are only transiently released by cells of the vessel wall and thus not detectable in the ex vivo studies. Moreover, a more detailed molecular analysis of the various phosphodiesterases in both platelets and vascular tissues may reveal differences that could be exploited to achieve adequate platelet selectivity.

2. Von Willebrand Factor Antagonists and Inhibitors of Platelet Adhesion

Receptors expressed only on the surface of platelets and megakaryocytes and mediating platelet functions essential for thrombus formation are also attractive targets for antiplatelet therapy. Glycoproteins have been identified on the platelet surface that are functionally involved in the first step required for thrombus formation, i.e., platelet adhesion. Most prominent among these adhesion receptors is glycoprotein Ib, which binds subendothelial von Willebrand factor and, particularly at high shear rates, anchors platelets to the subendothelial matrix (Fig. 10). Indeed, platelets from patients with von Willebrand's disease (i.e., lacking functionally active von Willebrand factor) and patients with the Bernard-Soulier

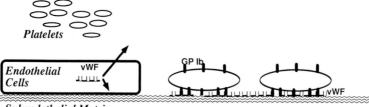

Figure 10 Platelet adhesion mediated by von Willebrand factor. At high shear rates von Willebrand factor (vWF) secreted by endothelial cells into the subendothelial matrix and into the circulating blood binds to glycoprotein Ib (GP Ib) on the platelet surface. This specific platelet–vessel wall interaction anchors individual platelets to the subendothelial matrix exposed at the site of vascular injury.

syndrome (i.e., with a deficiency of glycoprotein Ib) show a significantly decreased adhesion to subendothelium and a reduced thrombus formation in in vitro studies (89,90).

Monoclonal antibodies directed against von Willebrand factor or glycoprotein Ib (91–94) appear to suppress platelet adhesion and thus inhibit thrombus formation in animal models. Based on the identification of the glycoprotein Ib–binding domain of native human von Willebrand factor (95), a fragment of this protein representing the amino acid sequence from positions 445 to 733 has been produced as a recombinant protein. This recombinant fragment in concentrations of 1 to 3 μM prevents human platelet adhesion to von Willebrand factor attached to collagen matrix in vitro. In an in vivo model of recurrent thrombotic occlusions of the injured and stenosed carotid artery in pigs, this fragment inhibited arterial thrombus formation in a dose-related manner. (A clinical phase I study to evaluate this fragment in healthy volunteers has recently been completed.) Polymer aurin tricarboxylic acid binds to von Willebrand factor and thus inhibits the binding of von Willebrand factor to glycoprotein Ib. Significant antithrombotic activity of this agent has also been demonstrated in vivo in a dog model of recurrent coronary thrombosis.

These independent observations support the notion that von Willebrand factor participates importantly in the platelet–vessel wall interaction during arterial thrombus formation. Electron microscopic analysis of injured vascular segments demonstrated the presence of adherent platelets in pigs treated with a monoclonal antibody against von Willebrand factor in a dose that prevented occlusive arterial thrombus formation (96). This and additional findings (97,98) suggest that von Willebrand factor not only mediates platelet adhesion but may also be involved in platelet aggregation, at least at high shear rates.

Mechanisms of platelet adhesion independent of von Willebrand factor also have been identified, but their pathophysiological role remains to be established. Potential additional targets for inhibitors of platelet adhesion are glycoprotein IV (present in approximately 25,000 binding sites per platelet) as well as various members of the integrin family of adhesion receptors, such as receptors for collagen (glycoprotein complex Ia-IIa) (99), laminin (Ic-IIa), fibronectin (Ic-IIa), and vitronectin (α v-IIIa) (100). All are detectable on the platelet surface in a density of only 1000 or fewer receptors per platelet. However, severe bleeding problems, such as are known to occur in patients with deficient platelet adhesion, may be expected with potent, selective inhibition of platelet adhesion (93).

3. Fibrinogen Receptor Antagonists

The glycoprotein complex IIb-IIIa is the most prevalent member of the integrin family of adhesion receptors to be found on the platelet surface. The activation of platelets by all known physiological stimulators of platelet aggregation ultimately induces the calcium-dependent conversion of the glycoprotein complex IIb-IIIa into a receptor for fibrinogen, von Willebrand factor, or vitronectin. The multivalent adhesion molecules fibrinogen and von Willebrand factor are able to cross-link adjacent platelets by binding to these receptors on adjacent platelets (detectable in a density of up to 50,000 binding sites per activated platelet). The binding of fibrinogen to activated platelets has been shown to be initially reversible but subsequently irreversible. Platelets from patients with a substantial reduction of the number of, or with functional defects of, the glycoprotein complexes IIb-IIIa (Glanzmann's thrombasthenia) adhere to thrombogenic matrices and release the content of their granules, but they do not aggregate (101). The conversion of the glycoprotein complex IIb-IIIa to a binding site for fibrinogen and von Willebrand factor appears to be the final common pathway for all physiological mediators of platelet aggregation (Fig. 11). Whereas aspirin and ticlopidine suppress only thromboxane A_2- and ADP-mediated platelet aggregation, respectively, antagonists of fibrinogen or von Willebrand factor binding to the glycoprotein IIb-IIIa complex are expected to suppress platelet aggregation independently of the proaggregatory stimulus and intraplatelet signal transduction pathway(s) involved (Fig. 12).

This hypothesis has been evaluated using murine monoclonal antibodies that are directed against the glycoprotein IIb-IIIa complex and block fibrinogen binding to activated platelets (102). Fab_2 fragments of these antibodies potently inhibit both collagen- and ADP-induced platelet aggregation in human platelet-rich plasma and also suppress thrombus formation on a thrombogenic subendothelial matrix in vitro (103,104). Moreover, the fibrinogen receptor antagonism of these antibodies translates into a potent suppression of arterial platelet thrombus formation in various experimental models in vivo. Such antibodies

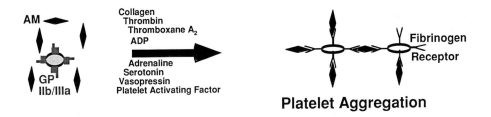

Platelet Aggregation

Fibrinogen Receptor Antagonist: ▲

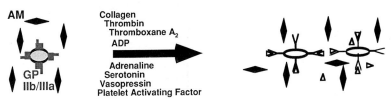

Figure 11 Fibrinogen binding to activated platelets is the final common pathway of platelet aggregation. Activation of platelets by proaggregatory stimuli triggers the conversion of the glycoprotein IIb-IIIa complex (GP IIb/IIIa) to a receptor for fibrinogen or von Willebrand factor. Binding of these multivalent adhesion molecules (AM) cross-links adjacent platelets into platelet aggregates. Fibrinogen receptor antagonists block the binding sites on GP IIb/IIIa and thus prevent platelet aggregation independently of the proaggregatory stimuli.

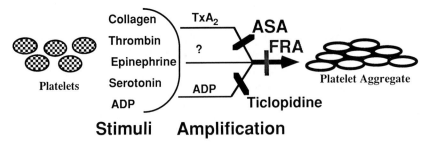

Stimuli   Amplification

Figure 12   Aspirin (ASA) and ticlopidine block only one of the multiple pathways of platelet aggregation. Binding of external stimuli (collagen, thrombin, etc.) triggers the different intraplatelet pathways of activation. Various factors including the specific vascular site and the time point of injury may determine the relevant pathway of platelet activation. Aspirin and ticlopidine inhibit only thromboxane A_2 (TxA_2)- and adenosine diphosphate (ADP)-mediated platelet aggregation, respectively, and thus may be insufficient for an effective prevention of platelet-dependent thrombosis. FRA = fibrinogen receptor antagonist.

prevented thrombotic occlusions in injured and severely stenosed coronary arteries of dogs (105,106). They also inhibited thrombus formation in damaged and moderately stenosed arteries of primates without profoundly affecting the bleeding time (107). The antibodies reduced platelet deposition in an arteriovenous shunt model in baboons in a dose-dependent manner (108). They also substantially enhanced the in vivo activity of thrombolytic agents, as indicated by a decreased time to reperfusion of occluded arteries, effective prevention of reocclusion, and reduction of the doses of thrombolytic agents required for successful lysis (109–111).

One of these antibodies (7E3) has already been investigated in humans (112). Injection of this antibody as an intravenous bolus (0.05–0.2 mg/kg) in 16 patients with unstable angina inhibited platelet aggregation ex vivo in a dose-dependent manner and did not cause major bleeding problems despite a profound prolongation of the bleeding time (113). In addition to these and other promising results (114), further clinical experience is required with regard to immunological effects of the antibody treatment (especially antibody-induced thrombocytopenia) and the relatively long duration of platelet inhibition due to an almost irreversible high-affinity binding of the antibodies to human platelets (115). Large clinical trials have been started evaluating the Fab fragment of a chimeric antibody that integrates the variable regions of the murine antibody (7E3) and the constant regions of a human antibody.

The unique antithrombotic potency to be expected from specific, direct antagonists of the platelet fibrinogen receptor has stimulated the search for functionally similar agents other than antibodies. Snake venoms, especially from vipers, contain proteins (5000 to 20,000 molecular weight) such as echistatin (116), kistrin (117), trigramin (118,119), bitistatin (120,121), and applagin (122,123), all of which belong to the disintegrins. Disintegrins bind with high affinity to activated platelets and inhibit human platelet aggregation in vitro (116–118,120,122,123). Furthermore, they potently suppress thrombus formation in vivo (117,119–121). However, the selectivity of these disintegrins for the various integrins has not been established.

Disintegrins and adhesive proteins, such as fibrinogen, von Willebrand factor, fibronectin, and vitronectin, which bind to the glycoprotein IIb-IIIa complex on activated platelets, contain the tripeptide arginine-glycine-aspartic acid (RGD) sequence (124). The conservation of this sequence suggests a functional role for RGD in the interaction between the RGD-containing adhesion molecule or disintegrin as ligand and the receptors. Indeed, RGD-containing small peptides ($\leq$7 amino acids) antagonize fibrinogen binding to activated platelets (125) and inhibit platelet aggregation (126,127), although they are approximately 500 to 1000 times less potent than disintegrins. However, these peptides are far less specific than antibodies for platelet glycoprotein IIb-IIIa and interfere with the binding of adhesive proteins to their receptors. A whole family of adhesion receptors composed of noncovalently associated $\alpha\beta$ heterodimers of transmembrane glycoproteins has been identified and termed integrins (128,129). Integrins and their multiple ligands mediate cell–cell and cell–matrix interactions. They are not only involved in hemostasis but may participate in the regulation of cell growth, development, and differentiation. The ubiquity of RGD-dependent inter-actions explains the broad biological profile of RGD-containing peptides, which have been shown to block the adhesion of human endothelial cells to a vitronectin matrix (130), to interfere with bone resorption by osteoclasts (131,132), and to suppress both tumor cell metastasis in animal models and tumor cell invasion in vitro (133,134).

Based on this lack of specificity of small linear RGD peptides for the platelet fibrinogen receptor and on the discovery of a lysine-glycine-aspartic acid (KGD)-containing disinteg-rin, barbourin (135), modified cyclic peptides have been designed to selectively antagonize the binding of fibrinogen to the glycoprotein IIb-IIIa complex. Such a peptide has already been tested in healthy volunteers, in whom a half-life of only a few minutes has been established. Treatment with this peptide appears to almost completely prevent platelet aggregation ex vivo in doses that do not prolong the bleeding time. It is expected that synthetic nonpeptide fibrinogen-receptor antagonists with high platelet specificity, excellent potency, and perhaps even oral activity may enter clinical development to substantially improve the efficacy of the established antiplatelet drugs.

B. Modulation of Platelet–Vessel Wall Interaction

The fine-tuning of local thrombus growth specifically at the interface between the blood and the damaged vessel wall apparently involves efficient communication between activated platelets and the cells of the adjacent vessel wall. Modulation of such "cross-talk" limited to the site of thrombus formation offers an attractive approach for pharmacological inter-ference confined both locally to this site and temporally to the duration of platelet activation.

Arachidonic acid metabolites such as thromboxane A_2 and prostacyclin have been identified as important mediators in the regulation of thrombosis. The availability of sensitive techniques for the analysis of their inactive metabolites thromboxane B_2 and 6-keto-PGF$_{1\alpha}$ in samples of circulating blood taken from patients with thromboembolic disease has greatly contributed to the misconception of the role of thromboxane and prostacyclin as circulating hormones determining the balance between hemostasis and thrombosis (136). Endothelial cells convert the endoperoxides prostaglandin G_2 (PGG$_2$) and PGH$_2$ to prostacyclin (137). Stimulation of platelets (prelabeled with ^{3}H-arachidonic acid) in the presence of endothelial cells (prelabeled ^{14}C-arachidonic acid) results in substantial formation of prostacyclin (138) completely derived from the ^{3}H-arachidonic acid of the platelets. This observation demonstrates the close cooperation between activated platelets generating endoperoxides and the endothelial cells synthesizing prostacyclin from these endoperoxides. More recently, prostacyclin synthesis utilizing the endoperoxides released from activated platelets has also been demonstrated for cultured human smooth muscle cells (139). This transcellular cooperation establishes a very efficient feedback mechanism whereby vascular cells automatically adjust the formation of prostacyclin and other anti-thrombotic prostaglandins to the extent of platelet stimulation in the near vicinity and no longer depend on the limited availability of endogenous arachidonic acid as source for the prostacyclin synthesis (Fig. 4). This hypothesis of local platelet–vessel wall feedback cooperation is corroborated by findings in an experimental model of thrombosis in dogs (140). In healthy volunteers the local formation of biologically effective concentrations of prostacyclin has been demonstrated at the site of a bleeding wound (141). An almost complete inhibition of local prostacyclin generation parallel to the inhibition of thromboxane A_2 synthesis in healthy volunteers at 12 h after the last oral dose of only 35 mg/day aspirin for 7 days is also consistent with the hypothesis of platelet-derived prostacyclin (142). Increased levels of prostacyclin have been reported for patients with severe atherosclerosis (143) or β-thalassemia (144), supporting the pathophysiological relevance of this antithrombotic feedback mechanism.

By virtue of cyclooxygenase inhibition, aspirin suppresses the generation of endoperoxides by activated platelets and thus abolishes the substrate for prostacyclin generation, thereby blocking this local antithrombotic feedback mechanism. In contrast, specific inhibition of thromboxane synthetase activity is expected to amplify this antithrombotic mechanism, as has been demonstrated in experimental models in vivo (140). Potent thromboxane synthetase inhibitors have been evaluated in small clinical trials in patients with coronary or peripheral vascular disease but failed to show substantial antithrombotic efficacy (145). However, an interpretation of these disappointing results is difficult, as none of the tested regimens fulfilled the basic requirement for a therapeutically relevant inhibition of thromboxane formation, i.e., to continuously inhibit thromboxane synthetase by at least 95% (146). Only recently, ridogrel (147,148), a potent thromboxane synthetase inhibitor, has been found to eliminate thromboxane A_2 formation adequately in volunteers (148) as well as in patients (149,150). Doses of at least 2.5 mg/kg of intravenous ridogrel were required to prevent formation of an occlusive platelet thrombus both in an everted segment of the coronary artery in dogs more potently than aspirin (151) and in a canine model of deep intimal injury of the coronary artery (152). At such high doses ridogrel not only inhibits thromboxane synthetase activity but also has thromboxane A_2 receptor–antagonistic activity, which is apparently required to block the prothrombotic activity of endoperoxides accumulating in response to the thromboxane synthetase inhibition. These experimental findings support the suggestion (153) that in an ideal agent both activities should be balanced (Fig. 13).

Ridogrel has been also evaluated in healthy volunteers (148), and first results from patients indicate its safety and pharmacological activity (149,150).

C. Anticoagulants

Antithrombotic efficacy has been unequivocally established for heparin treatment in the prevention of venous thrombosis and pulmonary embolism, thus supporting a pivotal role of thrombin for venous thromboembolism. However, the clinical data needed to substantiate this key role for thrombin in arterial thrombosis as well remain elusive.

Animal models of both arterial thrombosis and reocclusion after arterial thrombolysis demonstrate only a limited antithrombotic activity for unfractionated heparins. An improved understanding of the molecular mechanisms involved in the local regulation of heparin's activities (release of heparin-neutralizing factors by activated platelets; protection of matrix- and clot-bound thrombin from inactivation by heparin–antithrombin III; etc.) might help to

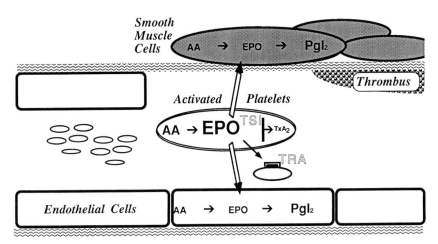

Figure 13 Combined inhibition of thromboxane synthetase and blockade of the prostaglandin endoperoxide/thromboxane A_2 receptor. Selective inhibition of the thromboxane synthetase (TSI) with continued cyclooxygenase activity induces the accumulation of prostaglandin endoperoxides (EPO) in activated platelets. In the presence of a prostaglandin endoperoxide/thromboxane A_2 receptor antagonist (TRA) the endoperoxides lose their prothrombotic potential. Importantly, they are converted by endothelial and vascular smooth muscle cells to prostacyclin (PGI_2) and other antithrombotic prostaglandins in the microenvironment of the injured vessel wall. Thus, the combination of TRA with TSI enhances prostaglandin generation locally to inhibit thrombus formation while avoiding the dose-limiting side-effects of systemically infused prostaglandins.

explain this limitation. However, only the clinical evaluation of novel thrombin inhibitors will unambiguously clarify the role of thrombin in arterial thrombosis (Fig. 14).

1. Hirudin and Synthetic Analogues

Leeches have long been used in medical practice and still provide an effective approach for the local treatment of hematoma after microsurgery. At the end of the last century, the anticoagulant properties of leech extracts were first described (154). Hirudin, a 65-amino-acid peptide stabilized by three intramolecular disulfide bridges (155), has since been identified by Markwardt (156) as an active principle in leech saliva, and several isoforms of this peptide were subsequently characterized (157). Recently, hirudin became available as a recombinant protein produced by bacteria or yeast but lacking the sulfation of the tyrosine in position 63 found in natural hirudin (158,159).

Hirudin is a direct tight-binding inhibitor highly specific for thrombin having a dissociation constant of approximately 10^{-11} M as determined for the stoichiometric complex of hirudin with human α-thrombin (160,161). Thus, hirudin is capable of displacing thrombin from its binding site on platelets (162). Hirudin's biological activity critically depends on the three intramolecular disulfide bridges and the resultant tertiary structure composed of three domains: the central core (composed of residues 3–30, 37–46, and 56–57), the finger (residues 31–36), and the flexible C-terminal tail (residues 50–65). X-ray analysis of thrombin-hirudin complexes (163,164) reveals that this tight binding is achieved by interaction not only at the active site of thrombin, but also at the anion binding "exosite" of thrombin, which extends as a long groove from the active site, binds the C-terminal tail of hirudin, and is involved in the substrate recognition (Fig. 15).

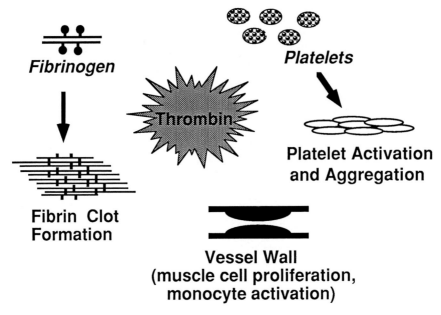

Figure 14 Thrombin: a pivotal mediator of arterial thrombosis? Thrombin's enzymatic activity is required for the final step of coagulation, i.e. the conversion of fibrinogen to the fibrin clot. Thrombin is also a highly potent activator of platelets and may also be involved in vascular repair mechanisms.

Potent antithrombotic properties of natural as well as of recombinant hirudin have been observed in in vivo models of both arterial and venous thrombosis in rats or rabbits (165). Inhibition of arterial thrombus formation required doses of hirudin at least ten times higher in comparison with models of venous thrombosis, but even these doses apparently did not affect the bleeding time. Hirudin treatment reduced the deposition of both platelet and fibrin in response to ballooning-induced deep injury (simulating angioplasty) of the carotid

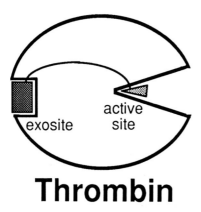

Figure 15 Hirudin and Hirulog. Hirudin and its synthetic analogue hirulog block not only the active site of thrombin but also the "exosite" essential for substrate recognition. These multiple sites of interaction with thrombin explain the excellent specificity of these potent thrombin inhibitors.

artery more efficiently than unfractionated heparin (166,167) and aspirin (168). In addition, hirudin was highly efficient in an in vivo model of coronary occlusion as an adjunct to thrombolytic therapy (169).

Pharmacokinetic studies in human volunteers indicate very similar parameters for native and recombinant hirudin. Plasma half-lifes of $t_{1/2\alpha} = 0.2$ h and $t_{1/2\alpha} = 1.8$ h have been estimated for recombinant hirudin injected intravenously (165). Hirudin is also bioavailable after subcutaneous administration, and it appears to have only weak immunogenic properties in man. However, the frequency of antibody formation will be adequately assessed only after long-term treatment in a large number of patients.

The elucidation of the above-mentioned molecular details of the hirudin-thrombin interaction has stimulated the design of synthetic peptides. In hirulog a catalytic site–inhibiting phenylalanine-proline-arginyl portion is connected via a flexible spacer of four glycine residues with the anion-binding "exosite" recognition moiety of hirudin. This synthetic hirudin analogue potently prolongs the activated partial thromboplastin time with an identical dose-response relationship in human plasma in vitro in the absence and the presence of platelet releasate, whereas platelet releasates neutralize heparin. Hirulog inhibits clot-bound (as opposed to soluble) thrombin not only much more potently than heparin but even slightly more effectively than the almost three times larger hirudin. Hirulog prevents arterial thrombosis in pigs as well as reocclusion after successful arterial thrombolysis more potently than does heparin. It reduces the deposition of platelets and fibrin more effectively than heparin in an arteriovenous shunt in baboons. Hirulog is safe and pharmacologically active in humans, as demonstrated in a phase I study in volunteers. Promising first results have been reported for the use of hirulog in patients.

The hirugens represent another family of hirudin-derived peptides binding to the anion-binding "exosite" of thrombin but without blocking the active site (170,171). A tyrosine-sulfated synthetic peptide of residues 53–64 of hirudin competitively inhibits the proteolytic cleavage of fibrinogen but does not interfere with the cleavage of synthetic chromogenic substrates by thrombin. It suppresses the formation of fibrin-rich thrombi in low-shear regions of venous-type flow conditions but not platelet thrombus deposition in an arteriovenous shunt in baboons in vivo (172). The lack in these experiments of any effect on bleeding time with hirugen in doses as high as 75 mg/kg/40 min by intravenous infusion suggests an extraordinary hemostatic safety margin for such inhibitors that selectively occupy the anionic binding "exosite" of thrombin. Moreover, these different antithrombotic activities of hirudin and hirugen support the hypothesis of a pivotal role for thrombin not only in fibrin formation, but also in platelet activation in arterial thrombosis.

2. Synthetic Thrombin Inhibitors

An independent line of evidence for the key role of thrombin in arterial thrombus formation has been generated in experiments using synthetic thrombin inhibitors, such as D-phenylalanine-L-proline-L-arginyl chloromethyl ketone (PPACK). This agent directly and irreversibly inhibits thrombin with high potency and specificity (173). In contrast to heparin, PPACK dose-dependently suppressed platelet deposition at high shear rates in an arteriovenous shunt model in baboons (174). This superiority of PPACK to heparin has been confirmed in another heparin-resistant model (175). Because of its systemic toxicity and its very short half-life (176), the use of PPACK may be feasible only for local treatment. Boroarginine peptides related to PPACK have recently been characterized as a new class of potent, slow-binding inhibitors of thrombin with good selectivity evidenced by poor inhibition of plasma kallikrein, plasmin, and tissue-type plasminogen activator (177,178).

These observations on PPACK's antithrombotic activity have helped to revive interest in other synthetic, but reversible and less toxic, thrombin inhibitors such as argatroban. Argatroban, an arginine derivative, competitively inhibits thrombin with a K_i of approximately 20 nM (PPACK: $K_i \approx 32$ nM) and with excellent selectivity (179). It effectively suppressed arterial thrombus formation in doses that prolonged the activated partial thromboplastin time approximately twofold in rabbits (180,181) as well as in dogs (182). In contrast to heparin, argatroban is beneficial both in reducing the time to reperfusion and in preventing the reocclusion of dog coronary arteries in models of tissue-type plasminogen activator–induced thrombolysis (183,184). Argatroban is only parenterally active and has been approved for clinical use in Japan. In healthy human volunteers argatroban dose-dependently prolonged coagulation parameters and did not further increase bleeding time when given alone or in combination with aspirin (185).

3. Thrombin Receptor Antagonists

The ability to inhibit thrombin-induced activation of vascular cells (especially platelets and vascular smooth muscle cells) without affecting the coagulatory functions of thrombin potentially offers an effective and safe strategy for the prevention of both acute arterial thrombosis and long-term restenosis following angioplasty. Specific thrombin receptor antagonists that do not inhibit thrombin's enzymatic activity are needed to test this attractive hypothesis. Peptide analogues have been described that suppress thrombin-induced platelet activation but without inhibition of thrombin's enzymatic activity (186). However, these compounds still have a weak agonistic activity and can affect endothelial cell function nonselectively (187).

Recently, a new thrombin receptor has been cloned, and the mechanism of its activation has been elucidated (188,189). Thrombin binds via its anion binding "exosite" to this receptor, cleaves it, and thus exposes a new N-terminus to autoactivate the receptor (Fig. 16). Peptides with the sequence of this neoterminus bind to the thrombin receptor and are sufficient to activate cells, including platelets, and lack procoagulant activity. This intriguing observation should finally help to identify specific antagonists of thrombin receptor–mediated cell activation (190,191) and to evaluate their biological profile.

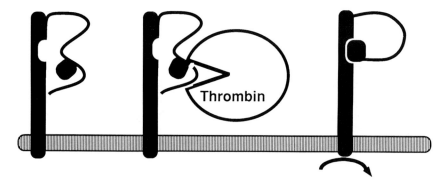

Figure 16 Activation of the thrombin receptor. Thrombin-induced proteolytic cleavage of the thrombin receptor on the cell surface exposes a "neoterminus." This portion of the receptor serves as ligand to autoactivate the thrombin receptor.

4. *Inhibitors of Thrombin Formation*

Thrombin is not only required for the final step of coagulation and activation of factor XIII to irreversibly cross-link fibrin. It is also of key importance for the activation and aggregation of platelets. Moreover, thrombin potentiates the rate of its own formation both by activating coagulation factors V and VIII and by stimulating platelets to release more factor V and to assemble the ternary coagulation complexes on the cellular surface (Fig. 17). These latter mechanisms allow for an explosive local generation of thrombin molecules. Instead of stoichiometrically neutralizing the activity of these thrombin molecules, it might be more attractive to modulate these highly efficient mechanisms for thrombin generation in order to reduce the rate of thrombin generation. Such an approach should result in superior thrombin inhibition. At least on a theoretical basis, this approach should avoid excessive thrombin inhibition, with its potential bleeding problems, and still maintain responsiveness to potent prothrombotic stimuli.

This type of servomechanism appears to be active in the regulation of hemostasis (192). Thrombin generated in response to a vascular injury is bound to thrombomodulin, a glycoprotein on the surface of endothelial cells (Fig. 18). This interaction probably induces a conformational change in thrombin, thereby changing its substrate specificity. Thus, thrombomodulin-bound thrombin preferentially activates plasma protein C. Activated protein C in concert with protein S binds to factor Va and VIIIa to rapidly inactivate them by proteolytic cleavage. Both protein C and protein S are vitamin K–dependent proteins and thus may assemble with either factor Va or factor VIIIa on the surface of activated cells in a mechanism similar to those ternary complexes (prothrombinase and tenase complex) required for an efficient formation of thrombin. The fate of patients with a homozygous

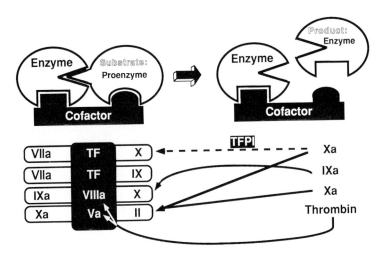

Figure 17 Assembly of coagulation complexes. This scheme summarizes the ternary complexes assembled on the surface of stimulated cells to activate coagulation factors X and IX as well as prothrombin with extraordinary high efficiency. The cooperation between coagulation factor VIIa and tissue factor (TF) is thought to initiate the activation of factor X required for thrombin formation. Tissue factor pathway inhibitor (TFPI) in concert with factor Xa regulates this step. The generation of factor IXa may contribute to an adequate rate of factor Xa formation to overcome the inhibitory activity of TFPI. Thrombin activates coagulation factors V and VIII and thus helps to further accelerate its own formation.

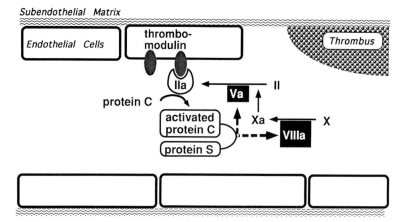

Figure 18 Feedback mechanism for the inactivation of factors Va and VIIIa. Thrombin bound to thrombomodulin specifically activates protein C. Activated protein C in concert with protein S efficiently cleaves and thus inactivates coagulation factors VIIIa and Va, which are required for the assembly of the ternary complexes to accelerate thrombin generation (see Fig. 17). This potent feedback mechanism may be essential to confine thrombin generation to only severely injured, deendothelialized parts of the blood vessel.

protein C deficiency, who die within a few years after birth, indicates the importance of this antithrombotic feedback.

The effects of native and recombinant human activated protein C have recently been evaluated in baboons. Platelet deposition on prosthetic vascular grafts in an arteriovenous shunt was dose-dependently reduced by up to 70% in these animals (193–195), and even the highest dose of activated protein C did not affect the template bleeding time. These promising results have been confirmed in the same experimental model of thrombosis when low doses of thrombin were infused to activate endogenous protein C. The production of amounts of functional recombinant activated protein C sufficient for therapeutic use may be feasible despite the complex post-translational modifications required for its biological activity. Circulating activated protein C has a half-life of approximately 20 minutes in vivo (196). It is slowly inactivated by binding to serine protease inhibitors, preferentially by protein C inhibitor (197).

Another essential prerequisite for thrombin generation is the enzymatic activity of factor Xa required for the prothrombinase complex. A few Xa molecules are sufficient to generate biologically effective concentrations of thrombin. Thus, strong inhibition of factor Xa should provide efficient antithrombotic therapy. The disappointingly weak antithrombotic activities observed for heparin fractions with a high specific anti-Xa activity have challenged this hypothesis. However, high-affinity binding and steric hindrance could protect Xa assembled in the prothrombinase complex from heparin-mediated inactivation. Synthetic low-molecular-weight inhibitors of Xa have to overcome similar limitations. Recently, inhibitors specific for factor Xa and characterized by tight-binding and K_i values below 1 nmol/L have been isolated from salivary glands of ticks (198), leeches (199), and the black fly (200). For such potent inhibitors of factor Xa, suppression of arterial thrombus formation has been reported for doses that do not prolong the cutaneous bleeding time. The crucial role of factor Xa activity in the prothrombinase complex is further emphasized by experiments with recombinant factor Xa, which lacks enzymatic activity (in response either to active-site inhibition by pretreatment with L-glutamine-L-glycine-L-arginyl chloromethylketone or to site-directed mutagenesis of the catalytic site) and thus competitively antagonizes the binding of enzymatically active factor Xa to the prothrombinase complex with excellent specificity. These inhibitors dose-dependently inhibit the formation of venous thrombi in rabbits without affecting the activated thromboplastin time. This pharmacological approach, i.e., active-site inhibition of an activated coagulation factor, has been also used to evaluate the role of the intrinsic "tenase" complex in thrombosis. Active site–inhibited factor IXa prevents the growth of an electrically induced thrombus in the dog coronary artery without prolongation of the cutaneous bleeding time or blood loss (201).

These findings with different pharmacological tools corroborate the pivotal role of the assembly of the ternary coagulation complexes for thrombus formation. The specific inhibition of the assembly of these complexes is the mechanism of action of a novel anticoagulant that has been initially isolated from human umbilical arteries (202). This protein, called vascular anticoagulant (VAC), binds with high affinity ($K_d < 10^{-10}$ M) and in a Ca^{2+}-dependent manner to negatively charged phospholipids. The cloning of this protein revealed that it is identical with placental protein 4 [PP4; (203)] and placental anticoagulant protein I [PAP-I; (204)]. This protein is a member of the annexin family of phospholipid- and Ca^{2+}-binding proteins (205) and thus called annexin V. Recently, it has been demonstrated that annexin V prevents thrombus formation in a rat model in intravenous doses as low as 0.3 and 1.0 mg/kg, which do not prolong bleeding time (206);. The pathophysiological relevance of this protein (abundant in endothelial cells) as well as its potential for safe and efficient antithrombotic therapy remains to be established.

The factor VIIa–tissue factor complex appears to be of key importance in the initiation of the coagulation cascade. Injury of the vessel wall exposes the blood to tissue factor, an integral membrane protein that is constitutively expressed in subendothelial tissues (207,208). Ternary complexes of tissue factor, factor VIIa, and factor X or factor IX efficiently activate the latter two factors (209). A plasma protein, also released from thrombin-stimulated platelets (210), termed tissue factor pathway inhibitor (TFPI) (formerly called extrinsic pathway inhibitor or lipoprotein-associated coagulation inhibitor) binds in concert with factor Xa to the factor VIIa–tissue factor complex. In this quaternary complex the enzymatic activity of factor VIIa is inhibited. This specific cooperation between factor Xa and TFPI to suppress further activity of the factor VIIa–tissue factor complexes represents an intriguing feedback mechanism to prevent excessive thrombin generation. These interactions have also stimulated the revision of the classical "waterfall" hypothesis of the coagulation cascade and redefined the role of the coagulation factors of the "intrinsic" pathway (211). This role of factor VIIa–tissue factor complex as the trigger of coagulation suggests that efficient inhibition of this complex should translate into potent antithrombotic activity. Indeed, recombinant TFPI has been shown to prevent arterial reocclusion after thrombolysis (212).

IV. SUMMARY

Thromboembolic disease in its various forms remains a primary cause of morbidity and mortality in the most developed countries. The pharmacological strategies currently available for the treatment of both venous and arterial thrombosis are limited, and innovative new approaches are urgently required. This need has fostered intensive basic research aimed at understanding the process of vascular repair and thrombus formation. From such research, a highly complex system involving an intimate interaction and communication between the vascular wall and components of the blood is emerging. This system is characterized by positive feedback mechanisms that permit a fast response to vascular damage, as well as negative feedback mechanisms to prevent inappropriate and dangerous thrombus development. Such a complex and highly regulated process offers numerous therapeutic possibilities of effecting change in the system to protect the patient from harmful thrombus formation, and a variety of these promising strategies have been outlined. Despite the variety of therapeutic approaches that might be successfully exploited, it is certain that those approaches taking into account (and possibly taking advantage of) the feedback mechanisms of the blood–vessel wall interaction have the best chance of making significant inroads in the treatment of thromboembolic disease.

REFERENCES

1. Weiss HJ, Aledort LM, Kochwa S. The effect of salicylates on the hemostatic properties of platelets in man. J Clin Invest. 1968; 47:2169–80.
2. O'Brien JR. Effects of salicylates on human platelets. Lancet 1968; 1:779–83.
3. Roth GJ, Stanford N, Majerus PW. Acetylation of prostaglandin synthase by aspirin. Proc Natl Acad Sci USA 1975; 72:3073–76.
4. Hamberg M, Svensson J, Samuelsson B. Thromboxanes: a new group of biologically active compounds derived from prostaglandin endoperoxides. Proc Natl Acad Sci USA 1975; 72: 2944–8.
5. Clarke RJ, Mayo G, Price P, FitzGerald GA. Suppression of thromboxane A_2 but not of systemic prostacyclin by a controlled-release aspirin. N Engl J Med 1991; 325:1137–41.
6. De Gaetano G, Cerletti C. Prolongation of bleeding time by aspirin: a dual mechanism. Thromb Res 1988; 50:907–12.
7. Owens MR, Cimino CD. The inhibitory effects of sodium salicylate on the synthesis of factor VII by the perfused rat liver. Thromb Res 1980; 18:839–45.
8. Loew D, Vinazzer H. Dose-dependent influence of acetylsalicylic acid on platelet functions and plasmatic coagulation factors. Haemostasis 1976; 5:239–49.
9. Roncaglioni MC, Ulrich MMW, Muller AD, Soute BAM, de Boer-van den Berg MAG, Vermeer C. The vitamin K-antagonism of salicylate and warfarin. Thromb Res 1986; 42: 727–36.
10. Moroz LA. Increased blood fibrinolytic activity after aspirin ingestion. N Engl J Med 1977; 296:525–9.
11. Bjornsson TD, Schneider DE, Berger H Jr. Aspirin acetylates fibrinogen and enhances fibrinolysis. Fibrinolytic effect is independent of changes in plasminogen activator levels. J Pharmacol Exp Ther 1989; 250:154–61.
12. Levin RL, Harpel PC, Weil D, Chang TS, Rifkin DB. Aspirin inhibits vascular plasminogen activator activity in vivo. Studies utilizing a new assay to quantify plasminogen activator activity. J Clin Invest 1984; 74:571–80.
13. Sinzinger H, Kaliman J, Fitscha P, O'Grady J. Diminished platelet residence time on active human atherosclerotic lesions in vivo—evidence for an optimal dose of aspirin. Prostagl Leukot Essent Fatty Acids 1988; 34:89–93.
14. The Dutch TIA Trial Study Group. A comparison of two doses of aspirin (30 mg vs. 283 mg a day) in patients after a transient ischemic attack or minor ischemic stroke. N Engl J Med 1991; 325:1261–6.
15. Graham DY, Smith JL. Aspirin and the stomach. Ann Intern Med 1986; 104:390–8.
16. The SALT Collaborative Group. Swedish Aspirin Low-dose Trial (SALT) of 75 mg aspirin as secondary prophylaxis after cerebrovascular ischaemic events. Lancet 1991; 338:1345–9.
17. Antiplatelet Trialists' Collaboration. Secondary prevention of vascular disease by prolonged antiplatelet treatment. Br Med J 1988; 296:320–31.

18. Samter M, Beers RF Jr. Intolerance to aspirin. Clinical studies and consideration of its pathogenesis. Ann Intern Med 1968; 68:975–83.

19. Thun MJ, Namboodiri MM, Heath CW Jr. Aspirin use and reduced risk of fatal colon cancer. N Engl J Med 1991; 325:1593–6.

20. Paganini-Hill A, Chao A, Ross RK, Henderson BE. Aspirin use and chronic diseases: a cohort study of the elderly. Br Med J 1989; 229:1247–50.

21. Harker LA, Kadatz RA. Mechanism of action of dipyridamole. Thromb Res 1983; (suppl IV): 39–46.

22. McElroy FA, Philip RB. Relative potencies of dipyridamole and related agents as inhibitors of cyclic nucleotide phosphodiesterases: possible explanation of mechanism of inhibition of platelet function. Life Sci 1975; 17:1479–93.

23. Dresse A, Chevolet C, Delapierre D, Masset H, Weisenberger H, Bozler G, Heinzel G. Pharmacokinetics of oral dipyridamole (Persantine®) and its effect on adenosine uptake in man. Eur J Clin Pharmacol 1982; 23:229–34.

24. Crutchley DJ, Ryan US, Ryan JW. Effects of aspirin and dipyridamole on the degradation of adenosine diphosphate by cultured cells derived from pulmonary artery. J Clin Invest 1980; 66:29–35.

25. Sollevi A, Ostergren J, Hjemdahl P, Fredholm BB, Fagrell B. The effect of dipyridamole on plasma adenosine levels and skin micro-circulation in man. J Clin Chem Clin Biochem 1982; 20:420–1.

26. Haslam RJ, Rosson GM. Effects of adenosine on levels of adenosine cyclic $3',5'$-monophosphate in human blood platelets in relation to adenosine incorporation and platelet aggregation. Mol Pharmacol 1975; 11:528–44.

27. Jacobs KH, Saur W, Johnson RA. Regulation of platelet adenylate cyclase by adenosine. Biochim Biophys Acta 1979; 583:409–21.

28. Eisert WG, Müller TH. Dipyridamole—evaluation of an established antithrombotic drug in view of modern concepts of blood cell–vessel wall interactions. Thromb Res 1990; (suppl XII): 65–72.

29. Sullivan JM, Harken DE, Gorlin R. Pharmacologic control of thromboembolic complications of cardiac valve replacement. N Engl J Med 1971; 284:1391–4.

30. Akaishi Y, Sakuma I, Fukao M, Makita M-A, Kobayashi T, Yasuda H. Dipyridamole potentiates the anti-aggregating effect of endothelium-derived relaxing factor (abstr.). Circulation 1989; 80(suppl 2):125.

31. Bult H, Fret HRL, Jordaens FH, Herman AG. Dipyridamole potentiates the antiaggregating and vasodilator activity of nitric oxide. Eur J Pharmacol 1991; 199:1–8.

32. Weber E, Haas TA, Müller TH, Eisert WG, Hirsh J, Richardson M, Buchanan MR. Relationship between vessel wall 13-HODE synthesis and vessel wall thrombogenicity following injury: influence of salicylate and dipyridamole treatment. Thromb Res 1990; 57:383–92.

33. Sinzinger H, O'Grady J, Fitscha P. Platelet deposition on human atherosclerotic lesions is decreased by low-dose aspirin in combination with dipyridamole. J Int Med Res 1988; 16: 39–43.

34. Hess H, Mietaschk A, Deichsel G. Drug-induced inhibition of platelet function delays progression of peripheral occlusive arterial disease: a prospective double-blind arteriographically controlled trial. Lancet 1985; 1:415–9.

35. The ESPS Group. The European Stroke Prevention Study (ESPS). Lancet 1987; 2:1351–4.

36. Sanz and GESIC Group G. Prevention of early aortocoronary bypass occlusion by low dose aspirin and dipyridamole. Circulation 1990; 82:765–73.

37. FitzGerald GA. Dipyridamole. N Engl J Med. 1987; 316:1247–56.

38. Thébault JJ, Blatrix CE, Blanchard JF, Panak EA. Effects of ticlopidine, a new platelet aggregation inhibitor in man. Clin Pharmacol Ther 1975; 18:485–90.

39. O'Brien JR, Etherington MD, Shuttleworth RD. Ticlopidine—an antiplatelet drug: effects in human volunteers. Thromb Res 1978; 18:245–54.

40. Feliste R, Delebassee D, Simon MF, Chap H, Defreyn G, Vallee E, Douste-Blazy L, Maffrand

JP. Broad spectrum antiplatelet activity of ticlopidine and PCR 4099 involves the suppression of the effects of released ADP. Thromb Res 1987; 48:403–15.

41.   Driot F, Defreyn G, Cazenave JP, Maffrand JP. Ticlopidine and SR 25990C selectively suppress platelet adenylate cyclase (AC) inhibition by ADP. Thromb Haemost 1989 (abstr.); 62:99.

42.   DiMinno G, Cerbone AM, Mattioli PL, Turco S, Iovine C, Mancini M. Functionally thrombasthenic state in normal platelets following the administration of ticlopidine. J Clin Invest 1985; 75:328–38.

43.   Majerus PW, Broze GJ Jr, Miletich JP, Tollefsen DM. Anticoagulant, thrombolytic and antiplatelet drugs. In: Goodman and Gilman's, The pharmacological basis of therapeutics (pp. 1311–1331). New York: Pergamon Press.

44.   Hardisty RM, Powling MJ, Nokes TJC. The action of ticlopidine on human platelets. Thromb Haemost 1990; 64:150–5.

45.   Hass WK, Easton JD, Adams HP Jr, Pryse-Phillips W, Molony BA, Anderson S, Kamm B. A randomized trial comparing ticlopidine hydrochloride with aspirin in the prevention of stroke in high-risk patients. N Engl J Med 1989; 321:501–7.

46.   Gent M, Easton JD, Hachinsky VC, Blakely JA, Ellis DJ, Harbison JW. The Canadian American Ticlopidine Study (CATS) in thromboembolic stroke. Lancet 1989; 1:1215–1220.

47.   Gryglewski RJ, Szceklik A, Nizankowski R. Anti-platelet action of intravenous infusion of prostacyclin in man. Thromb Res 1978; 13:153–63.

48.   Aiken JW, Gorman RR, Shebuski RJ. Prevention of blockage of partially obstructed coronary arteries with prostacyclin correlates with inhibition of platelet aggregation. Prostaglandins 1979; 17:483–94.

49.   Coppe D, Sobel M, Seamans L, Levine F, Salzman E. Preservation of platelet function and number by prostacyclin during cardiopulmonary bypass. J Thorac Cardiovasc Surg 1981; 81: 274–8.

50.   Sinzinger H, Silberbauer K, Horsch AK, Gall A. Decreased sensitivity of human platelets to PGI_2 during long-term intraarterial prostacyclin infusion in patients with peripheral vascular disease—a rebound phenomenon? Prostaglandins 1981; 21:49–51.

51.   Jaschonek K, Faul C, Schmidt H, Renn W. Desensitization of platelets to iloprost. Loss of specific binding sites and heterologous desensitization of adenylate cyclase. Eur J Pharmacol 1988; 147:187–96.

52.   Jaschonek K, Karsch KR, Weisenberger H, Tidow S, Faul C, Renn W. Platelet prostacyclin binding in coronary artery disease. J Am Coll Cardiol 1988; 8:259–66.

53.   Kahn NN, Mueller HS, Sinha AK. Impaired prostaglandin E_1/I_2 receptor activity of human blood platelets in acute ischemic heart disease. Circ Res 1990; 66:932–940.

54.   Szceklik A, Gryglewski RJ, Nizankowski R, Musial J, Pieton R, Mruk J. Circulatory and antiplatelet effects of intravenous prostacyclin in healthy men. Pharmacol Res Commun 1978; 10:545–56.

55.   Mann KG, Jenny RJ, Krishnaswamy S. Cofactor proteins in the assembly and expression of blood clotting enzyme complexes. Annu Rev Biochem 1988; 57:915–56.

56.   Mann KG, Neesheim ME, Church WR, Haley P, Krishnaswamy S. Surface-dependent reactions of the vitamin K–dependent enzyme complexes. Blood 1990; 76:1–16.

57.   Nesheim ME, Taswell JB, Mann KG. The contribution of bovine factor V and factor Va to the activity of prothrombinase. J Biol Chem 1979; 254:10952–62.

58.   Rosing J, Trans G, Govers-Riemslag JWP, Zwaal RFA, Hemker HC. The role of phospholipids and factor Va in the prothrombinase complex. J Biol Chem 1980; 255:274–83.

59.   Loeliger EA. Oral anticoagulation in patients surviving myocardial infarction. A new approach to old data. Eur J Clin Pharmac 1984; 26:137–41.

60.   Loeliger EA. Anticoagulant therapy in acute myocardial infarction. Am Heart J 1985; 110:1322–3.

61.   Smith P, Arnesen H, Holme I. The effect of warfarin on morbidity and reinfarction after myocardial infarction. N Engl J Med 1990; 323:3004–5.

62. Peterson P, Boysen G, Godtfredson J, Andersen ED, Andersen B. Placebo controlled, randomized trial of warfarin and aspirin for prevention of thromboembolic complications in chronic arterial fibrillation: the Copenhagen AFASAK study. Lancet 1989; 1:175–9.

63. Furie B, Liebman HA, Blanchard RA, Coleman MS, Kruger SF, Furie BC. Comparison of the native prothrombin antigen and the prothrombin time for monitoring oral anticoagulant therapy. Blood 1984; 64:445–51.

64. Furie B, Diuguid CF, Jacobs M, Diuguid DL, Furie BC. Randomized prospective trial comparing the native prothrombin antigen with the prothrombin time for monitoring oral anticoagulant therapy. Blood 1990; 75:344–9.

65. Pauli RM, Lian JB, Mosher DF, Suttie JW. Association of congenital deficiency of multiple vitamin K–dependent coagulation factors and the phenotype of the warfarin embryopathy: clues to the mechanism of teratogenicity of coumarin derivatives. Am J Hum Gen 1987; 41: 566–83.

66. Price PA. Role of vitamin K–dependent proteins in bone metabolism. Annu Rev Nutr 1988; 8: 565–83.

67. Fiore CE, Tamburino C, Foti R, Grimaldi D. Reduced axial bone mineral content in patients taking an oral anticoagulant. South Med J 1990; 83:538–42.

68. Busch C, Owen WG. Identification in vitro of an endothelial cell surface cofactor for antithrombin III. Parallel studies with isolated perfused rat hearts and microcarrier cultures of bovine endothelium. J Clin Invest 1982; 69:726–9.

69. Choay J, Petitou M, Lormeau JC, Sinay P, Casu BJ, Gatti G. Structure-activity relationship in heparin: a synthetic pentasaccharide with high affinity for antithrombin III and eliciting high antifactor Xa activity. Biochem Biophys Res Comm 1983; 116:492–9.

70. Beguin S, Lindhout T, Hemker HC. The mode of action of heparin in plasma. Thromb Haemost 1988; 60:457–62.

71. Ofosu FA, Sie P, Modi GJ, Fernandez F, Buchanan MR, Blajchman MA, Hirsh J. The inhibition of thrombin-dependent positive feedback reactions is critical to the expression of the anti-coagulant effect of heparin. Biochem J 1987; 243:579–88.

72. Hirsh J. Heparin. N Engl J Med 1991; 324:1565–74.

73. Bar-Shavit R, Eldor A, Vlodavsky I. Binding of thrombin to subendothelial extracellular matrix. Protection and expression of functional properties. J Clin Invest 1989; 84:1096–1104.

74. Hogg PJ, Jackson CM. Heparin promotes the binding of thrombin to fibrin polymer. J Biol Chem 1990; 265:241–7.

75. Weitz JI, Hudoba M, Massel D, Maraganore J, Hirsh J. Clot-bound thrombin is protected from inhibition by heparin–antithrombin III but is susceptible to inhibition by antithrombin III–independent inhibitors. J Clin Invest 1990; 86:385–91.

76. Lijnen HR, Hoylaerts M, Collen D. Heparin binding properties of human histidine-rich glycoprotein. Mechanism and role in the neutralization of heparin in plasma. J Biol Chem 1983; 258:3803–8.

77. Lane DA, Flynn AM, Pejler G, Lindahl U, Choay J, Preissner KT. Structural requirements for the neutralization of heparin-like saccharides by complement S protein/vitronectin. J Biol Chem 1987; 262:16343–8.

78. Denton J, Lane DA, Thunberg L, Slater AM, Lindahl U. Binding of platelet factor 4 to heparin oligosaccharides. Biochem J 1983; 209:455–60.

79. Lane DA, Denton J, Flynn AM, Thunberg L, Lindahl U. Anticoagulant activities of heparin oligosaccharides and their neutralization by platelet factor 4. Biochem J 1984; 218:752–732.

80. Barzu T, Molho P, Tobelem G, Petitou H, Caen JP. Binding of heparin and low molecular weight heparin fragments to human vascular endothelial cells in culture. Nouv Rev Fr Hematol 1984; 26:243–7.

81. Mahadoo J, Heibert L, Jaques LB. Vascular sequestration of heparin. Thromb Res 1978; 12:79–90.

82. Sandset PM, Abildgaard U, Larsen ML. Heparin induces release of extrinsic coagulation pathway inhibitor (EPI) Thromb Res 1988; 50:803–13.

83. Novotny WF, Palmier M, Wun TC, Broze GJ Jr, Miletich JP. Purification and properties of heparin-releasable lipoprotein-associated coagulation inhibitor. Blood 1991; 78:394–400.

84. Morabia A. Heparin doses and major bleedings. Lancet 1986; 1:1278–1279.

85. Yett HS, Skillman JJ, Salzman EW. The hazards of aspirin plus heparin. N Engl J Med 1975; 298:1092.

86. Hirsh J, Ofosu F, Buchanan M. Rationale behind the development of low molecular weight heparin derivatives. Semin Thromb Hemost 1985; 11:13–16.

87. Salzmann EW, Rosenberg RD, Smith MH, Linton JN, Favreau L. Effects of heparin and heparin fractions on platelet aggregation. J Clin Invest 1980; 65:64–73.

88. Warkentin TE, Kelton JG. Heparin-induced thrombocytopenia. Annu Rev Med 1989; 40:31–44.

89. Weiss HJ, Turitto VT, Baumgartner HR. Effect of shear rate on platelet interaction with subendothelium in citrated and native blood. I. Shear rate dependent decrease of adhesion in von Willebrand's disease and the Bernard-Soulier syndrome. J Lab Clin Med 1978; 92:750–64.

90. Turitto VT, Weiss HJ, Baumgartner HR. Platelet interaction with rabbit subendothelium in von Willebrand's disease: altered thrombus formation distinct from defective platelet adhesion. J Clin Invest 1984; 74:1730–41.

91. Stel HV, Sakariassen KS, Scholte BJ, Veerman ECI, van der Kwast TM, de Groot PG, Sixma JJ, van Mourik JA. Characterization of 25 monoclonal antibodies to factor VIII–von Willebrand factor. Relationship between ristocetin-induced platelet aggregation and platelet adherence to subendothelium. Blood 1984; 63:1408–15.

92. Bellinger DA, Nichols TC, Read MS, Reddick RL, Lamb MA, Brinkhous KM, Evatt BL, Griggs TR. Prevention of occlusive coronary artery thrombosis by a murine monoclonal antibody to porcine von Willebrand factor. Proc Natl Acad Sci USA 1987; 84:8100–4.

93. Takami H, Nichols WL, Kaese SE, Bowie JW. Infusion study of monoclonal antibodies against porcine platelet membrane GPIb and GP IIb/IIIa: differential effect on platelet function and bleeding time. Blood 1987 (abstr.); 70(suppl 1):344a.

94. Cadroy Y, Kelly A, Marzec U, Evatt B, Harker L, Hanson S, Ruggeri Z. Comparison of the antihemostatic and antithrombotic effects of monoclonal antibodies (MoA) against von Willebrand factor (vWF) and platelet (P) glycoprotein IIb/IIIa (GPIIb/IIIa). Circulation 1989 (abstr.); 80:II-24.

95. Fujimura Y, Titani K, Holland LZ, Russel SR, Roberts JR, Elder JH, Ruggeri ZM, Zimmerman TS. Von Willebrand factor. A reduced and alkylated 52/48 kD fragment beginning at amino acid residue 449 contains the domain interacting with platelet glycoprotein Ib. J Biol Chem 1986; 261:381–5.

96. Nichols TC, Bellinger DA, Reddick RL, Read MS, Koch GG, Brinkhous KM, Griggs TR. Role of von Willebrand factor in arterial thrombosis. Studies in normal and von Willebrand disease pigs. Circulation 1991; 83:IV-56–IV-64.

97. Fujimoto T, Ohara S, Hawiger J. Thrombin-induced exposure and prostacyclin inhibition of the receptor for factor VIII/von Willebrand factor on human platelets. J Clin Invest 1982; 69:1212–22.

98. Ruggeri ZM, Bader R, DeMarco L. Glanzmann's thrombasthenia: deficient binding of von Willebrand factor to thrombin-stimulated platelets. Proc Natl Acad Sci USA 1982; 79:6038–41.

99. Staaz WD, Rajpara SM, Wayner EA, Carter WG, Santoro SA. The membrane glycoprotein Ia-IIa (VLA-2) complex mediates the Mg^{++}-dependent adhesion of platelets to collagen. J Cell Biol 1989; 108:1917–24.

100. Thiagarajan P, Kelly KL. Exposure of binding sites for vitronectin on platelets following stimulation. J Biol Chem 1988; 263:3035–8.

101. George JN, Nurden AT, Phillips DR. Molecular defects in interactions of platelets with the vessel wall. N Engl J Med 1984; 311:1084–98.

102. Coller BS, Peerschke EI, Scudder LE, Sullivan CA. A murine monoclonal antibody that completely blocks the binding of fibrinogen to platelets produces a thrombasthenic-like state in normal platelets and binds to glycoproteins IIb and/or IIIa. J Clin Invest 1983; 72:325–38.

103. Eldor A, Vlodavsky I, Martinowicz U, Fuks Z, Coller BS. Platelet interaction with subendothelial extracellular matrix: platelet-fibrinogen interactions are essential for platelet aggregation but not for the matrix induced release reaction. Blood 1985; 65:1477–83.

104. Kaplan AV, Leung LL-K, Leung WH, Grant GW, McDougall IR, Fischell TA. Roles of thrombin and platelet membrane glycoprotein IIb/IIIa in platelet-subendothelial deposition after angioplasty in an ex vivo whole artery model. Circulation 1991; 84:1279–88.

105. Coller BS, Folts JD, Scudder LE, Smith SR. Antithrombotic effect of a monoclonal antibody to the platelet glycoprotein IIb/IIIa receptor in an experimental animal model. Blood 1986; 68: 783–6.

106. Mickelson JK, Simpson PJ, Lucchesi BR. Antiplatelet monoclonal F(ab')$_2$ antibody directed against the platelet GP IIb/IIIa receptor complex prevents coronary artery thrombosis in the canine heart. J Mol Cell Cardiol 1989; 21:393–405.

107. Coller BS, Folts JD, Smith SR, Scudder LE, Jordan R. Abolition of in vivo platelet thrombus formation in primates with monoclonal antibodies to the platelet GP IIb/IIIa receptor: correlation with bleeding time, platelet aggregation, and blockage of GPIIb/IIIa receptors. Circulation 1989; 80:1766–74.

108. Hanson SR, Pareti FI, Ruggeri ZM, Marzec UM, Kunicki TJ, Montgomery RR, Zimmerman TS, Harker LA. Effects of monoclonal antibodies against the platelet glycoprotein IIb/IIIa complex on thrombosis and hemostasis in the baboon. J Clin Invest 1988; 81:149–58.

109. Yasuda T, Gold HK, Fallon JT, Leinbach RC, Guerrero JL, Scudder LE, Kanke M, Shealy D, Ross MJ, Collen D, Coller BS. Monoclonal antibody against the platelet glycoprotein (GP) IIb/IIIa receptor prevents coronary artery reocclusion after reperfusion with recombinant tissue-type plasminogen activator in dogs. J Clin Invest 1988; 81:1284–91.

110. Gold HK, Coller BS, Yasuda T, Fallon JT, Guerrero JL, Leinbach RC, Ziskind AA, Collen D. Rapid and sustained coronary artery recanalization with combined bolus injection of recombinant tissue-type plasminogen activator and monoclonal antiplatelet GPIIb/IIIa antibody in a dog model. Circulation 1988; 77:670–7.

111. Mickelson JK, Simpson PJ, Cronin M, Homeister JW, Laywell LE, Kitzen J, Lucchesi BR. Antiplatelet antibody [7E3 F(ab')$_2$] prevents rethrombosis after recombinant tissue-type plasminogen activator-induced coronary artery thrombolysis in a canine model. Circulation 1990; 81:617–27.

112. Coller BS, Scudder LE, Berger HJ, Iuliucci JD. Inhibition of human platelet function in vivo with a monoclonal antibody: with observations on the newly dead as experimental subjects. Ann Intern Med 1988; 109:635–8.

113. Gold HK, Gimple LW, Yasuda T, Leinbach RC, Werner W, Holt R, Jordan R, Berger H, Collen D, Coller BS. Pharmacodynamic study of F(ab')$_2$ fragments of murine monoclonal antibody 7E3 directed against human platelet glycoprotein IIb/IIIa in patients with unstable angina. J Clin Invest 1990; 86:651–9.

114. Anderson HV, Revana M, Rosales O, Brannigan L, Stuart Y, Weisman H, Willerson JT. Intravenous administration of monoclonal antibody to the platelet GPIIb/IIIa receptor to treat abrupt closure during coronary angioplasty. Am J Cardiol 1992; 69:1373–6.

115. Coller BS. A new murine antibody reports an activation-dependent change in the conformation and/or microenvironment of the platelet GP IIb/IIIa complex. J Clin Invest 1985; 76:101–8.

116. Gan ZR, Gould RJ, Jacobs JW, Friedman PA, Polokoff MA. Echistatin: a potent platelet aggregation inhibitor from the venom of the viper, Echis carinatus. J Biol Chem 1988; 263: 19872–19832.

117. Dennis MS, Henzel WJ, Pitti RM, Lipari MT, Napier MA, Deisher TA. Platelet glycoprotein IIb-IIIa protein antagonists from snake venoms: evidence for a family of platelet-aggregation inhibitors. Proc Natl Acad Sci USA 1990; 87:2471–5.

118. Huang T-F, Holt JC, Lakasiewicz H, Niewiaroswski S. Trigramin. A low molecular weight peptide inhibiting fibrinogen interaction with platelet receptors expressed on glycoprotein IIb-IIIa complex. J Biol Chem 1987; 262:16157–63.

119. Cook JJ, Huang TF, Rucinski B, Strzyzewski M, Tuma RF, Williams JA. Inhibition of platelet hemostatic plug formation by trigramin, a novel RGD-peptide. Am J Physiol 1989; 256: H1038–H1043.

120. Shebuski RJ, Ramjit DR, Bencen GH, Polokoff MA. Characterization and platelet inhibitory activity of bitistatin, a potent arginine-glycine-aspartic acid containing peptide from the venom of the viper bitis arietans. J Biol Chem 1989; 264:21550–6.

121. Shebuski RJ, Stabilito IJ, Sitko GR, Polokoff MH. Acceleration of recombinant tissue-type plasminogen activator–induced thrombolysis and prevention of reocclusion by the combination of heparin and the Arg-Gly-Asp-containing peptide bitistatin in a canine model of coronary thrombosis. Circulation 1990; 82:169–77.

122. Chao BH, Jakubowski JA, Savage B, Chow EP, Marzec UM, Harker LA. Agkistrodon piscivorous platelet aggregation inhibitor: a potent inhibitor of platelet aggregation. Proc Natl Acad Sci USA 1989; 86:8050–4.

123. Savage B, Marzec UM, Chao BH, Harker LA, Maraganore JM, Ruggeri ZM. Binding of the snake venom–derived proteins applaggin and echistatin to the arginine-glycine-aspartic acid recognition site(s) on platelet glycoprotein IIb-IIIa complex inhibits receptor function. J Biol Chem 1990; 265:11766–72.

124. Ruoslahti E, Pierschbacher MD. New perspectives in cell adhesion: RGD and integrins. Science 1987; 238:491–7.

125. Gartner TK, Bennett JS. The tetrapeptide analogue of the cell attachment site of fibronectin inhibits platelet aggregation and fibrinogen binding to activated platelets. J Biol Chem 1985; 260:11891–4.

126. Plow EF, Pierschbacher MD, Ruoslahti E, Marguerie GA, Ginsberg MH. The effect of Arg-Gly-Asp-containing peptides on fibrinogen and von Willebrand factor binding to platelets. Proc Natl Acad Sci USA 1985; 82:8057–61.

127. Plow EF, Pierschbacher MD, Ruoslahti E, Marguerie G, Ginsberg MH. Arginyl-glycyl-aspartic acid sequences and fibrinogen binding to platelets. Blood 1987; 70:110–5.

128. Hynes RO. Integrins: versatility, modulation, and signalling in cell adhesion. Cell 1992; 69: 11–25.

129. Ruoslahti E. Integrins. J Clin Invest 1991; 87:1–5.

130. Preissner KT, Anders E, Grulich-Henn J, Müller-Berghaus G. Attachment of cultured human endothelial cells is promoted by specific association with S protein (vitronectin) as well as with the ternary S protein–thrombin–antithrombin III complex. Blood 1988; 71:1581–9.

131. Sato M, Sardana MK, Grasser WA, Garsky VM, Murray JM, Gould RJ. Echistatin is a potent inhibitor of bone resorption in culture. J Cell Biol 1990; 111:1713–23.

132. Horton MA, Taylor ML, Arnett TR, Helfrich MH. Arg-Gly-Asp (RGD) peptides and anti–vitronectin receptor antibody 23C6 inhibit dentine resorption and cell spreading by osteoclasts. Exp Cell Res 1991; 195:368–75.

133. Humphries MJ, Olden K, Yamada KM. A synthetic peptide from fibronectin inhibits experimental metastasis of murine melanoma cells. Science 1986; 233:467–70.

134. Gehlsen KR, Argraves WS, Pierschbacher MD, Ruoslahti E. Inhibition of in vitro tumor cell invasion by Arg-Gly-Asp-containing synthetic peptides. J Cell Biol 1988; 106:925–30.

135. Scarborough RM, Rose JW, Hsu MA, Phillips DR, Fried VA, Campbell AM, Nannizzi L, Charo IF. Barbourin. A GPIIB-IIIA-specific integrin antagonist from the venom of sistrurus M. Barbouri. J Biol Chem 1991; 266:9359–62.

136. Moncada S, Korbut R, Bunting S, Vane JR. Prostacyclin is a circulating hormone. Nature 1978; 273:767–8.

137. Needleman P, Wyche A, Raz A. Platelet and blood vessel arachidonate metabolism and interactions. J Clin Invest 1979; 63:345–50.

138. Chesterman CN, Owe-Young R, Macpherson J, Krilis SA. Substrate for endothelial prostacyclin production in the presence of platelets exposed to collagen is derived from platelets rather than the endothelium. Blood 1986; 67:1744–50.

139. Hechtman DH, Kroll MH, Gimbrone MA Jr, Schafer AI. Platelet interaction with vascular smooth muscle in the synthesis of prostacyclin. Am J Physiol 1991; 260:H1544–H1551.
140. Fitzgerald DJ, Fragetta J, FitzGerald GA. Prostaglandin endoperoxides modulate the response to thromboxane synthase inhibition during coronary thrombosis. J Clin Invest 1988; 82: 1708–13.
141. Nowak J, FitzGerald GA. Redirection of prostaglandin endoperoxide metabolism at the platelet-vascular interface in man. J Clin Invest 1989; 83:380–5.
142. Kyrle PA, Eichler HG, Jäger U, Lechner K. Inhibition of prostacyclin and thromboxane A_2 generation by low-dose aspirin at the site of plug formation in man in vivo. Circulation 1987; 75: 1025–9.
143. FitzGerald GA, Smith B, Pedersen AK, Brash AR. Increased prostacyclin biosynthesis in patients with severe atherosclerosis and platelet activation. N Engl J Med 1984; 310:1065–8.
144. Eldor A, Lellouche F, Goldfarb A, Rachmilewitz EA, Maclouf J. In vivo platelet activation in beta-thalassemia major reflected by increased platelet-thromboxane urinary metabolites. Blood 1991; 77:1749–53.
145. Fiddler GI, Lumley P. Preliminary clinical studies with thromboxane synthase inhibitors and thromboxane receptor blockers; a review. Circulation 1990; 81:I69–I78.
146. Reilly IAG, FitzGerald GA. Inhibition of thromboxane formation in vivo and ex vivo: Implications for therapy with platelet inhibitory drugs. Blood 1987; 69:180–6.
147. Clerk FD, Beetens J, de Chaffoy de Courcelle D, Freyne E, Janssen PA. R 68070: thromboxane synthetase inhibition and thromboxane A_2/prostaglandin endoperoxide receptor blockade combined in one molecule: I. Biochemical profile in vitro. Thromb Haemost 1989; 61:35–42.
148. Hoet B, Falcon C, DeReys S, Arnout J, Deckmyn H, Vermylen J. R68070, a combined thromboxane receptor antagonist and thromboxane synthase inhibitor, inhibits human platelet activation in vitro and in vivo: a comparison with aspirin. Blood 1990; 75:646–53.
149. Timmermans C, Vrolix M, Vanhaecke J, Stammen F, Piessens J, Vercammen E, DeGeest H. Ridogrel in the setting of percutaneous transluminal angioplasty. Am J Cardiol 1991; 68:463–6.
150. Rapold HJ, Van de Werf F, De Gest H, Arnout J, Sangtawesin W, Vercammen E, De Clerk F, Weber C, Collen D. Pilot study of combined administration of ridogrel and alteplase in patients with myocardial infarction. Coronary Artery Disease 1991; 2:455–63.
151. Yasuda T, Gold HK, Yaotia H, Guerrero JL, Holt RE, Fallon JT, Leinbach RC, Collen D. Antithrombotic effects of ridogrel, a combined thromboxane A_2 synthase inhibitor and prostaglandin endoperoxide receptor antagonist, in a platelet-mediated coronary artery occlusion preparation in the dog. Coronary Artery Disease 1991; 2:1103–10.
152. Vandeplassche L, Hermans C, Van de Water A, Xhonneux R, De Clerk F. Differential effect of TxA_2 synthetase inhibition, singly or combined with TxA_2/PgH_2 receptor antagonism (R68070), on thrombosis over endothelial cell damage or deep intimal injury in canine coronary arteries. Thromb Haemost 1989; 62:509.
153. Gresele P, Deckmyn H, Nenci GG, Vermylen J. Thromboxane synthetase inhibitors, thromboxane receptor antagonists and dual blockers in thrombotic disorders. Trends Pharmacol Sci 1991; 12:158–163.
154. Haycraft JB. Über die Einwirkung eines Secretes des officinalen Blutegels auf die Gerinnbarkeit des Blutes. Naunyn-Schmiedebergers Arch Exp Pathol Pharmakol 1884; 18:209–17.
155. Dodt J, Seemüller U, Maschler R, Fritz H. The complete covalent structure of hirudin. Localization of the disulfide bonds. Biol Chem Hoppe-Seyler 1985; 366:379–85.
156. Markwardt F. Die Isolierung und chemische Charakterisierung des Hirudins. Z Physiol Chem 1957; 308:147–56.
157. Scharf M, Engels J, Tripier D. Primary structures of new 'iso-hirudins'. FEBS Lett 1989; 255: 105–10.
158. Fortkamp E, Rieger M, Heisterberg-Moutses G, Schweizer S, Sommer R. Cloning and expression in Escherichia coli of a synthetic DNA for hirudin, the blood coagulation inhibitor in the leech. DNA 1986; 5:511–7.

159. Harvey RP, Degryse E, Stefani L, Schamber F, Cazenave JP, Courtney M, Tolstoshev P, Lecocq JP. Cloning and expression of cDNA coding for the anticoagulant hirudin from the bloodsucking leech, Hirudo medicinalis. Proc Natl Acad Sci USA 1986; 83:1084–8.

160. Markwardt F, Walsmann P. Die Reaktion zwischen Hirudin und Thrombin. Z Physiol Chem 1958; 348:85–9.

161. Dodt J, Müller HP, Seemüller U, Chang J-Y. The complete amino acid sequence of hirudin, a thrombin specific inhibitor. FEBS Lett 1984; 165:180–4.

162. Tam SW, Fenton JW, Detwiler TC. Dissociation of thrombin from platelets by hirudin. Evidence for receptor processing. J Biol Chem 1979; 254:8723–5.

163. Grütter MG, Priestle JP, Rahuel J, Grossenbacher H, Bode W, Hofsteenge J, Stone SR. Crystal structure of the thrombin-hirudin complex: a novel mode of serine protease inhibition. EMBO J 1990; 9:2361–5.

164. Rydel TJ, Ravichandran KQ, Tulinsky A, Bode W, Huber R, Roitsch C, Fenton JW. The structure of a complex of recombinant hirudin and human α-thrombin. Science 1990; 249: 277–80.

165. Markwardt F. Hirudin and derivatives as anticoagulant agents. Thromb Haemost 1991; 66: 141–52.

166. Heras M, Chesebro JH, Penny WJ, Bailey KR, Badimon L, Fuster V. Effects of thrombin inhibition on the development of acute platelet-thrombus deposition during angioplasty in pigs: heparin versus recombinant hirudin, a specific thrombin inhibitor. Circulation 1989; 79: 657–65.

167. Heras M, Chesebro JH, Webster MWI, Mruk JS, Gill DE, Penny WJ, Bowie EJW, Badimon L, Fuster V. Hirudin, heparin, and placebo during deep arterial injury in the pig. The in vivo role of thrombin in platelet-mediated thrombosis. Circulation 1990; 82:1476–84.

168. Lam JYT, Chesebro JH, Steele PM, Heras M, Webster MWI, Badimon L, Fuster V. Antithrombotic therapy for deep arterial injury by angioplasty. Efficacy of common platelet inhibition compared with thrombin inhibition in pigs. Circulation 1991; 84:814–20.

169. Haskel EJ, Prager NA, Sobel BE, Abendschein DR. Relative efficacy of antithrombin compared with antiplatelet agents in accelerating coronary thrombolysis and preventing early reocclusions. Circulation 1991; 83:1048–56.

170. Maraganore JM, Chao B, Joseph ML, Jablonski J, Ramachandran KL. Anticoagulant activity of synthetic hirudin peptides. J Biol Chem 1989; 264:8692–8.

171. Naski MC, Fenton JW II, Maraganore JM, Olson ST, Shafer JA. The COOH-terminal domain of hirudin. An exosite-directed competitive inhibitor of the action of α-thrombin on fibrinogen. J Biol Chem 1990; 265:13484–9.

172. Cadroy Y, Maraganore JM, Hanson SR, Harker LA. Selective inhibition by a synthetic hirudin peptide of fibrin-dependent thrombosis in baboons. Proc Natl Acad Sci USA 1991; 88: 1177–81.

173. Kettner C, Shaw E. D-Phe-Pro-ArgCH2Cl—a selective affinity label for thrombin. Thromb Res 1979; 14:969–73.

174. Hanson SR, Harker LA. Interruption of the acute platelet-dependent thrombosis by the synthetic antithrombin D-phenylalanyl-L-prolyl-L-arginyl chloromethyl ketone. Proc Natl Acad Sci USA 1988; 85:3184–8.

175. Krupski WC, Bass A, Kelly AB, Marzec UM, Hanson SR, Harker LA. Heparin resistant thrombus formation by endovascular stents in baboons. Interruption by a synthetic antithrombin. Circulation 1990; 81:570–7.

176. Collen D, Matsuo O, Stassen JM, Kettner C, Shaw E. In vivo studies of a synthetic inhibitor of thrombin. J Lab Clin Med 1982; 99:76–83.

177. Kettner C, Mersinger L, Knabb R. The selective inhibition of thrombin by peptides of boroarginine. J Biol Chem 1990; 265:18289–97.

178. Knabb RM, Kettner CA, Timmermans PBMWM, Reilly TM. In vivo characterization of a new synthetic thrombin inhibitor. Thromb Haemost 1992; 67:56–9.

179. Kikumoto R, Tamao Y, Tezuka T, Tonomura S, Hara H, Ninomiya K, Hijikata A, Okamoto S.

Selective inhibition of thrombin by (2R,4R)-4-methyl-1-(N2-((3-methyl-1,2,3,4-tetrahydro 8-quinolinyl) sulfonyl)-L-arginyl))-2-piperidinecarboxylic acid. Biochemistry 1984; 23: 85–90.

180. Müller TH, Gerster U, Eisert WG. Synthetic thrombin inhibitors (argipidine, PPACK) are more effective than heparin in a model of arterial reocclusion. Thromb Haemost 1989 (abstr.); 62:533.

181. Jang IK, Gold HK, Ziskind AA, Leinbach RC, Fallon JT, Collen D. Prevention of platelet-rich arterial thrombosis by selective thrombin inhibition. Circulation 1990; 81:219–25.

182. Eidt JF, Allison P, Noble S, Ashton J, Golino P, McNatt J. Thrombin is an important mediator of platelet aggregation in stenosed canine coronary arteries with endothelial injury. J Clin Invest 1989; 84:18–27.

183. Fitzgerald DJ, FitzGerald GA. Role of thrombin and thromboxane A$_2$ in reocclusion following coronary thrombolysis with tissue-type plasminogen activator. Proc Natl Acad Sci USA 1989; 86:7585–9.

184. Yasuda T, Gold HK, Yaoita H, Leinbach RC, Guerrero JL, Jang IK. Comparative effects of aspirin, a synthetic thrombin inhibitor and a monoclonal antiplatelet glycoprotein IIb/IIIa antibody on coronary reperfusion, reocclusion and bleeding with recombinant tissue type plasminogen activator in a canine preparation. J Am Coll Cardiol 1990; 16:714–22.

185. Clarke RJ, Mayo G, FitzGerald GA, Fitzgerald DJ. Combined administration of aspirin and a specific thrombin inhibitor in man. Circulation 1991; 83:1510–8.

186. Ruda EM, Petty A, Scrutton MC, Tuffin DP, Manley PW. Identification of small peptide analogues having agonist and antagonist activity at the platelet thrombin receptor. Biochem Pharmacol 1988; 37:2417–26.

187. Ruda EM, Scrutton MC, Tuffin DP, Manley PW, Tuffin DP. Thrombin receptor antagonists. Structure-activity relationships for the platelet thrombin receptor and effects on prostacyclin synthesis by human umbilical vein endothelial cells. Biochem Pharmacol 1990; 39:373–81.

188. Vu T-KH, Hung DT, Wheaton VI, Coughlin SR. Molecular cloning of a functional thrombin receptor reveals a novel proteolytic mechanism of receptor activation. Cell 1991; 64:1057–68.

189. Vu T-KH, Wheaton VI, Hung DT, Charo I, Coughlin SR. Domains specifying thrombin-receptor interaction. Nature 1991; 353:674–7.

190. Hung DT, Vu T-KH, Wheaton VI, Charo IF, Nelken NA, Esmon N, Esmon CT, Coughlin SR. "Mirror image" antagonists of thrombin-induced platelet activation based on thrombin receptor structure. J Clin Invest 1992; 89:444–50.

191. Hung DT, Vu T-KH, Wheaton VI, Ishii K, Coughlin SR. Cloned platelet thrombin receptor is necessary for thrombin induced platelet activation. J Clin Invest 1992; 89:1350–3.

192. Esmon CT. The roles of protein C and thrombomodulin in the regulation of blood coagulation. J Biol Chem 1989; 264:4743–6.

193. Gruber A, Griffin JH, Harker LA, Hanson SR. Inhibition of platelet-dependent thrombus formation by human activated protein C in a primate model. Blood 1989; 73:639–42.

194. Gruber A, Hanson SR, Kelly AB, Yan BS, Bang NU, Griffin JH, Harker LA. Inhibition of thrombus formation by activated recombinant protein C in a primate model of arterial thrombosis. Circulation 1990; 82:578–85.

195. Gruber A, Harker LA, Hanson SR, Kelly AB, Griffin JH. Antithrombotic effects of combining activated protein C and urokinase in nonhuman primates. Circulation 1991; 84:2454–62.

196. Comp PC, Jacocks RM, Ferrell GL, Esmon CT. Activation of protein C in vivo. J Clin Invest 1982; 70:127–34.

197. Suzuki K, Nishioka J, Hashimoto S. Protein C inhibitor. Purification from human plasma and characterization. J Biol Chem 1983; 258:163–8.

198. Waxman L, Smith DE, Arcuri KE, Vlasuk GP. Tick anticoagulant peptide (TAP) is a novel inhibitor of blood coagulation factor Xa. Science 1990; 248:593–6.

199. Condra C, Nutt E, Petroski CJ, Simpson E, Friedman PA, Jacobs JW. Isolation and structural characterization of a potent inhibitor of coagulation factor Xa from the leech Haementeria ghilianii. Thromb Haemost 1989; 61:437–41.

200. Jacobs JW, Cupp EW, Sardana M, Friedman PA. Isolation and characterization of a coagulation factor Xa inhibitor from black fly salivary glands. Thromb Haemost 1990; 64:235–8.
201. Benedict CR, Ryan J, Wolitzky B, Ramos R, Gerlach M, Tijburg P, Stern D. Active site-blocked factor IXa prevents intravascular thrombus formation in the coronary vasculature without inhibiting extravascular coagulation in a canine thrombosis model. J Clin Invest 1991; 88:1760–5.
202. Reutelingsperger CPM, Hornstra G, Hemker HC. Isolation and partial purification of a novel anticoagulant from arteries of human umbilical cord. Eur J Biochem 1985; 151:625–30.
203. Iwasaki A, Suda M, Nakao H, Nagoya T, Saino Y, Arai K, Mizoguchi T, Sato F, Yoshizaki H, Hirata M, Murata M, Maki M. Structure and expression of cDNA for an inhibitor of blood coagulation from human placenta: a new lipocortin-like protein. J Biochem 1989; 102: 1261–73.
204. Tait JF, Sakata M, McMullen BA, Miao CH, Funakoshi T, Hendrickson LE, Fujikawa K. Placental anticoagulant proteins: isolation and comparative characterization of four members of the lipocortin family. Biochemistry 1988; 27:6268–76.
205. Crompton MR, Moss SE, Crumpton MJ. Diversity in the lipocortin/calpactin family. Cell 1988; 55:1–3.
206. Römisch J, Seiffge D, Reiner G, Paques E-P, Heimburger N. In-vivo antithrombotic potency of placental protein 4 (annexin V). Thromb Res 1991; 61:93–104.
207. Wilcox JH, Smith KM, Schwartz SM, Gordon D. Localization of tissue factor in the normal vessel wall and in the atherosclerotic plaque. Proc Natl Acad Sci USA 1989; 86:2839–43.
208. Weiss HJ, Turitto VT, Baumgartner HR, Nemerson Y, Hoffmann T. Evidence for the presence of tissue factor activity on subendothelium. Blood 1989; 73:968–75.
209. Komiyama Y, Pedersen AH, Kisiel W. Proteolytic activation of human factors IX and X by recombinant human factor VIIa: effects of calcium, phospholipids, and tissue factor. Biochemistry 1990; 29:9418–25.
210. Novotny WF, Girard TJ, Miletich JP, Broze GJ Jr. Platelets secrete a coagulation inhibitor functionally and antigenically similar to the lipoprotein-associated coagulation inhibitor. Blood 1988; 72:2020–5.
211. Gailani D, Broze GJ Jr. Factor XI activation in a revised model of blood coagulation. Science 1991; 253:909–12.
212. Haskel EJ, Torr SR, Day KC, Palmier MO, Wun TC, Sobel BE, Abendschein DR. Prevention of arterial reocclusion after thrombolysis with recombinant lipoprotein associated coagulation inhibitor.; Circulation 1991; 84:821–7.

II
TECHNOLOGY

The technology used in the evaluation of the patient with a suspected systemic embolization, or in the evaluation of a condition that may predispose to the development of a systemic embolization, is discussed in this section. Tests are directed at identifying intracardiac sources for systemic embolization as well as sources in the aorta and carotid vessels and, in the case of the patient with a suspected paradoxical embolus, in the peripheral venous circulation.

This section will deal with the fundamentals of ultrasound, radionuclide imaging techniques, impedance plethysmography, magnetic resonance imaging, and ultrafast computed tomography scans, as well as invasive angiographic and venographic techniques.

7

Cardiac and Peripheral Ultrasound

Michael D. Ezekowitz
Yale University School of Medicine, West Haven Veterans Affairs, and Cardiovascular Thrombosis Research Laboratory, New Haven, Connecticut

Ira S. Cohen
Yale University School of Medicine and West Haven Veterans Affairs, New Haven, Connecticut

Lynwood W. Hammers
Yale University School of Medicine, New Haven, Connecticut

I. INTRODUCTION

Ultrasound has a frequency beyond the range detectable by the human ear ($>20,000$ cycles per second). For application in medicine, frequencies in the megahertz range ($\geqslant 1,000,000$ cycles per second) are routinely used. To date, the use of ultrasound for medical imaging is without known adverse biological effects. Its primary diagnostic limitation, particularly important in transthoracic cardiac imaging, is its inability to penetrate air (lung) and bone. Accurate interpretation of studies is critically dependent on the quality of the examination.

Clinical ultrasound imaging equipment relies, fundamentally, on the application of the property of certain crystals (e.g., quartz) to change shape when an electric current passes through them and to return to their original shape when current flow stops (piezoelectric effect) (Fig. 1). Rapid, alternating application and withdrawal of current causes the crystal to oscillate and thereby generate alternating compressions and rarefactions of air, i.e., sound waves. Reflection of these waves back to the crystal from interfaces of tissues with different acoustic impedance causes the crystal to generate an electrical impulse. These impulses are time-gated and integrated to produce an image that can be displayed in a variety of formats including A-mode, M-mode, and B-mode.

For cardiac and peripheral vascular imaging, the objectives of the ultrasound examination are to define anatomy and to characterize blood flow patterns and velocities.

Anatomy is defined using both M-mode and cross-sectional imaging. Characterization of flow is achieved using Doppler echocardiography. The ability to obtain high-quality echocardiographic recordings is the most important factor in determining the usefulness of the subsequent images. Examinations are standardized to avoid omissions and to facilitate routine systematic evaluation. Examination must also be customized, to some extent, for each patient to ensure that information critical to the particular clinical problem is obtained. Thus a high level of sophistication and an understanding of the physiology and pathophysiol-

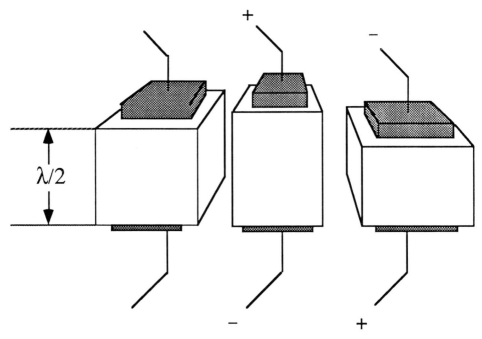

Figure 1   Sketch of a crystal that has piezoelectric properties. The crystal changes shape as the surrounding electrical field is reversed. The wavelength (λ) of the emitted ultrasound is a function of the size of crystal. (From: Feigenbaum H. Echocardiography. 3d ed. Philadelphia: Lea & Febiger, 1981. Reprinted with permission.)

ogy of the process being evaluated are required to successfully complete a comprehensive, individually tailored examination.

M-mode echocardiography uses a single-element transducer that generates a single M-mode ultrasound beam (Fig. 2). Use of a single element allows high-frequency sampling of the area (typically 1000 cps as opposed to 30 cps for the two-dimensional beam), providing greater resolution and accuracy of measurement. Thus M-mode echocardiography is the ultrasound method of choice both for obtaining dimensions of cardiac structures and for timing of events. An oscilloscopic display (no longer used clinically) plots the amplitudes of the echoes reflected at tissue interfaces as moving point sources of light to produce an A-mode display (A = amplitude of motion of the echoes). Amplitude is plotted on the y axis; depth from the chest wall on the x axis. The A mode display is projected onto a thin, linear cathode ray tube juxtaposed to a sheet of moving light-sensitive paper on which the electrocardiogram (ECG) and time lines are also projected as point sources of light. This format produces a "time-motion" display or "strip chart" recording. The term adopted for this type of presentation is "M-mode," where M stands for "motion," or, more appropriately, "TM" or "time-motion" mode (Fig. 3).

The major disadvantage of M-mode echocardiography is that it obtains an "ice pick" view or ultrasound "biopsy" of the heart, which is then assumed to be accurately representative of the structure being imaged. To deal with this problem, reproducible measurements are obtained by using the mitral valve and chordae tendineae as landmarks. The limitations of this approach are particularly apparent when attempting to identify localized intracardiac

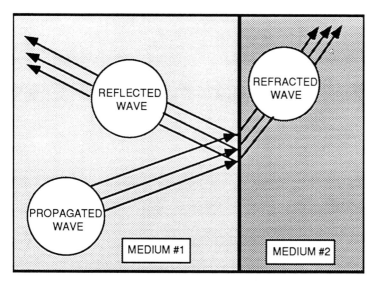

Figure 2 Ultrasound is reflected and refracted by an interface between two media of different acoustic impedance. (From: Feigenbaum H. Echocardiography. 3d ed. Philadelphia: Lea & Febiger, 1981. Reprinted with permission.)

masses or thrombi or to quantify ventricular function when regional wall motion abnormalities are present, as in ischemic heart disease.

To overcome the sampling problem, cross-sectional or two-dimensional echocardiographic imaging was developed (Fig. 4). The two-dimensional ultrasound transducer (or probe) consists of a series of piezoelectric crystal elements sequentially activated to generate an ultrasound beam along a single plane that can be aimed at the structure to be imaged. Two cross-sectional technologies are currently in use: phased-array imaging, which employs multiple-element transducers (typically 48–128 elements per probe) electronically steered and sequentially activated so as to sweep over an interrogating sector plane typically encompassing a 90° arc. The second technology involves mechanical sector scanning, in which one to three crystal elements are rapidly oscillated or rotated over a plane to provide similar tomographic two-dimensional imaging. The spatial orientation provided by this approach has, to a large extent, overcome many limitations of M-mode echocardiographic imaging. It also provides the spatial orientation necessary for more reproducible M-mode measurements and for more accurate assessment of global ventricular function. In cardiac imaging, anatomic measurements are generally obtained using two-dimensionally guided M-mode technique. The M-mode beam is electronically selected by the ultrasonographer from those in the two-dimensional probe so that the area of interest within the two-dimensional echo image can be selected for M-mode interrogation.

The second function of the ultrasound examination is the determination of the direction and quantification of velocity of blood flow through the heart and blood vessels. This approach employs the Doppler principle, first described by Johann Christian Doppler in 1842. As applied to cardiac and vascular imaging, the Doppler principle states that if an ultrasound beam is directed toward a moving target, the sound reflected by that target will change in frequency (the Doppler shift) in direct proportion to the velocity of the moving target. If the target is moving toward the beam, the reflected frequency will increase, and

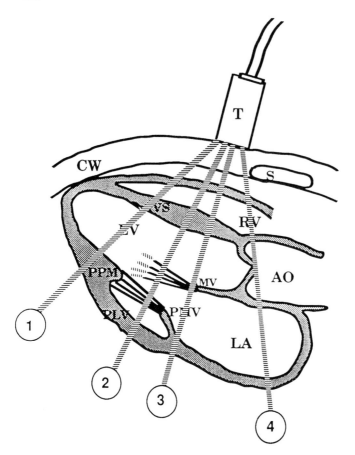

Figure 3 A cross-section of the heart showing the structures through which the ultrasonic beam passes as it is directed from the apex toward the base of the heart. CW = chest wall; T = transducer; S = sternum; ARV = anterior right ventricular wall; RV = right ventricular cavity; IVS = interventricular septum; LV = left ventricle; PPM = posterior papillary muscle; PLV = posterior left ventricular wall; AMV = anterior mitral valve leaflet; AO = aorta; LA = left atrium; 1–4 = intercostal spaces 1–4. (From Feigenbaum H. Echocardiography. 3d ed. Philadelphia: Lea & Febiger, 1981. Reprinted with permission.)

if the target is moving away, it will decrease relative to the sound frequency transmitted to interrogate the target (carrier frequency). Thus analysis of the Doppler frequency shift allows determination of both the direction and the velocity of flow.

Three forms of Doppler interrogation are currently in clinical use: pulsed-wave (PW), color-flow (CF), and continuous-wave (CW) Doppler. Pulsed-wave Doppler allows sampling of flow patterns at specific sites within the two-dimensional cardiac image. The vascular structure of interest is imaged and, typically, a controlling roller ball is moved to place a sampling volume indicator on the image at a site of interest for flow analysis. The ultrasound instrument measures the distance of that site from the transducer, calculates the time necessary for the ultrasound to reach that site (determined by the velocity of ultrasound in tissue, 1540 cm/s). The frequency shifts displayed are limited to those occurring within the time window required for sound to travel from the transducer to the sampling site and back to the transducer (time-gating technique). This allows, for example, interrogation

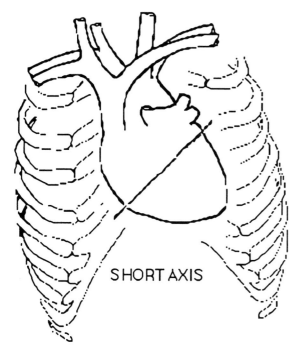

SHORT AXIS

Figure 4 Illustration of the short axis of the heart. (From: Feigenbaum H. Echocardiography. 3d ed. Philadelphia: Lea & Febiger, 1981. Reprinted with permission.)

of the left atrium above the mitral valve plane to determine whether retrograde systolic flow, diagnostic of mitral regurgitation, is present in the atrium.

Color Doppler is a modification of pulsed-wave Doppler. Sampling generally involves a wider imaging area, often including one or more cardiac chambers, within an operator-designated area of interest displayed on the two-dimensional image. The detected velocities are shown in the format of a color display superimposed on the two-dimensional image, flow toward the probe being coded in orange and flow away in blue, with the shades becoming brighter and lighter as the velocity and number, respectively, of red cells increase. This format allows rapid screening of abnormal flow patterns, which at times are quite localized and therefore both difficult and time-consuming to detect by pulsed-wave mapping alone.

Both pulsed and color Doppler imaging are limited by the delay imposed by the need to wait for the beam to reach the site or sites of interest, return, and be analyzed as described above. The highest frequency that can be resolved is equal to half the rate of interrogation that can be achieved at the sampling depth of interest—the Nyquist limit. This limitation on sampling frequency creates a technical problem known as "aliasing." In pulsed-wave Doppler, the inability to resolve frequencies beyond the Nyquist limit results in a "wrap-around" of the displayed frequencies, creating a band of unresolved frequencies that totally obliterate the frequency display. In color-flow Doppler, aliasing results in a wrap-around in colors displayed, so that oranges turn blue and, with higher velocities, back to orange, resulting in a mosaic display that can become quite confusing but that identifies areas of turbulence indicative of abnormal flow.

Since high velocities are present at areas of valvular or vascular stenosis, and since a simple mathematic relationship exists between the measured velocity and the pressure gradient across an obstruction (peak instantaneous pressure gradient $= 4$ [peak velocity]^2), it is important to overcome the Nyquist limit if accurate estimates of pressure gradient are to be made. This is accomplished by the use of continuous-wave Doppler techniques. Within a continuous-wave Doppler probe are two ultrasound elements whose field of interrogation is overlapped by the use of an acoustic lens. Thus one element constantly pulses ultrasound while the other constantly receives the reflected sound within the same area of interest. This enables the accurate measurement of very high frequencies extending well beyond the upper limits of velocities encountered clinically in areas of stenosis.

II. DIAGNOSTIC CONSIDERATIONS BASED ON THE PHYSICS OF ULTRASOUND

For two-dimensional and M-mode imaging the optimal study is obtained by imaging as perpendicularly as possible to the structure of interest. The resolution of the ultrasound image is a function of the wavelength of the sound beam used for interrogation. Transducers using higher frequencies have shorter wavelengths that can be reflected by smaller structures and provide superior resolution. However, these shorter wavelengths are better reflected by *all* acoustic interfaces, so that the ultrasound beam is rapidly attenuated by structures in the near field, including the chest wall itself. As a result, high-frequency transducers have a decreased penetration into tissue and are generally unable to reach the 10- to 20-cm depths needed for adult imaging. A compromise is made in adults by the use of 2.25- or 2.5-MHz transducers, with the occasional small individual or female patient being imaged by a 3.5-MHz probe. In children 3.5- or 5.0-MHz probes are used, and babies are routinely imaged with a 5.0-MHz probe. The markedly superior imaging provided by transesophageal echocardiography is largely due to two factors: proximity of the transducer to the structures being imaged and the ability to use a 5.0-MHz probe in adults.

For optimal Doppler studies imaging as parallel as possible to the blood flow pattern of interest is essential, because the accuracy of the flow velocity estimation is proportional to the cosine of the angle of incidence of the probe to the flow. Since the cosine of 30° is 0.866, attempts should be made to align the probe at an angle less than 30° to the flow pattern. Color-flow imaging demonstrates that flow patterns are often discordant to those that might be anticipated from anatomic considerations. This is particularly true in patients with deformed valves and associated regurgitant flow. The use of color Doppler facilitates more accurate alignment in some patients, but it has not been particularly helpful in the approach to aortic stenosis.

For any flow velocity the Doppler shift is directly proportional to the interrogating frequency. Thus for any given velocity of flow the Doppler shift will be greater for a 5-MHz probe than for a 2.25-MHz probe. In accordance with the limitations imposed by the Nyquist limit, the ability to resolve the Doppler shift will be greater for lower-frequency probes. Therefore, in contrast to anatomic imaging, low-frequency probes are preferable to high-frequency probes for Doppler studies. As a consequence, dedicated Doppler probes routinely use a carrier frequency of 1.9 or 2.0 MHz or lower. Despite the recent availability of steerable continuous-wave Doppler probes, higher-quality Doppler signals are often obtained using a nonimaging dedicated Doppler probe. These probes have a smaller "footprint," or contact surface, allowing better insertion both into intercostal spaces and into the suprasternal notches. They remain the standard for comprehensive Doppler assessment, particularly in aortic stenosis.

III. CARDIAC ULTRASOUND

The clinical application of ultrasound techniques is discussed in detail in Part III. The following is a brief outline of the general approach taken in obtaining cardiac ultrasound images using the techniques already described above. For additional information, the reader should consult a standard echocardiographic text.

A. Transthoracic Echocardiography

In general, the optimal initial patient position for transthoracic echocardiography, regardless of the ultrasound modality used, is the left lateral decubitus position with the subject's left hand behind the head so as to expose the left thorax more fully. A three-lead ECG channel is connected to the machine, and the gain and position are adjusted to provide an adequate tracing for the timing of the cardiac cycle. A commercially available acoustic gel is placed either on the chest or on the probe. The experienced echocardiographer will initially place the probe in thoracic positions as outlined below (Fig. 5), but will then freely use additional interrogation sites and patient positions in an attempt to locate optimal interrogation windows for the structure of interest. These may include positioning the patient in supine, right lateral decubitus, and/or sitting positions while placing the probe in standard left thoracic positions as well as in the right parasternal intercostal spaces and additional

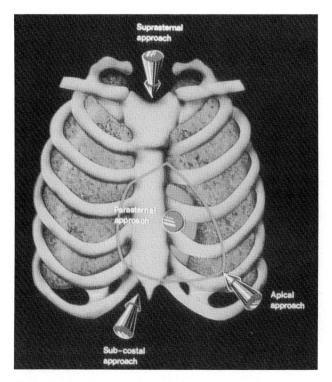

Figure 5 Echocardiographic approaches to the heart. (From: *An Introduction to Echocardiography*, 2nd Series, Unit 1: "Two Dimensional Echocardiography in the Normal Heart." Eds. Graham Leech and Joseph Kisslo, Medi-Cine Ltd., London, UK, 1981. Reprinted with permission.)

subcostal and suprasternal positions. Occasionally the presence of pleural fluid may provide additional imaging windows, including posterior thoracic approaches. In the latter situation care should be taken not to misinterpret a collapsed lung segment as a hilar mass, as a similar picture may occur with both.

1. M-Mode Techniques

If a dedicated M-mode probe is used, it is initially positioned in the third or fourth intercostal space 1–2 cm lateral to the sternum (Fig. 3). The position is adjusted until a site is located from which a high-quality mitral echocardiogram is obtained with the probe as perpendicular as possible to the chest wall. The probe is then angled superiorly and medially to obtain a recording of the aortic root and valve cusps and left atrium. It is then angled through the mitral valve inferolaterally to image the basal septal and posterior wall segments of the left ventricle and the right ventricle at a mitral substructure level immediately below the leaflet tips. A sweep from the aorta through the mitral plane to the left ventricular plane should be made (Fig. 6). In a correctly performed study the anterior aortic root and interventricular septum, the posterior aortic root and anterior mitral leaflet, and the posterior atrial wall and epicardial surface of the left ventricle are at three different but approximately equidistant depths from the chest wall. Measurements of cardiac dimensions and high-frequency motion of valves and chambers are best assessed using M-mode techniques, which have a higher sampling rate than two-dimensional real-time imaging. Current equipment provides two-dimensionally guided M-mode capability. A parasternal long-axis view of the left ventricle is obtained. The probe is rotated to a short-axis view (Fig. 4) and angled sequentially through the aortic valve, mitral valve, and mitral substructure planes with the

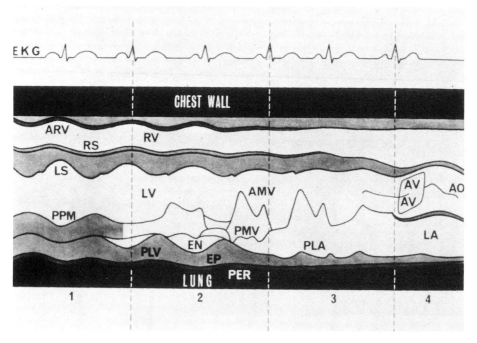

Figure 6 Sweep from the left ventricle to aorta and left atrium. (From: Feigenbaum H. Echocardiography. 3d ed. Philadelphia: Lea & Febiger, 1981. Reprinted with permission.)

selected M-mode transducer element positioned to bisect the chamber imaged. This technique provides the spatial orientation to allow acquisition of reproducible measurements.

2. Two-Dimensional Echocardiography

With the patient in the left lateral decubitus position, the probe is first positioned in the third or fourth intercostal space 1–2 cm lateral to the left sternal border and perpendicular to the chest wall to obtain a parasternal long-axis view of the heart. The basal structures and basal portions of the ventricles are visualized in this way (Fig. 7). The apex is not normally seen in a true parasternal long-axis plane.

The probe is then rotated 90° to obtain a short-axis view (Fig. 8). Angulation superiorly and medially will image the aorta, right and left atria, tricuspid valve, right ventricular outflow tract, and pulmonary artery. On occasion, slight inferolateral angulation and rotation of the probe will demonstrate the pulmonary artery bifurcation or left atrial appendage (Fig. 9). The probe is then angled inferiorly and laterally to sequentially image the mitral valve and left ventricular outflow tract, the mitral substructure and left ventricle in cross section, and, finally, the short axis of the left ventricle at the level of the papillary muscles.

The apical cardiac impulse is then palpated and the probe placed at the apical impulse or slightly superior and medial to it, in order to obtain apical views (Fig. 10). Apical views are essential for evaluation of ischemic disease, since the apex receives the most distal coronary blood flow and is at high risk for ischemic injury. The absence of apical and/or other segmental wall motion abnormality in a technically good-quality study (showing clear apical endocardial borders) essentially excludes transmural infarction. Regional wall motion abnormalities are commonly absent in subendocardial infarction. The two-dimensional echocardiographic technique is the preferred screening modality for the detection of potential cardiac embolic sources. It is our practice to use the transthoracic approach routinely and to consider the transesophageal approach only when the transthoracic study is not adequate to address the diagnostic question.

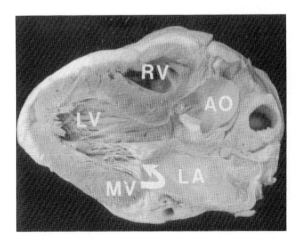

Figure 7 Anatomical section through the long axis—parasternal orientation. RV = right ventricle; LV = left ventricle; MV = mitral valve; LA = left atrium. (From: *An Introduction of Echocardiography*, 2nd Series, Unit 1: "Two Dimensional Echocardiography in the Normal Heart." Eds. Graham Leech and Joseph Kisslo, Medi-Cine Ltd., London, UK, 1981. Reprinted with permission.)

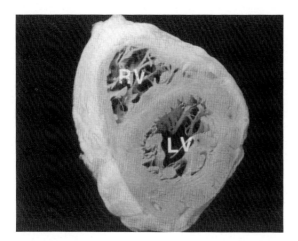

Figure 8 Anatomical section through the short axis at papillary muscle level—parasternal orientation. RV = right ventricle; LV = left ventricle. (From: *An Introduction to Echocardiography*, 2nd Series, Unit 1: "Two Dimensional Echocardiography in the Normal Heart." Eds. Graham Leech and Joseph Kisslo, Medi-Cine Ltd., London, UK, 1981. Reprinted with permission.)

3. Doppler Echocardiography

As discussed above, for optimal Doppler study the interrogating beam should be aligned as closely as possible parallel to the direction of the flow of interest. In general, the apical view is used for aortic, mitral, and tricuspid valve flow and the short-axis view at the aortic plane for the pulmonic valve. However, the use of nonparallel views is often diagnostically

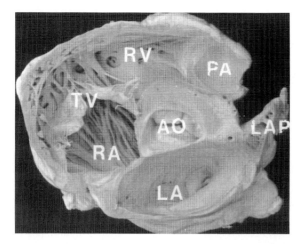

Figure 9 Anatomical section through the short axis at aortic valve level—parasternal orientation. RV = right ventricle; TV = tricuspid valve; RA = right atrium; AO = aorta; LA = left atrium; LAP = left atrial appendage; PA = pulmonary artery. (From: *An Introduction to Echocardiography*, 2nd Series, Unit 1: "Two Dimensional Echocardiography in the Normal Heart." Eds. Graham Leech and Joseph Kisslo, Medi-Cine Ltd., London, UK, 1981. Reprinted with permission.)

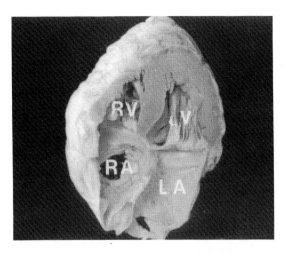

Figure 10 Anatomical section through the 4-chamber plane—apical orientation. RV = right ventricle; LV = left ventricle; RA = right atrium; L = left atrium. (From: *An Introduction to Echocardiography*, 2nd Series, Unit: "Two Dimensional Echocardiography in the Normal Heart." Eds. Graham Leech and Joseph Kisslo, Medi-Cine Ltd., London, UK, 1981. Reprinted with permission.)

useful as well. For example, the detection of a high-velocity aliased jet in the left ventricular outflow tract in diastole, identified by pulsed-wave or color-flow Doppler, implies the presence of aortic insufficiency. Furthermore, accurate measurement of the velocity of regurgitant jets is generally less important than is the determination of the area of distribution of the jet in the regurgitant chamber. These jets are occasionally best interrogated from a nonparallel view. Pulsed or color-flow Doppler mapping of the chamber to determine the area of distribution of the aliased regurgitant flow can be more useful than parallel velocity interrogation.

B. Transesophageal Echocardiography

Transesophageal echocardiographic techniques evolved over the course of the last decade when first M-mode (in 1976) (1), then two-dimensional (1981), and finally color Doppler phased-array (1988) (2) capabilities were successfully incorporated into this instrumentation. After initial use during open heart surgery for the evaluation of intraoperative ischemia and for assessment of the adequacy of heart valve repair and replacement, diagnostic outpatient use has been growing in the United States in response to the European experience. The first performance of the technique in outpatients in the United States was probably by Ezekowitz et al. (3) at the University of Oklahoma in 1981. The transesophageal technique takes advantage of the close anatomic relationship of the esophagus to the heart and aorta (Fig. 11).

In essence the transesophageal echocardiographic probe is a gastroscope modified by replacing the fiberoptic elements with an ultrasound probe (Fig. 12). Probe design specifics vary by manufacturer. The initial single-plane probes allowed visualization in the horizontal plane; later probes (biplanar) include a second vertical imaging plane, and more recently, totally rotatable (multiplanar) probes are commercially available that permit a much more comprehensive analysis. The proximity of the probe to the structures imaged permits the

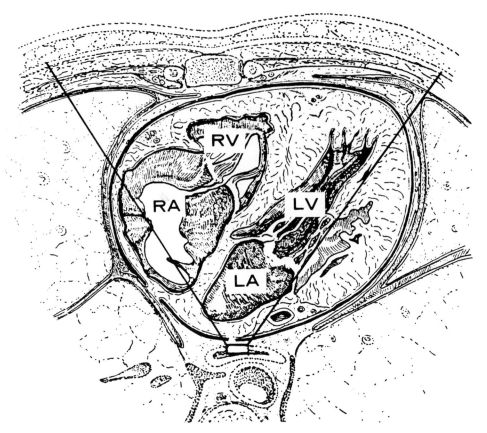

Figure 11 Transesophageal probe in the esophagus showing close proximity to left atrium (LA). LV = left ventricle; RA = right atrium; RV = right ventricle.

use of a high-frequency 3.5- to 7.5-MHz probe (providing a short wavelength and higher resolution), with 5MHz being the standard. Most probes have color Doppler capability, and both biplanar and multiplanar probes have steerable continuous-wave Doppler capability as well. The ability to use a higher-frequency probe in close proximity to the structures of diagnostic interest permits superior imaging. As currently configured, the single-plane and biplanar systems have limitations related to the restricted mobility of the probe in the esophagus. This limitation is largely obviated by the multiplanar probe. However, the left atrial appendage is generally quite well seen, as is the mitral valve and its substructure as well as the interatrial septum, the fossa ovalis, both atria, (upper) pulmonic veins, the tricuspid valve, pulmonary arteries, and the septum and posterior left ventricular walls. Anteflexion of the probe allows visualization of the aortic valve in the short axis. A transgastric short-axis view provides visualization of the circumference of the left ventricle and is commonly used for intraoperative monitoring of cardiac function (Fig. 13). Using a single plane, the apex of the heart is the least well seen structure, and the pulmonic valve is often difficult to image. Both areas are generally well seen with vertical (biplanar) imaging. The ascending aorta, the aortic arch in the transverse section, and the descending aorta are seen as well as they can be with any other currently available technology. The presence of

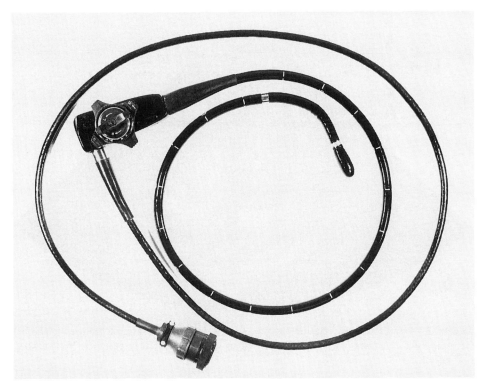

Figure 12 Modified gastroscope, prototype of early transesophageal probe, made for Dr. Ezekowitz by Varian Co. in 1980.

atheromata in the aorta is readily detected. Because of its superior resolution and the proximity of the probe to basal cardiac structures and the aorta, transesophageal echocardiography has emerged as an excellent imaging modality for the determination of an intracardiac source of thrombus.

A cardiologist wishing to perform transesophageal echocardiography must first be fully trained as an echocardiographer, preferably with at least 6 months of dedicated hands-on experience. Training should include comprehensive familiarization with the indications for and interpretation and recording of M-mode, two-dimensional Doppler, and color-flow Dopper echocardiographic techniques, all of which are generally utilized during the transesophageal examination. Performance of transesophageal studies require initial experience with the blind passage of an endoscope under the tutelage of either a gastroenterologist or a trained cardiologist. A minimum of 40 passages before unsupervised passage of the probe has been suggested (2).

Critical to the performance of a study, and often the most time-consuming portion of the procedure, is adequate preparation of the patient. Patients generally have considerable anxiety about swallowing the probe. Older patients tend to be more accepting of the procedure and can often undergo the procedure with topical oropharyngeal anesthesia alone. Greater acceptance of the procedure may be a function of an age-related reduction in the intensity of the gag reflex. Younger patients are more likely to require additional short-acting intravenous anesthesia with or without ancillary narcotics. Appropriate physiological

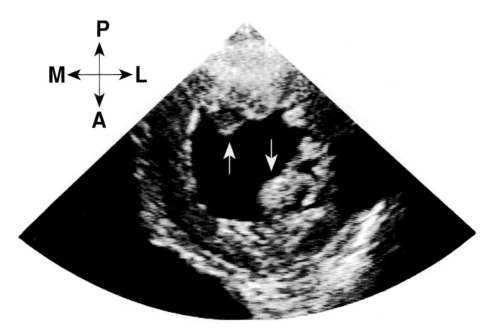

Figure 13 Transesophageal echo of the left ventricle in short axis as seen from an anteflexed transgastric view. Arrows indicate papillary muscles. A = anterior; P = posterior; M = medial; L = lateral.

monitoring of blood pressure and oxygen saturation, nasal oxygen, suction equipment, and cardiopulmonary resuscitation equipment must also be immediately available.

The patient is placed in the left lateral decubitus position. The neck is flexed to facilitate passing the probe beyond the trachea into the esophagus. There are two general approaches to introduction after topical anesthesia has been achieved: first, the use of two fingers to guide the probe while displacing the tongue anteriorly, and second, the initial introduction of a bite guard before insertion with either blind passage thereafter or use of a single finger, introduced outside the guard, to provide additional guidance. The latter is the preferred initial approach in a patient with a small oropharynx.

The major discomfort associated with the procedure occurs at the zone of transition from striated to smooth muscle, 18–20 cm from the incisors, at the level of the cricopharyngeus muscle. At this position the probe tip will often elicit a gag response despite determined efforts at topical anesthesia. We have found the use of the disposable flexible spray tip manufactured by Astra to be particularly useful in anesthetizing this area. If the patient is asked to swallow when the probe tip reaches about 18 cm, and/or the patient can voluntarily suppress the urge to gag, the probe will pass readily into the esophagus. The gag reflex may remain intact at this depth even with deeper levels of sedation. We have found that supplemental meperidine has a potent effect in relieving anxiety in patients with a persistently active gag reflex. Once the probe is passed beyond 20 cm the patient is asked to concentrate on taking deep slow breaths as a means of focusing attention away from the probe. In general, patients become calm at this point and will feel no significant further discomfort. A dental sucker attached to a source of low-intensity intermittent suction may be a helpful adjunct for an occasional patient with excessive salivation. Imaging is then begun. Images are recorded on a videotape recorder throughout the procedure. Most imaging is performed at depths of 25–40 cm from the incisors. The aortic arch lies in a plane close to the cricopharyngeal region and should be imaged last, just before completion of the study, as gagging is again more likely at this position.

A recent report from a European study of 10,419 transesophageal echocardiographic examinations showed a remarkable safety record. Ten clinically significant complications occurred. A single death related to the procedure was reported, occurring when an undiagnosed pulmonary cancer that had invaded the esophagus was traumatized, causing severe hemorrhage during the procedure. The patient died during palliative surgery unrelated to the transesophageal study (4).

Imaging for specific entities with embolic potential is discussed in further detail in Chapters 12, 13, and 14.

IV. PERIPHERAL ULTRASOUND

Each vascular laboratory should have standard imaging protocols for Doppler color-flow imaging (DCFI) that have been validated with angiography or venography to insure accuracy and reproducibility of the examination. Doppler color-flow imaging combines high-resolution real-time imaging with qualitative real-time evaluation of blood flow, displayed as a color flow on an anatomic image, and quantitative assessment of blood flow (direction and velocity) by duplex Doppler or time-velocity analyses (Fig. 14). Duplex Doppler combines B-mode imaging and pulsed Doppler ultrasound. Color Doppler equipment with high-frequency transducers (5, 7.5, or 10 MHz) should be utilized.

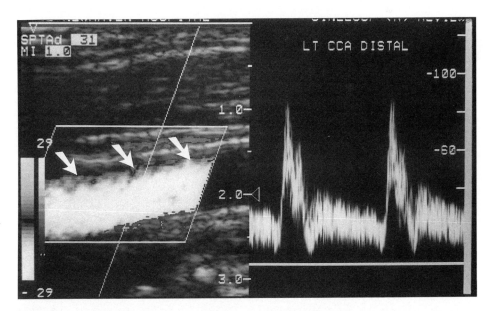

Figure 14 Longitudinal Doppler color-flow imaging demonstrates high-resolution gray-scale image of the common carotid artery with nondisturbed color flow (arrow) displayed in black and white and Doppler-measured absolute velocities. Doppler indicates low-impedance flow of a normal common carotid artery.

A. Carotid Arteries

For the evaluation of the carotid arteries, the patient is placed in a supine position with the head turned away from the side to be examined. The patient is asked to lower the ipsilateral shoulder to enhance exposure of the neck. The common carotid artery (CCA) examination begins at the CCA/subclavian artery bifurcation and extends to the carotid bifurcation, an area predisposed to atherosclerosis, and to the proximal internal carotid artery (ICA) and external carotid artery (ECA). The examination is usually recorded on videotape and/or hard copy film.

The first objective is to define anatomy. The ICA is directed posterolaterally, while the ECA is directed anteromedially. The ICA is larger than the ECA and does not have extracranial branches. The ICA is a low-impedance (high diastolic flow) system (Fig. 15), while the ECA is a high-impedance (relatively low diastolic flow) system (Fig. 16). Approximately 70% of the CCA flow to the head is directed to the ICA. The CCA is a low-impedance system, similar to the ICA (Fig. 15). The examination must be performed both longitudinally and transversely. Plaque should be defined as to its location, size, and imaging characteristics (5–8), i.e., whether it is homogeneous or heterogeneous. Plaque is categorized according to its internal echocardiographic characteristics as hypoechoic, isoechoic, or hyperechoic. Calcification in the plaque creates acoustic shadowing, which may obscure the vessel lumen. The plaque surface may appear smooth, irregular, or ulcerated. Intraplaque hemorrhages, which appear as hypoechoic, heterogeneous plaque, are more common in symptomatic patients. Imperato et al. (6) reported that a high percentage of symptomatic patients, who had stenoses, also had intraplaque hemorrhage. The recognition of ulceration is important because of the associated higher incidence of embolization (9,10). Bassiouny et al. (11) reported that large plaques are more likely to be

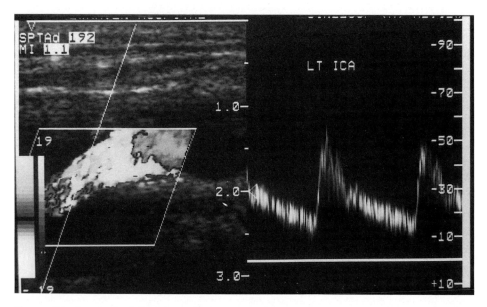

Figure 15 Longitudinal Doppler color-flow imaging (displayed in black and white) of normal internal carotid artery, with absolute velocities measured by pulse-wave Doppler. Approximately 70% of common carotid artery flow is to the low-impedance internal carotid artery.

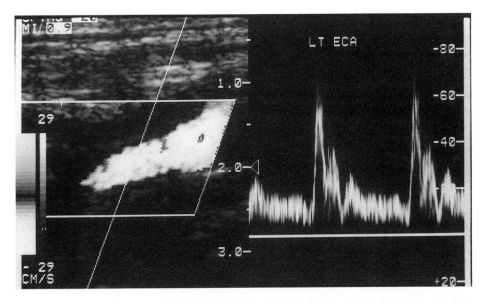

Figure 16 Longitudinal Doppler color-flow imaging (displayed in black and white) of the relatively high-resistance external carotid artery. Note the lower diastolic flow when compared to the common carotid artery (Fig. 14) and internal carotid artery (Fig. 15).

ulcerated. An assessment of the degree of stenosis should be made using gray-scale images (Fig. 17).

Characterization of flow patterns is achieved with color-flow imaging (12–14). Normal CCA and ICA flow is continuous for constant brain perfusion. The high-resistance ECA has reduced flow in diastole. With mild stenosis, swirling or turbulent flow is noted distal to the stenosis. With severe stenosis, the turbulent jet becomes elongated and chaotic (Figs. 18a and 18b). Significant stenoses are recognized by marked turbulence, which is seen even when extensive calcified plaque limits imaging of the stenotic area. When total occlusions are present, flow is absent distal to the occlusion (Figs. 19a and 19b).

Color flow is qualitative, whereas the Doppler analysis is quantitative (15–19). The point of greatest hemodynamic changes is identified by color flow and quantified by conventional Doppler. A peak systolic velocity (PSV) of 120 cm/s or greater corresponds to 50% stenosis. Stenoses of less than 50% are not considered hemodynamically significant. Velocities between 120 and 210 cm/s correspond to stenosis of 50–80% (Fig. 20). Stenoses of more than 80% typically have velocities greater than 220 cm/s. Velocities greater than 250 cm/s correlate with high-grade stenoses of more than 90% (Fig. 21). When the PSV of the ICA is 120 cm/s, the PSV of the CCA is typically no greater than 60 cm/s, creating a 2:1 ratio. The use of this ratio has proved invaluable, particularly in cases of low cardiac output, where the PSV within the lumen of the ICA may be 100 cm/s, while the CCA may be only 30 cm/s. The ratio would suggest a 50% stenosis, even though an absolute PSV of 120 cm/s in the ICA was not obtained. This ratio is also useful when the ICA is obstructed unilaterally. The nonoccluded ICA carries the entire flow to the brain. A PSV ratio of the ICA to the CCA of more than 2:1 represents a 50% stenosis or greater. High-impedance time-velocity Doppler waveforms of the CCA may signify severe stenosis or occlusion of the ICA. The waveforms of both CCAs should be compared. Low PSV may signify cardiac disease.

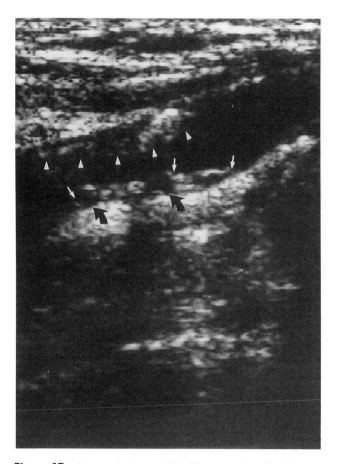

Figure 17 Gray-scale image identifies smooth-walled heterogenous plaque (arrowheads) and irregular-walled heterogeneous plaque (white arrows). Hypoechoic areas represent intraplaque hemorrhage or ulceration (in curved black arrows). The stenosis is greater than 50%.

At the conclusion of the carotid artery study, the final interpretation should correlate anatomical imaging with color-flow and conventional Doppler assessment (Figs. 22a–d).

As might be expected, there are pitfalls in the evaluation of the carotid vessels (20). Clearly study quality is the primary determinant of its utility. The most common error made clinically is the misidentification of the ICA and ECA. It is important to note that the ICA is posteriorly directed, has no extracranial branches, and has low-impedance flow. Without color-flow imaging, hypoechoic occlusive plaque within the ICA may be missed. Exclusive reliance on color-flow imaging to assess degrees of narrowing can provide misinformation, because plaques can attenuate the signal and result in underestimation of the degree of stenosis. In addition, color-flow imaging has a "ballooning effect" that may make the lumen appear larger (Figs. 22a, 18b).

Doppler color-flow imaging complements angiography. Angiography is an invasive test, carrying a definite morbidity and mortality. Stenotic lesions are accurately identified when at least two views are obtained. Doppler color-flow imaging is noninvasive and provides assessment of lumen narrowing and lumen surface quality and characterization of the plaque. It provides information comparable to that obtained by angiography with

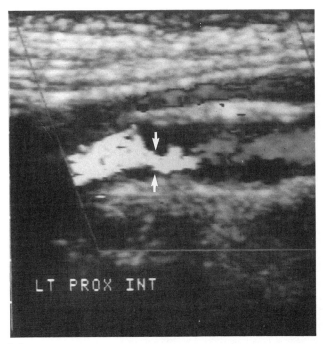

(a)

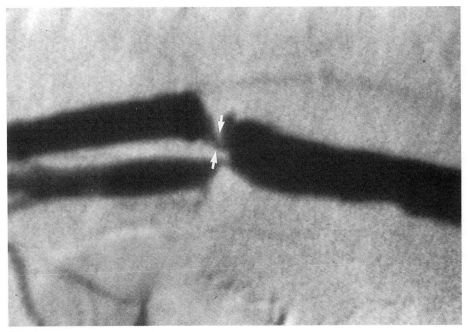

(b)

Figure 18 (a) Longitudinal image of the carotid bifurcation with a severe stenosis (arrows) of the internal carotid artery (> 80%) with chaotic flow. Color flow (displayed in black and white) makes the lumen appear wider than the angiogram (Fig. 18b), demonstrating the "ballooning effect." (b) Corresponding angiogram confirms high-grade stenosis (arrows) of the internal carotid artery.

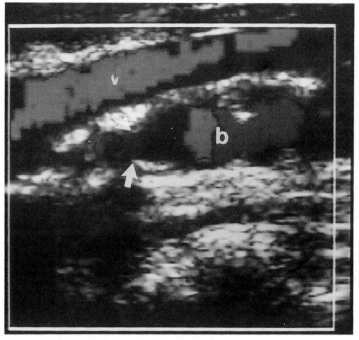

(A)

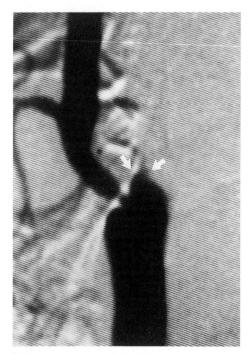

(B)

Figure 19   (A) Longitudinal flow image of the (common) carotid bulb (b) and internal jugular vein
(V). There is no flow in the internal carotid artery (arrows), which is totally occluded. (B) Angiogram
confirms complete occlusion of the internal carotid artery (arrows).

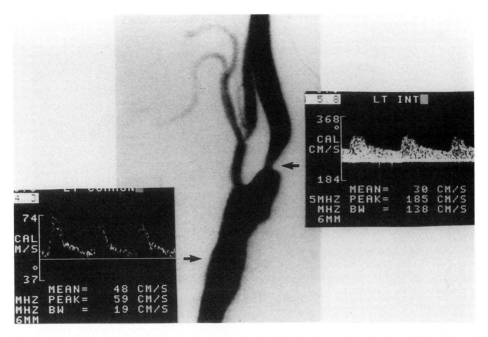

Figure 20 Montage of pulsed-wave determined velocities (peak systolic velocity = 185 cm/s) and carotid angiogram demonstrates a 50–80% stenosis.

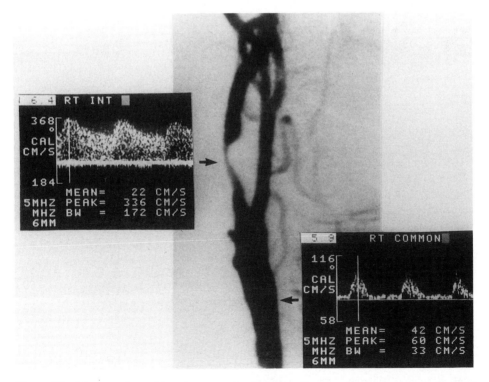

Figure 21 Montage of carotid angiogram and pulsed-wave Doppler of a severe stenosis (> 90%) of the internal carotid artery, with increased peak systolic velocities of 336 cm/s.

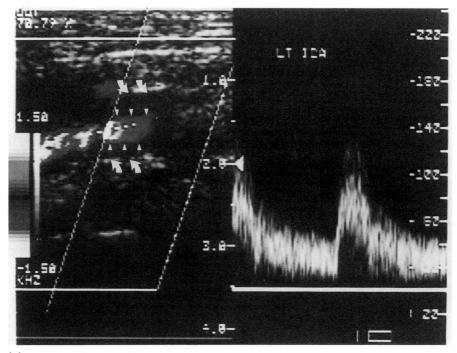

(a)

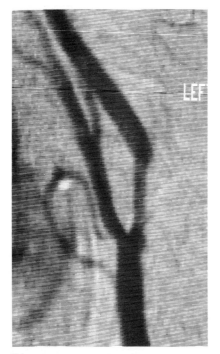

(b)

Figure 22   (a) Doppler color-flow image (displayed in black and white) of a 50% narrowing of the left internal carotid artery lumen (small arrowheads) compared with the outer wall of the vessel (curved arrows). Turbulent color flow is present. Peak systolic velocity of 140 cm/s is consistent with a 50–80%

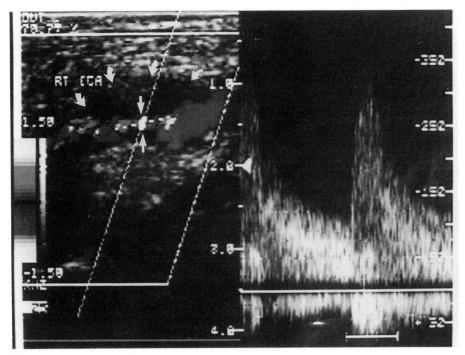

(c)

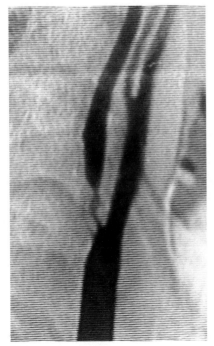

(d)

stenosis. (b) Angiogram verifies a 50–80% stenosis. (c) Doppler color-flow images of a narrowed lumen of the right internal carotid artery (straight arrows) at the interrogation site. Turbulent flow is present. Curved arrows mark a hypoechoic plaque. Doppler peak systolic velocities of 350 cm/s are consistent with a >90% stenosis. (d) Angiogram verifies severe stenosis.

regard to assessment of the extent of disease at the carotid bifurcation. Angiography is the test of choice in the evaluation of intracerebral vessels. Doppler color-flow imaging provides greater information regarding the composition of the plaque and the possible complications, such as intraplaque hemorrhage (Fig. 22). Both procedures are highly accurate in evaluating the severity of disease, but angiography remains the "gold standard."

B. Deep Venous Thrombosis of the Lower Extremity

Evaluation of the deep veins of the lower extremity involves defining both anatomy and flow (21–28). Evaluation of patients suspected of acute deep venous thrombosis (DVT) requires a high-resolution linear-array (5, 7.5, and 10 MHz) transducer. Phased-array (2.25 MHz) and curved-array (3.5 MHz) transducers are used in obese patients. The lowest possible pulse repetition frequency should be used because of the low velocities of venous blood. Color Doppler gain threshold settings should be maximized, and wall filters should be set at their lowest level to improve sensitivity.

The deep veins examined as part of a routine evaluation are the common femoral vein (CFV), the superficial femoral vein (SFV), and the popliteal vein. The proximal trifurcation of the tibial and peroneal trunks should also be assessed (Figs. 23a and 23b). The patient is scanned in the supine position for evaluation of the CFV and SFV. The popliteal vein is scanned with the patient in the decubitus position with a slight bend of the knee or in a prone position with the knee slightly bent and supported at the ankle. In patients unable to assume a prone or decutibus position, the popliteal vein is scanned with the knee bent and supported laterally.

Longitudinal color-flow examination allows evaluation of flow patterns. However, the transverse examination is the most useful. The veins are scanned transversely, with moderate compression of the vein at approximately 1-cm intervals. Blood flow, depicted by the color format, should fill the entirety of the lumen. The femoral, superficial femoral, and popliteal arteries should all be visualized to ensure that anatomical errors are minimized (Figs. 24a and 24b). A major effort should be made to define the proximal extent of the thrombus. Interior vena cava and common iliac vein thrombosis should be explored proximally if the CFV is involved. This is particularly important in patients with anticipated inferior vena cava filter replacement.

Inability to compress the vein completely (Figs. 25a and 25b), the direct visualization of intraluminal thrombus (Figs. 26a and 26b), failure to augment flow with calf compression, and lack of spontaneous flow have been used as criteria for the diagnosis of DVT. Noncompressibility is the most important of these criteria, with the others providing complementary information (23,24). When interpreting an examination the morphologic, hemodynamic, and Doppler information must be correlated. If the examination is technically limited or if information is not concordant, a venogram may be necessary.

The time-velocity profile in the Doppler examination can substitute for the color format (29). In a normal patient, there are phasic changes in venous flow as a result of cardiorespiratory effects. A nonphasic pattern may indicate a proximal thrombosis, external compression, or cardiac disease (Figs. 27a and 27b).

The saphenofemoral junction must be evaluated, as superficial venous thrombosis may propagate into the deep system. The distal SFV in the adductor canal requires special attention because it is often difficult to compress the vein in this region (30). Minimal pressure behind the knee with the nonscanning hand displaces the SFV anteriorly, where it can be compressed. The complementary criteria discussed above are of value in this location, with visualizing of the clot and flow patterns using the "color mode" after manual compression of the calf being a particularly useful adjunct.

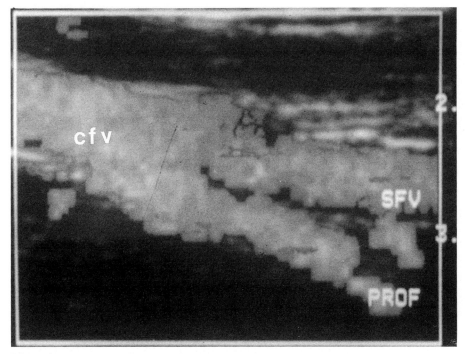

(a)

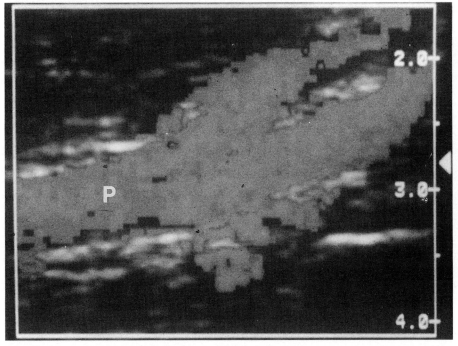

(b)

Figure 23 (a) Longitudinal image of normal common femoral vein (cfv), superficial femoral vein (SFV) and profunda femoris vein (PROF). (b) Longitudinal image of normal common femoral vein and trifurcation of the popliteal vein (P).

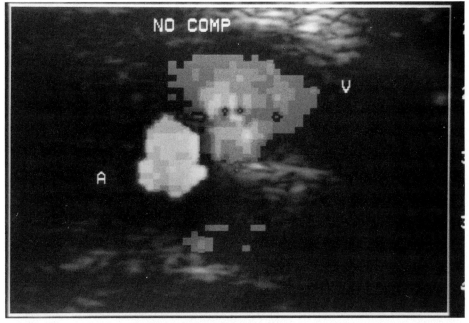

(a)

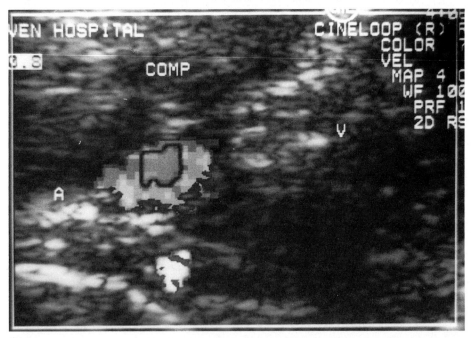

(b)

Figure 24   (a) Transverse image of common femoral vein (V) and artery (A). No compression was applied. (b) Transverse image of common femoral vein (V) and artery (A) with compression applied. There is total obliteration of the venous lumen indicating absence of thrombus.

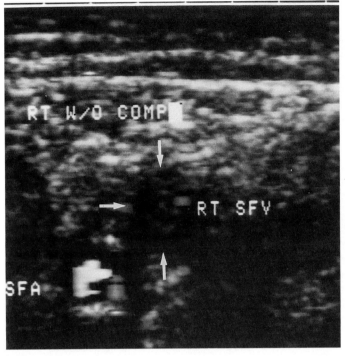

(a)

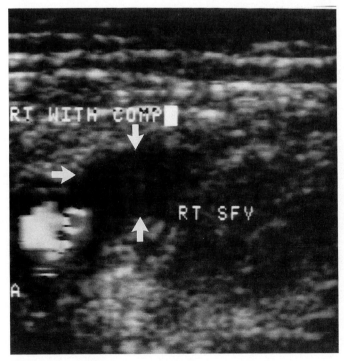

(b)

Figure 25 Transverse image of common femoral vein demonstrates an occlusive superficial vein thrombosis (arrows), (a) without and (b) with compression.

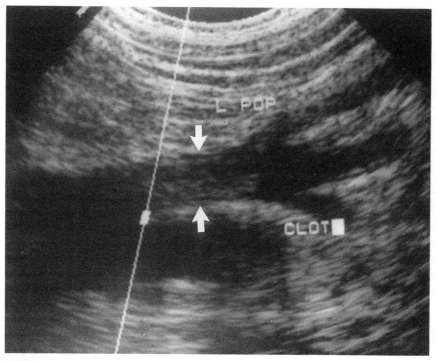

(a)

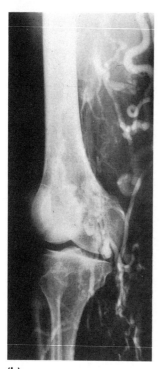

(b)

Figure 26   (a) Longitudinal image of echogenic occlusive thrombus (arrows) in the popliteal vein. (b) Venogram confirms occlusion of deep venous system with collaterals.

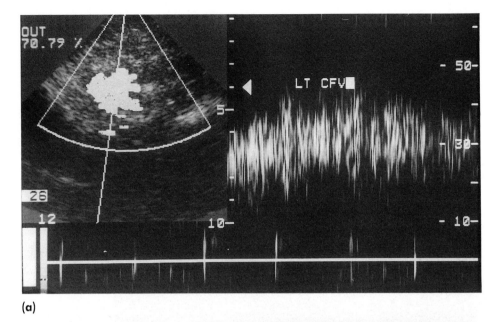

(a)

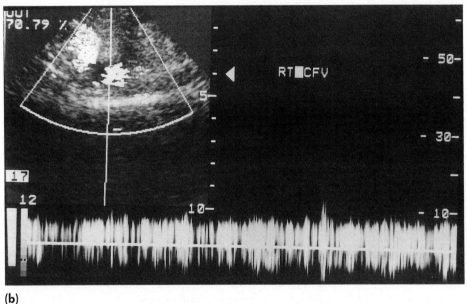

(b)

Figure 27 (a) Normal Doppler derived velocities from asymptomatic left common femoral veins with normal phasic variation. (b) Abnormal right common femoral vein velocity profile with loss of phasic changes in a patient with an ovarian mass compressing the right iliac vein.

Calf veins can usually be identified at the trifurcation and, with much more difficulty, distally (31). The portions within the muscles of the calf are not easily scanned. At our institution calf veins are not scanned routinely. Serial studies can be performed to document progression of thrombus into the popliteal vein.

It is difficult to differentiate acute thrombus from subacute or chronic thrombus (32,33). In each case the vein is noncompressible. Echogenicity of the clot has not proved to be of

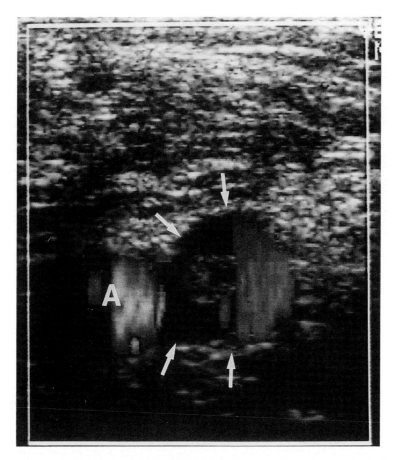

Figure 28   Transverse common femoral vein of a nonocclusive popliteal vein thrombosis (arrows). Adjacent is the popliteal artery (A).

value in differentiating old from new clot. If the vein appears dilated the thrombus is likely to be acute. Acute soft thrombus may be deformable. Chronic thrombi are firm and more difficult to deform. Platelet scanning may distinguish acute from chronic thrombus.

The major technical pitfalls are inexperience and nonfamiliarity with venous anatomy (29). Color flow has been helpful in the rapid assessment of patients with suspected venous thrombosis (Fig. 28). Compressibility is the most reliable parameter for assessment of venous thrombosis and can be achieved without color-flow capabilities. The adductor canal remains the major area of error.

Doppler color-flow imaging has been proved highly accurate in the evaluation of lower extremity DVT and has virtually replaced venography at many institutions in the diagnosis of lower extremity DVT (21,28,34).

V.   SUMMARY

Ultrasound has wide application in the study of both cardiac and peripheral arterial and venous disease. To date, the use of ultrasound for medical imaging is without known biologic adverse effects. In general, the objectives of the ultrasound examination are to define anatomy and characterize blood flow patterns and velocities. By so doing, it is possible to identify disease processes that are associated with embolic potential in the heart and also identify atherosclerotic disease in the aortic arch and carotid vessels. For the diagnosis of venous disease, it is particularly accurate for proximal vein thrombosis.

REFERENCES

1. Frazin L, Talano JV, Stephanides L, Loeb HS, Kopel L, Gunnar RM. Esophageal echocardiography. Circulation 1976; 54:102–108.
2. Lancee CT, deJong N, Bom N. Design and construction of an esophageal phased array probe. Med Prog Technol 1988; 13:139.
3. Ezekowitz MD, Wilson DA, Smith EO, Kanaly PJ, Parker DE. Two dimensional echocardiography and indium-111 platelet scintigraphy in the diagnosis of left ventricular thrombi—competitive or complementary. In: Rijsterburgh H, ed. Echocardiography. Martinus Nijhoff, 1981:75–79.
4. Daniel WG, Erbel R, Kasper W, et al. Safety of transesophageal echocardiography: a multicenter survey of 10,419 examinations. Circulation 1991; 83:817–21.
5. Bluth EI, Kay D, Merritt CRB, et al. Sonographic characterization of carotid plaque: detection of hemorrhage. AJNR 1986; 7:311–5.
6. Imparato AM, Riles TS, Gorstein F. The carotid bifurcation plaque: pathologic findings associated with cerebral ischemia. Stroke 1979; 10:238–45.
7. Lusby RJ, Ferrell LD, Ehrenfeld WK, Stoney RJ, Wylie EJ. Carotid plaque hemorrhage: its role in production of cerebral ischemia. Arch Surg 1982; 117:1479–88.
8. Imperato AM, Riles TS, Mintzer R, Bauman FG. The importance of hemorrhage in the relationship between gross morphologic characteristics and cerebral symptoms in 376 carotid artery plaques. Ann Surg 1983; 197:195–203.
9. O'Leary DH, Holen J, Ricotta JJ, Roe S, Schenk EA. Carotid bifurcation disease: prediction of ulceration with B-mode ultrasound. Radiology 1987; 162:523–5.
10. Bluth EI, McVay LV, Merritt CRB, Sullivan MA. The identification of ulcerative plaque with high-resolution duplex carotid scanning. J Ultrasound Med 1988; 7:73–6.
11. Bassiouny HS, Davis H, Massawa N, Gewertz BL, Glagov S, Zarins CK. Critical carotid stenoses: morphological and chemical similarity between symptomatic and asymptomatic plaques. J Vasc Surg 1989; 9:202–12.
12. Polak JF, Dobkin GR, O'Leary DH, Wang AM, Cutler SS. Internal carotid artery stenosis: accuracy and reproductibility of color-Doppler-assisted duplex imaging. Radiology 1989; 173: 793–8.
13. Merritt CRB. Doppler color flow imaging. J Clin Ultrasound 1987; 15:591–7.
14. Middleton WD, Foley WD, Lawson TL. Color-flow Doppler imaging of carotid artery abnormalities. AJR 1988; 150:419–25.
15. Blackshear WM, Phillips DJ, Chikos PM, Harley JD, Thiele BL, Strandness DE. Carotid artery velocity patterns in normal and stenotic vessels. Stroke 1980; 154:385–91.
16. Garth KE, Carroll BA, Sommer FG, Oppenheimer DA. Duplex ultrasound scanning of the carotid arteries with velocity spectrum analysis. Radiology 1983; 147:823–7.
17. Carroll BA. Carotid sonography. Radiology 1991; 178:303–13.
18. Nicholls SC, Strandness DE. Noninvasive diagnosis of cerebrovascular insufficiency. Int Surg 1984; 69:199–206.
19. Taylor D, Strandness DE. Carotid artery duplex scanning. J Clin Ultrasound 1987; 15: 605–13.
20. Zwiebel WJ, Crummy AB. Sources of error in Doppler diagnosis of carotid occlusive disease. AJR 1981; 137:1–12.
21. Foley WD, Middleton WD, Lawson TL, Erickson S, Quiroz FA, Macrander S. Color Doppler ultrasound imaging of lower extremity venous disease. AJR 1989; 152:371–6.

22. Appelman PT, De Jong TE, Lampmann LE. Deep venous thrombosis of the leg: US findings. Radiology 1987; 163:743–6.

23. Cronan JJ, Dorfman GS, Scola FH, Schepps B, Alexander J. Deep venous thrombosis: US assessment using vein compression. Radiology 1987; 162:191–4.

24. Cronan JJ, Dorfman GS, Grusmark J. Lower extremity deep venous thrombosis: further experience with and refinements of US assessment. Radiology 1988; 168:101–7.

25. Raghavendra BN, Rosen RB, Lam S, Riles T, Horii SC. Deep venous thrombosis: detection by high-resolution real-time ultrasonography. Radiology 1984; 152:789–93.

26. Killewich LA, Bedford GR, Beach KW, Strandness DE. Diagnosis of deep venous thrombosis: a prospective study comparing duplex scanning to contrast venography. Circulation 1989; 79: 810–4.

27. Killewich LA, et al. Duplex scanning in the diagnosis of deep venous thrombosis: limitations and methods for improving diagnostic accuracy. Dyn Cardiovasc Imag 1989; 2:33–8.

28. Rose SC, Zwibel WJ, Nelson BD, Priest DL, Knighton RA, Brown JW, Lawrence PF, Stults BM, Reading JC, Miller FJ. Symptomatic lower extremity deep venous thrombosis: accuracy limitations and role of color duplex flow imaging in diagnosis. Radiology 1990; 175:639–44.

29. Moneta GL, et al. Duplex ultrasound assessment of venous diameters, peak velocities and flow patterns. J Vasc Surg 1988; 8:286–91.

30. Wright DJ, Shepard AD, McPharlin M, Ernst CB. Pitfalls in lower extremity venous duplex scanning. J Vasc Surg 1990; 11:657–79.

31. Polak JF, Cutler SS, O'Leary DH. Deep veins of the calf: assessment with color Doppler flow imaging. Radiology 1989; 171:481–5.

32. Murphy TP, Cronan JJ. Evolution of deep venous thrombosis: a prospective evaluation with US. Radiology 1990; 177:543–8.

33. Killewich LA, Bedford GR, Beach KW, Strandness DE. Spontaneous lysis of deep venous thrombi. J Vasc Surg 1990; 11:62–9.

34. Vaccaro JP, Cronan JJ, Dorfman GS. Outcome analysis of patients with normal compression US examinations. Radiology 1990; 175:645–9.

Radionuclide-Based Imaging Techniques for Thrombus Detection

Michael D. Ezekowitz
Yale University School of Medicine, West Haven Veterans Affairs, and Cardiovascular Thrombosis Research Laboratory, New Haven, Connecticut

Holley M. Dey
Yale University School of Medicine and West Haven Veterans Affairs, New Haven, Connecticut

Mathew L. Thakur
Thomas Jefferson University Hospital, Philadelphia, Pennsylvania

I. HISTORIC PERSPECTIVE

Developing and evaluating thrombus imaging agents has been a major challenge in the field of nuclear medicine for more than a quarter of a century. This chapter will cover successful agents and will include a discussion of promising agents currently under evaluation (1–4). The tempo and direction of the field is best illustrated by the development of fibrinogen, platelet, and antibody-labeling techniques.

The earliest radionuclide technique developed for detecting thrombosis used ^{125}I fibrinogen for detection of venous thrombosis in the legs (5,6). This test was a nonimaging, count-based technique. For optimal diagnostic accuracy, monitoring occurred over several days, making the technique slow and time-consuming. The test required the intravenous injection of ^{125}I fibrinogen. Initially, there was a significant risk of inducing hepatitis and/or allergic/anaphylactic reactions (7,8). Because of careful selection of plasma donors, no cases of hepatitis or any other adverse reactions were reported after 1984. The use of ^{123}I, an agent suitable for imaging, was considered impractical because of its short half-life (13.3 h) and the lack of a steady commercial supply, particularly in times of emergency. Despite its disadvantages, ^{125}I fibrinogen, with its 92% sensitivity and 87% specificity for detecting distal (calf) venous thrombi, was used extensively for two decades. This agent is no longer commercially available in the United States.

There has been interest in platelet labeling for over 30 years. This technique relies on the ability to tag platelets without altering their physiological function. In the early evolution of this technology, several radioactive compounds have been used as platelet labels for the study of platelet kinetics (9–14). None of these was entirely satisfactory as a physiological label, and none was suitable for imaging. In 1975, an expert panel on diagnostic applications of radioisotopes recommended that ^{51}Cr be considered the only satisfactory agent for platelet labeling and the study of platelet kinetics in humans (15). Chromium 51, however, has significant limitations. Only 10% of the emissions are useful gamma photons. Also, the half-life of 27.8 days is long in comparison with the survival of platelets (8–10 days). Thus, patients are exposed to a significant amount of nonuseful radiation. Additionally, the physical characteristics of the radionuclide make it unsuitable for imaging studies, and the low labeling efficiency necessitates the acquisition of large volumes of blood to harvest a sufficient number of platelets for labeling. This last factor precludes its use in seriously ill or hemodynamically compromised patients.

McAfee and Thakur, working at Hammersmith Hospital in London, first chelated indium 111 with the 8-hydroxyquinoline complex and obviated many of the difficulties that are associated with ^{51}Cr–labeled platelets (16). Indium 111 is a cyclotron-produced isotope with a short half-life (2.8 days) and gamma photon energies of 173 and 247 keV, with gamma yields of 84% and 94%, respectively. These physical characteristics allow the study of platelet kinetics (17–20) and, most important, also allow the imaging of platelet deposition using standard camera systems (21–25). There is evidence that ^{111}In disturbs the in vivo behavior of platelets very little (16;26–31). Furthermore, successful labeling requires platelets derived from only 26–43 ml of blood, thus allowing study in seriously ill patients. In vitro experiments have shown that the ^{111}In 8-hydroxyquinoline label is complexed to soluble proteins within the platelet cytosol (32,33) and that minimal release of ^{111}In from human platelets occurs during aggregation induced with collagen (16,31,32,34,35), adenosine diphosphate (32,35,36), epinephrine (34), and thrombin (32,34,35) or with storage (34,37). "Tagged" platelets retain physiological function both in vitro (aggregation, morphologic studies [29,31,34,35]) and in vivo (survival of 8–10 days [16,31,35,38]). Thus, this technique affords a unique opportunity not available with any other technique, invasive or noninvasive, to detect and localize active thrombotic lesions in all viscera in the body in stable as well as hemodynamically compromised patients (39). The success of this technique depends on the ability to prepare physiologically active labeled platelets that when injected into the patient migrate selectively to sites of active thrombosis. The field advanced along three lines. First, labeling techniques were modified and improved. Second, feasibility studies were performed in animals, and last, clinical trials were instituted. This is considered in further detail below (see "Cell Labeling").

II. FUNDAMENTALS OF THE TECHNOLOGY

The successful detection of thrombus with radiolabeled tracers depends on the biochemical nature of the compound to be labeled and second on the radioactive label itself. Ideally, the tracer must specifically localize in the clot against a low background from the blood pool (Table 1).

Radioactive isotopes are defined as elements with unstable nuclei. These nuclei emit

Table 1   Characteristics of Ideal Thrombus-Imaging Agent

- High affinity to substrate
- Rapid clearance from blood pool
- No elution of radiolabel from parent molecule or cell
- Nontoxicity

radiation, or decay, in order to reduce mass and attain stability. The time required for one-half of the atoms in a sample of isotope to decay is called the half-life of that isotope. Each radioisotope can be characterized by its half-life and mode of decay. Most nuclei decay through emission of alpha, beta, or gamma radiation. Only radioisotopes that emit gamma radiation are suitable for detection or imaging with standard nuclear medicine equipment.

Gamma emissions consist of short-wave electromagnetic radiation released from the atomic nucleus. No change in the number of protons or neutrons results. The general equation describing this process is: $^A_Z X^*_\gamma \; ^A_Z X_\gamma + \delta$ (40). The energy of emitted gamma rays varies over a wide range and is specific to a given isotope. Technetium 99m, for example, emits a 140-keV photon that is ideally suited to imaging with a standard nuclear medicine gamma camera. Indium 111 releases photons of higher energy, including one at 247 keV, that are less well resolved by the gamma camera, adversely affecting image quality.

The choice of radiopharmaceutical for thrombus imaging depends in part on the proposed duration of imaging. Technetium 99m has a half-life of 6 h. The combined effects of radioactive decay and biological excretion of tracer limits imaging to approximately the first 24 h after isotope injection using ^{99m}Tc. Indium 111, however, has a half-life of 2.8 days. Imaging of radiotracer distribution can therefore be continued for several days after administration. Selection of a radiopharmaceutical for thrombus imaging therefore requires a compromise between image resolution and the need to image for several days after intravenous injection of the isotope.

A. The Gamma Camera

The Anger gamma camera was first developed by Hal Anger in 1957. The early camera consisted of a sodium iodide detector crystal coupled to 19 photomultiplier tubes (41). Substantial modifications have been made to the Anger system since the original camera was designed. The Anger gamma camera is the most frequently used instrument in nuclear medicine. Its design and performance are discussed below.

The essential components of the working gamma camera are the collimator, the detector crystal, the photomultiplier tubes, the amplifiers, the pulse height analyzer, and the position circuitry. A diagram of the camera design is shown in Figure 1 (42).

The purpose of the collimator is to focus emitted gamma rays onto the crystal face so that these photons can be detected and displayed. The collimator consists of a number of holes drilled in a dense material such as lead or tungsten. If a gamma ray passes through one of the collimator holes, the photon interacts with the crystal and is counted as a decay event. If, however, a gamma ray strikes the collimator lead septum, then that photon may either be absorbed, penetrate the material, or be scattered off the septum and strike the crystal at a lower energy level. Both penetrated and scattered photons contribute to image background and reduce contrast. The goal of collimator design is to maximize detection of photons traveling parallel to the collimator holes, while minimizing the effects of penetration (42).

The collimator used to filter photons emitted by both ^{99m}Tc and ^{111}In is the parallel hole collimator. This device is equal in diameter to the scintillation crystal, and provides a constant sensitivity and image size at any distance from the object of interest. The collimator can be modified to accommodate gamma rays of varied energies by increasing the thickness of the lead septae or the diameter or length of the holes. Because ^{111}In emits higher energy photons, the appropriate collimator would have thicker septae and longer holes than the collimator used to image ^{99m}Tc (42).

Those photons that successfully pass through the collimator interact with the thallium-

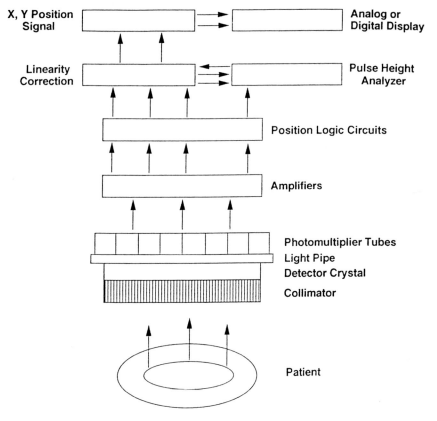

Figure 1   Basic design of the Anger gamma camera (42).

activated sodium iodide scintillation crystal. This interaction can be photoelectric, with photon absorption within the crystal; or the photon can Compton scatter and be all or partially consumed. For lower-energy gamma rays, including [99mTc], the interaction is primarily photoelectric. Gamma photons impinging on the crystal are absorbed, emitting photons of light. As the gamma ray energy increases, the Compton effect predominates, and the number of scattered photons increases. As scattered photons may be detected at a point in the crystal remote from the site of origin, spatial resolution is degraded (42).

Arrayed behind the sodium iodide crystal, the photomultiplier tubes convert light photons emitted by the crystal to electronic pulses. These pulses are amplified both within the photomultiplier tubes and by specific preamplifiers. The electronic signal is then checked by the pulse height analyzer to ensure that the energy of the signal falls within the range expected for a photon of [99mTc] (or other isotope). Photons within the proper energy range are corrected for nonlinearity in the crystal and displayed on the cathode ray tube and/or on film at the correct x,y position (42).

The overall performance of any camera system is no better than its weakest link. In the case of the Anger gamma camera, significant design improvements have been made over the past several years. The weak link is now the collimator. Poor counting statistics and scattered decay events contribute to the loss of spatial resolution attributable to collimation (42).

B. Single Photon Emission Computed Tomography (SPECT)

The sensitivity of radionuclide imaging can in some cases be improved by acquisition of tomographic data. The advantage of tomography is the removal of overlying and underlying activity that may mask a thrombus site. The disadvantage is the poor count statistics associated with SPECT.

SPECT can be performed with a rotating Anger gamma camera. The detector passes through a 360° arc around the camera bed with stepwise acquisition of data every few degrees. The acquired data are filtered and back-projected to produce axial tomographs that can be reoriented and displayed in multiple planes.

C. Nuclear Medicine Computers

Most modern day gamma cameras are interfaced to dedicated computers. These computers can be used to acquire, display, analyze, and store data. Each computer system consists of a central processing unit, memory bank, external storage unit (floppy disk drive or other), camera interface, and display system. Advances in computer hardware have been extensive, and powerful nuclear medicine computers with expanded memory are now available at a reasonable cost (43).

Use of interfaced computers is limited only by the relative lag in nuclear medicine software development. With the purchase of a dedicated computer, basic operational and data acquisition/analysis software is provided. Generally this software supports static and dynamic data acquisition and basic image processing, and may permit reconstruction and display of tomographic image sets. However, the specialized needs of nuclear medicine imaging require continuous revision and updating of software to speed and enhance complex quantitative analysis of acquired images. To date, software design has not kept pace with the demand for new applications, and many nuclear medicine specialists write their own user-specific software (43).

D. Radiation Protection

The use of radioisotopes in diagnostic imaging requires an appreciation of the potential hazards of radiation exposure. Any proposed diagnostic use of radioactivity should be prescreened for clinical appropriateness and offer clear medical benefit to the patient. If use of radioactivity is considered necessary, then every effort should be made to limit exposure to the patient, staff, and general public.

The patient can best be protected by limiting the administered dose of radioisotope to that required to give a diagnostic result. Exposure can also be reduced by encouraging rapid biologic excretion of isotope. For example, unchelated ^{99m}Tc is excreted through the urinary tract. By encouraging the patient to void frequently, the whole-body and bladder radiation dose can be minimized.

The ALARA (as low as reasonably achievable) concept of radiation protection also applies to radiation workers. Staff must be instructed to limit exposure through the principles of time, distance, and shielding. By definition, radiation exposure decreases with time because of isotope decay. Standing at least 3 feet from a radioactive source (for example, the patient) will also minimize exposure, as will use of appropriate lead shielding. In all cases, staff must wear radiation exposure badges on the body and on the hands to permit radiation exposure to be monitored and reviewed.

Exposure to the general public can be limited by restricting access to radiation areas and through safety education.

E. Dosimetry

Radiopharmaceuticals currently used in diagnostic nuclear medicine procedures generally impart a small whole-body radiation dose. The absorbed dose is a function not only of the physical nature of the isotope, but also of the biodistribution and excretion of the labeled drug. The radiation absorbed dose to the whole body and to critical organs such as the bone marrow must be determined for each administered radiopharmaceutical. This information should be used by the physician in prescribing a diagnostic dose of radioactivity.

In general, absorbed dose is a function of the effective half-life (combined biologic and physical half-lives) of the radiopharmaceutical in the body and the quality of the emitted radiations. Radiopharmaceuticals with high energy emissions and long residence times will impart a larger radiation dose. For example, ^{111}In platelets give a whole-body dose of 0.6 rad/ mCi and a dose to the spleen of 33.5 rad/mCi (44). The same platelets labeled with ^{99m}Tc will give a significantly lower exposure because of the short half-life and low-energy gamma ray emission of the isotope.

III. CELL LABELING

Several groups of investigators have successfully demonstrated that platelets could be centrifugally extracted from venous blood, passively labeled with a chelated ^{111}In-oxine complex during a period of incubation in a physiological medium (45), and then reinjected into the donor (46–57). Using gamma camera scintigraphy, tagged platelets were seen to selectively accumulate at sites of active thrombosis both in animals (47;58–60) and in humans (50;61–66) (Figs. 2–4). These images were obtained using a camera fitted with a medium-energy collimator and set on both photopeaks of ^{111}In with a 20% window. The potential value of this marker of active thrombosis is summarized in Table 2.

A. Modifications of Labeling Techniques

Since the early report of platelet labeling (67), several attempts have been made to improve the labeling technique:

1. Alterations in the incubation medium
    a. Saline (50,51)
    b. Acid citrate dextrose (ACD):saline (51,57,58)
    c. Tyrode buffer (54,57)
    d. Plasma (69,73)
2. Alterations in centrifugation forces for harvesting and washing (37,70)
3. Different chelates
    a. oxine (51,52,58,59)
    b. tropolone (59,71)
    c. acetylacetone (72)
    d. mercaptopyridine-n-oxide (73)
4. Alterations in incubation duration (48,53,69), temperature (48,53,57,69), and chelate concentration (57,69)
5. Alteration in the anticoagulant–ACD:saline ratio (69,73)

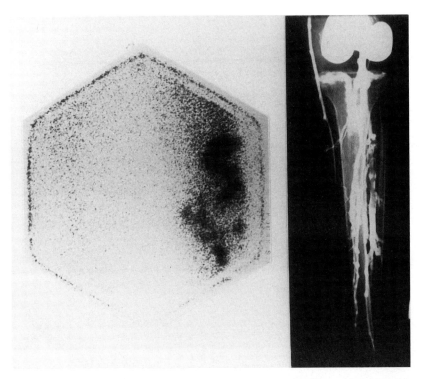

Figure 2 The panel on the left is an ^{111}In scintiphoto obtained 24 h after injection of the platelet suspension. Both calves are in the scintiphoto. The tortuous area of increased activity seen in the left calf is due to a fresh deep vein thrombosis. The corresponding venogram confirming the diagnosis is seen in the right panel. (From Ezekowitz MD et al. Indium-111 platelet imaging. In: Goldhaber SZ, ed. Pulmonary embolism and deep venous thrombosis. Philadelphia: W.B. Saunders, 1985:261–8.)

The best platelet preparation is achieved by using a modification of Heaton's method (51). The platelet suspension is incubated at room temperature (22°C) for 20 min using the desired activity of ^{111}In chloride in (0.01 M) HCl, complexed to 50 µl of 8-hydroxyquinoline (oxine) in absolute alcohol (1 mg/ml) diluted in 4 ml of a solution of ACD:saline (1:7), the pH of which is adjusted to 6.5–7.0. Centrifugation forces of 200 G × 15 min for platelet harvesting and 2000 G × 5 min for washing are used (45).

Of interest is a method developed by Hawker (36) that demands only 26 ml of blood for platelet harvesting and requires only 45 min from the initial drawing of blood to reinjection of the labeled platelet suspension. This halves both the volume of blood required and the procedural time of the more established methods while apparently preserving platelet physiological function. It therefore may be adopted as the preferred method for widespread use.

B. Technetium Labeling

Because of its shorter half-life and the broader availability of the generator system, ^{99m}Tc is potentially a preferable tracer for platelet scintigraphy. For other applications, such as

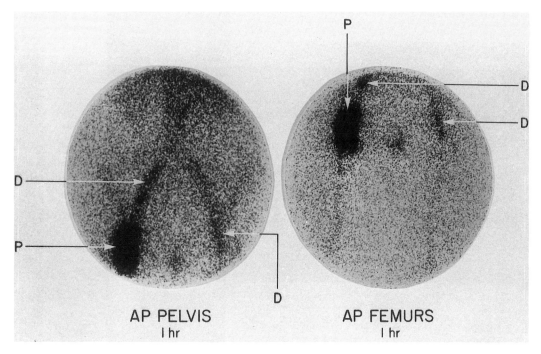

Figure 3   This is an ^{111}In scintiphoto, after angioplasty. P = the puncture site; D = increased platelet activity at the site of balloon dilation. (From Pope CF et al. Detection of platelet deposition at the site of peripheral balloon angioplasty using indium-111 platelet scintigraphy. Am J Cardiol 1985; 55:495–9.)

determination of platelet survival or kinetic studies, the half-life of 6 h is too short for its use, and ^{111}In is the preferred isotope. Numerous attempts to label platelets with ^{99m}Tc have been made, with modest success. Difficulties have been primarily attributed to the spontaneous elution of the radioactivity from the labeled platelets (74,75). In a recent case report, ^{99m}Tc hexamethyl propyleneamineoxine (^{99m}Tc HMPAO)–labeled platelets were used successfully to image a large intracardiac thrombus 2 h after injection (68). Although it is too early to assess the clinical applicability of this technique, it is clear that ^{99m}Tc platelet labeling technique does not eliminate the most undesirable aspect of platelet labeling, the in vitro procedure.

IV. LABELING ELEMENTS OF THE COAGULATION CASCADE FOR IMAGING

Labeling fibrinogen with ^{99m}Tc is feasible, and preparations have been tested in humans by several investigators (76–80). Although ^{99m}Tc is an ideal radionuclide for imaging, there are two major disadvantages to its use. First, the long clearance time of fibrinogen from circulation causes high blood background for 8 to 10 h. By the following day, ^{99m}Tc would have decayed, making it impractical for acquisition of good-quality images. Investiga-

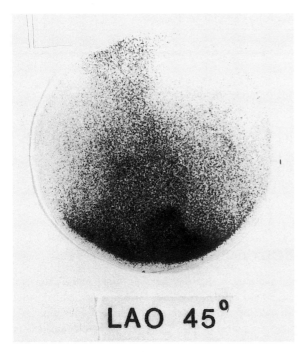

LAO 45°

Figure 4 Scintiphoto obtained 72 h after injection of platelet suspension. The top of the illustration is cephalad. The increased activity in the right lower quadrant of the panel is from the spleen. The activity in the lower left quadrant of the panel is from the liver. The arrow points to an area of increased activity within the left ventricle and represents typical active thrombi within large anteroapical left ventricular aneurysms. LAO = left anterior oblique. (From Ezekowitz MD et al. Diagnostic accuracy of indium-111 platelet scintigraphy in identifying left ventricular thrombi. Am J Cardiol 1983; 51: 1712–6.)

tors who acquired sufficient counts reported 73% sensitivity and 100% specificity for detection of deep vein thrombosis (81).

Streptokinase and urokinase are thrombolytic enzymes. These convert plasminogen to plasmin. Plasmin dissolves fibrin, promoting clot lysis. Iodine 131- and ^{99m}Tc-labeled streptokinase and urokinase have been used by several groups as potential thrombus-imaging agents. These radiopharmaceuticals (81–83) have rapid plasma clearance but offer variable and unpredictable thrombus-to-blood ratios, resulting in unreliable results in patients (79).

Table 2 The Potential Applications of ^{111}In Platelet Scintigraphy

Thrombus visualization at any site in the body
Monitoring thrombus formation, propagation, and migration for up to 7 days using a single injection of labeled platelets
Monitoring therapeutic efficacy over 7 days
An index of thrombus activity

Table 3 Radiolabeled Monoclonal Antibodies Specific for Platelets

Antibody	Specificity	Reference
B.79.7	Human platelet	Thakur et al., 1987 (97)
B.59.2	Human platelet	Thakur et al., 1987
	Glycoprotein IIb-IIIa (also interacts with rabbit, canine, and baboon platelets)	
P.256	Human platelet	Stuttle et al., 1988 (87)
P.256-F(ab')2	Glycoprotein IIb-IIIa	Stuttle et al., 1988 (87)
50H.19	Human platelet	Rhodes et al., 1988
5OH.19-F(ab')2	Glycoprotein IIb-IIIa	Som et al., 1986 (86)
50H.19-F(ab')	Interacts with rabbit and canine platelets	

V. MONOCLONAL ANTIBODY LABELING

The disadvantage of in vitro platelet labeling is the long labeling times and the fact that platelets remain within the cardiac blood pool, providing background against which thrombus detection is difficult. To obviate these limitations much work has been directed at labeling monoclonal antibodies (Table 3) against determinants on the platelet surface and against coagulation proteins.

Monoclonal antibodies specific for platelet surface glycoproteins have offered the opportunity to eliminate in vitro platelet labeling. Their role in imaging vascular lesions with intravenous administration of the radiolabeled proteins was first evaluated in animals and then tested in patients (84–89) (Tables 4 and 5).

Most of the antibodies tested recognize the fibrinogen-binding site, the glycoprotein IIb-IIIa complex, on the human platelet surface. Scintigraphic detection of experimental lesions in animals as well as in patients has been encouraging, not only because the agents clearly delineated vascular thrombi, but also because there was a rapid clearance of radioactivity from circulation (88). Normal platelets survive in circulation for up to 8 days. Radiolabeled platelets thus cause a high background and require successful imaging to be performed 2 to 5 days later, once the background has cleared. The direct injection of the antibody obviates this problem. The effect of anticoagulation is of practical importance. Heparin appears to interfere with the thrombus uptake of ^{111}In antibody 7E-3 (90). Imaging thrombi with radiolabeled antiplatelet antibody in patients receiving anticoagulant therapy may therefore carry a lower sensitivity.

Table 4 Imaging Deep Vein Thrombosis with [111]In 59D8-Fab

Author	No. of patients	Sensitivity (%)	Specificity (%)
Alavi et al., 1990 (98)	33	97	75
Defaucal et al., 1991	44	85	100
Jung et al., 1989 (99)	52	84	81
Lusiani et al. (100)	30	78	92

Table 5 Examples of Radiolabeled Monoclonal Antibodies Specific for Platelets

Antibody	Antigen	Studied In	Reference
In-111/Tc-99m-7.E.3	IIb-IIIa	Humans/animals	Coller et al. (84)
In-111-B.79.7	IIb-IIIa	Animals	Thakur et al. (85)
In-111/Tc-99m-50-H.19	IIb-IIIa	Humans/animals	Som et al. (86)
In-111/Tc-99m-P.256	IIb-IIIa	Humans	Stuttle et al. (87)
Tc-99m/S-12	GMP-140*	Animals/humans	Palabrica et al. (88)

*Platelet alpha granule membrane protein GMP-140.

The matrix of venous thrombi is composed largely of fibrin, a polymeric thread that forms from its soluble precursor fibrinogen and entangles platelets as well as other cells on thrombus formation. Anticoagulants such as heparin may not prevent binding of antifibrin antibodies to fibrin of the preformed thrombus. A large number of antibodies that recognize fibrin have been examined. These are given in Table 6 (91–95).

These antibodies are targeted for fibrin monomers formed by cleavage of fibrin peptide A or B, while others recognize the D-dimer region of fibrin.

A novel ^{99m}Tc-labeled antifibrin Fab′ murine monoclonal antibody, NH-1, is currently being evaluated in patients with suspected deep vein thrombosis, left atrial thrombi, and pulmonary emboli. This antibody is produced from a murine hybridoma cell line established by the fusion of a mouse myeloma cell line and splenocytes from antigen-free Balb-c mice that have been immunized with a suspension of cross-linked fibrin. Preliminary in vitro and in vivo studies seem promising, with a dissociation constant of 6.7×10^{-10} for cross-linked fibrin. The antibody does not recognize fibrinogen. Early studies suggest that it can be used safely in humans.

Fragment E_1, a 60-kD component of fibrin, has been radioiodinated. In experimental thrombi (96), ^{123}I-labeled fragment E_1 produced better thrombus-to-blood ratios with older (>20 h) thrombi than with fresh (1–6 h) thrombi. This will have obvious advantages in imaging deep vein thrombosis in patients (96).

The promise for the future for radionuclide imaging of thrombosis rests with the use of monoclonal antibodies that are directed against components of the coagulation process, bind tightly to their target, and are cleared rapidly from the circulation, thereby allowing easy detection.

Table 6 Antifibrin Antibodies for Imaging Vascular Thrombi

Antibody	Antigen	Studied in	Reference
I-131/In-111-CG-4	D region in fibrin	Animals	Rosebrough (91)
I-131/In-111-T$_2$-GI S	Alpha chain of fibrin	Animals	Kudryk et al. (92)
In-111/Tc-99m-59D8	Beta chain	Humans	Hui et al. (93)
Tc-99m-Y22	D-dimer region of fibrin	Animals	Rylatt et al. (94)
I-131-DG-1	D-dimer region of fibrin	Animals	Gargan et al. (95)

REFERENCES

1. Knight LC. Radiopharmaceuticals for thrombus detection. Semin Nucl Med 1990; 20:52.
2. Koblik PD, DeNardo G, Berger HJ. Current status of immunoscintigraphy in the detection of thrombosis and thromboembolism. Semin Nucl Med 1989; 19:221.
3. Schaible TF, Alavi A. Antifibrin scintigraphy in the diagnostic evaluation of acute deep venous thrombosis. Semin Nucl Med 1991; 21:313.
4. Ezekowitz MD, Zaret BL. Indium-111 platelet scintigraphy, a technique whose time has come. Int J Cardiol 1984; 5:11823.
5. Kakkar V. The diagnosis of deep vein thrombosis using the ^{125}I fibrinogen test. Arch Surg 1972; 104:152.
6. Kakkar V. Fibrinogen uptake test for detection of deep vein thrombosis—a review of current practice. Semin Nucl Med 1977; 7:229.
7. Krohn KA, Knight LC. Radiopharmaceuticals for thrombus detection: Selection, preparation and critical evaluation. Semin Nucl Med 1977; 7:219.
8. Clarke-Pearson DL, Coleman RE, Seigel R, et al. Indium-111 platelet imaging for the detection of deep venous thrombosis and pulmonary embolism in patients without symptoms after surgery. Surgery 1985; 98:98.
9. Mustard JF, Roswell HC, Smythe HA, Senyi A, Murphy EA. The effect of sulfinpyrazone on platelet economy and thrombus formation in rabbits. Blood 1967; 29:859.
10. Zucker MB, Ley AB, Mayer K. Studies on platelet life-span and platelet deposits by use of DFP-32. J Lab Clin Med 1961; 58:406.
11. Leeksma CHW, Cohen JA. Determination of the life-span of human blood platelets using labeled di-isopropylfluoro-phosphonate. J Clin Invest 1956; 35:964.
12. Firkin BG, William WJ: Incorporation of radioactive phosphorous into phospholipids of human leukemic leucocytes and platelets. J Clin Invest 1961; 40:423.
13. Grossman CM, Kohn R, Koch R. Possible errors in the use of 32-P-orthophosphate for the estimation of platelet life span. Blood 1963; 22:9.
14. Zucker MB, Hellman L, Zumoff B. Rapid disappearance of 14-C-labeled serotonin from platelets in patients with carcinoid syndrome. J Lab Clin Med 1964; 63:137.
15. Panel on Diagnostic Application of Radioisotopes in Hematology. International Committee for Standardization in Hematology: recommended methods for radioisotope platelet survival studies. Blood 1977; 50:1137.
16. Thakur ML, Welch MJ, Joist JH, Coleman RE. Indium-111 labeled platelets: studies on the preparation and evaluation of in vitro and in vivo functions. Thromb Res 1976; 9:345.
17. Scheffel U, Tsan MF, Mitchell TG, Camargo EE, Braine M, Ezekowitz MD, Nickoloff EL, Hill-Zobel R, Murphy E, McIntyre PA. Human platelets labeled with In-111 hydroxyquinoline: kinetics, distribution and estimates of radiation dose. J Nucl Med 1982; 23:149–56.
18. Snyder EL, Ezekowitz MD, Aster R, Murphy S, Ferri P, Smith E, Rzad L, Davisson W, Pope C, Rakaiya R, Bucholz DH. Extended storage of platelets in new plastic containers. II. In vivo response to infusion of platelets stored five days. Transfusion 1985; 25:209–14.
19. Snyder EL, Pope C, Ferri PM, Smith EO, Walter SD, Ezekowitz MD. The effect of mode of agitation and type of plastic bag on storage characteristics and in vivo kinetics of platelet concentrates. Transfusion 1986; 26:125–30.
20. Snyder EL, Ezekowitz MD, Malech P, Napychank A, Smith EO, Kiraly T, Gardner JP, Kalish RI. In vitro characteristics and in vivo viability of platelets contained in granulocyte-platelet apheresis concentrate. Transfusion 1987; 27:10–14.
21. Ezekowitz MD, Smith EO, Allen EW, Leonard JC, Smith CW Jr, Basmadjian GP, Taylor FB. Identification of left ventricular thrombi in humans using indium-111 labeled platelets. In: Thakur ML, Gottschalk A, eds. Indium-111 labeled neutrophils, platelets and lymphocytes. Trivirum, 1980:177–82.
22. Ezekowitz MD, Wilson DA, Smith EO, Kanaly PJ, Parker DE. Two dimensional echocardiogra-

phy and indium-111 platelet scintigraphy in the diagnosis of left ventricular thrombi—competitive or complementary. In: Rijsterburgh H., ed. Echocardiography. Martinus Nijhoff, 1981:75–9.

23. Ezekowitz MD, Eicher ER, Scatterday R, Elkins RC. Diagnosis of a persistent pulmonary embolus by indium-111 platelet scintigraphy with angiographic and tissue confirmation. Am J Med 1982; 72:839–42.

24. Ezekowitz MD, Wilson DA, Smith EO, Burow RD, Harrison LH Jr, Parker DE, Elkins RC, Peyton M, Taylor FH. Comparison of indium-111 platelet scintigraphy and two-dimensional echocardiography in the diagnosis of left ventricular thrombi. N Engl J Med 1982; 306:1509–13.

25. Desir G, Johnson M. Bia, Lange RC, Smith EO, Kashgarian M, Flye W, Schiff M, Ezekowitz MD. Detection of acute allograft rejection by indium-111 labeled platelet scintigraphy in renal transplant patients. Transplant Proc 1987; 19:1677–80.

26. Dewanjee MK, Fuster V, Kaye MP, Josa M. Imaging platelet deposition with 111-In-labeled platelets in coronary artery bypass grafts in dogs. Mayo Clin Proc 1978; 53:327.

27. Davis HH, Heaton WA, Siegel BA, Mathias CJ, Joist JH, Sherman LA, Welch MJ. Scintigraphic detection of atherosclerotic lesions and venous thrombi in man by indium-111 labeled autologous platelets. Lancet 1978; 1:1185.

28. Riba AL, Thakur ML, Gottschalk A, Zaret BL: Imaging experimental coronary artery thrombosis with indium-111 platelets. Circulation 1979; 60:767.

29. Goodwin DA, Bushberg JT, Doherty PW, Lipton MJ, Conley FK, Diamanti CI, Meares CF. Indium-111 labeled autologous platelets for location of vascular thrombi in humans. J Nucl Med 1978; 19:626.

30. Ezekowitz MD, Leonard JC, Smith EO, Allen EW, Taylor FB. Identification of left ventricular thrombi in man using indium-111 labeled autologous platelets. Circulation 1981; 63:803.

31. Heaton WA, Davis HH, Welch MJ, Mathias CJ, Joist JH, Sherman LA, Siegel BA. Indium-111: a new radionuclide label for studying human platelet kinetics. Br J Haematol 1979; 42:613.

32. Baker JRJ, Butler KD, Eakins MN, Pay GF, White AM. Subcellular localization of 111-indium in human and rabbit platelets. Blood 1982; 59:351.

33. Mathias CJ, Welch MJ. Labeling mechanism and localizing of indium-111 in human platelets (abstr). J Nucl Med 1979; 20:659.

34. Joist JH, Baker RK, Thakur ML, Welch MJ. Indium-111 labeled human platelets: uptake and loss of label and in vitro function of labeled platelets. J Lab Clin Med 1978; 92:829.

35. Hawker RJ, Hawker LM, Wilkinson AR. Indium (111-In)-labeled human platelets: improved method, efficacy and evaluation. J Nucl Med 1981; 22:381.

36. Thakur ML, Walsh L, Malech HL, Gottschalk A. Indium-111-labeled human platelets: improved method, efficacy and evaluation. J Nucl Med 1981; 22:381.

37. Joist JH, Baker RK. Loss of 111-indium as indicator of platelet injury. Blood 1981; 58:350.

38. Wistow BW, Grossman ZD, McAfee JG, Subramanian G, Henderson RW, Roskopf ML. Labeling of platelets with oxine complexes of Tc-99m and In-111. Part 1. In vitro studies and survival in the rabbit. J Nucl Med 1978; 19:483.

39. Scheffel U, Tsan M-F, Mitchell TG, Camargo EE, Braine H, Ezekowitz MD, Nickoloff EL, Hill-Zobel R, Murphy E, McIntyre PA. Human platelets labeled with In-111 8-hydroxy-quinoline: kinetics, distribution, and estimates of radiation dose. J Nucl Med 1982; 23:149.

40. Lange RC. Basic physics of nuclear medicine. In: Gottschalk A, Hoffer PB, Potchen EJ, eds. Diagnostic nuclear medicine. Baltimore: Williams & Wilkins, 1988:38.

41. Lindeman JF, Quinn JL. The history of nuclear medicine instrumentation and clinical procedures. In: Gottschalk A, Hoffer PB, Potchen EJ, eds. Diagnostic nuclear medicine. Baltimore: Williams & Wilkins, 1988:5.

42. Muehllehner G. The Anger scintillation camera. In: Gottschalk A, Hoffer PB, Potchen EJ, eds. Diagnostic nuclear medicine. Baltimore: Williams & Wilkins, 1988:71–81.

43. Royal HD, Parker A, Holman BL. Basic principles of computers. In: Gottschalk A, Hoffer PB, Potchen EJ, eds. Diagnostic nuclear medicine. Baltimore: Williams & Wilkins, 1988:82–107.

44. Bushberg JT. Radiation dosimetry. In: Gottschalk A, Hoffer PB, Potchen EJ, eds. Diagnostic nuclear medicine. Baltimore: Williams & Wilkins, 1988:201.

45. Scheffel U, McIntyre PA, Evatt B, et al. Evaluation of indium-111 as a new high photon yield gamma-emitting "physiological" platelet label. Johns Hopkins Med J 1977; 140:285.

46. McIlmoyle G, Davis HH, Welch MJ, et al: Scintigraphic diagnosis of experimental pulmonary embolism with In-111-labelled platelets. J Nucl Med 1977; 18:910.

47. Wistow BW, Grossman ZD, McAfee JG, et al. Labelling of platelets with oxine complexes of Tc-99m and In-111. Part I. In vitro studies and survival in the rabbit. J Nucl Med 1978; 19:483.

48. Dewanjee MK, Fuster V, Kaye MP, et al. Imaging platelet deposition with 111-In-labelled platelets in coronary artery bypass grafts in dogs. Mayo Clin Proc 1978; 53:327.

49. Goodwin DA, Bushberg JT, Doherty PW, et al. Indium-111-labelled autologous platelets for location of vascular thrombi in humans. J Nucl Med 1978; 19:626.

50. Heaton WA, Davis HH, Welch MJ, et al. Indium-111: A new radionuclide label for studying human platelet kinetics. Br J Haematol 1979; 42:613.

51. Knight LC, Primeau JL, Siegel BA, et al. Comparison of In-111-labelled platelets and iodinated fibrinogen for the detection of deep vein thrombosis. J Nucl Med 1978; 19:891.

52. Joist JH, Baker RK, Thakur ML, et al. Indium-111-labelled human platelets: uptake and loss of label and in vitro function of labelled platelets. J Lab Clin Med 1978; 92:829.

53. Hawker RJ, Hawker LM, Wilkinson AR. Indium (111-In)-labelled human platelets: optimal method. Clin Sci 1980; 58:243.

54. Heyns A DuP, Badenhorst PN, Pieters H, et al. Preparation of a viable population of indium 111–labelled human blood platelets. Thromb Haemost 1980; 42:1473.

55. Klonizakis I, Peters AM, Fitzpatrick ML, et al. Radionuclide distribution following injection of 111-indium-labelled platelets. Br J Haematol 1980; 46:595.

56. Ezekowitz MD, Leonard JC, Smith EO, et al. Identification of left ventricular thrombi in man using indium-111-labelled autologous platelets. Circulation 1981; 63:803.

57. Mathias CJ, Welch MJ. Labelling mechanism and localization of indium-111 in human platelets (abstr). J Nucl Med 1979; 20:659.

58. Baker JR, Butler KD, Eakins MN, et al. Subcellular localization of ^{111}In in human and rabbit platelets. Blood 1982; 59:351.

59. Fedullo PF, Moser KM, Moser KS, et al. Indium-111-labelled platelets: effect of heparin on uptake by venous thrombi and relationship to the activated partial thromboplastin time. Circulation 1982; 66:632.

60. Davis HH, Heaton WA, Siegel BA, et al. Scintigraphic detection of atherosclerotic lesions and venous thrombi in man by indium-111-labelled autologous platelets. Lancet 1978; 1:1185.

61. Davis HH, Siegel BA, Sherman LA, et al. Scintigraphic with ^{111}In labelled autologous platelets in venous thromboembolism. Radiology 1980; 136:203.

62. Fenech A, Hussey JK, Smith FW, et al. Diagnosis of deep vein thrombosis using autologous indium-111-labelled platelets. Br Med J 1981; 282:1020.

63. Grimley RP, Rafiqi E, Hawker RJ, et al. Imaging of ^{111}In-labelled platelets—a new method of the diagnosis of deep vein thrombosis. Br J Surg 1981; 68:714.

64. Ezekowitz MD, Eichner ER, Scatterday R, et al. Diagnosis of a persistent pulmonary embolus by indium-111 platelet scintigraphy with angiographic and tissue confirmation. Am J Med 1982; 72:839.

65. Sostman HD, Neumann RD, Loke J, et al. Detection of pulmonary embolism in man with ^{111}In-labelled autologous platelets. Am J Radiol 1982; 138:945.

66. Dewanjee MK, Rao SA, Rosemark JA, et al. Indium-111 tropolone, a new tracer for platelet labelling. Radiology 1982; 145:149.

67. Thakur ML, Welch MJ, Joist JM, Coleman RC. Indium-111 labeled platelets: studies on the preparation and evaluation of in vitro and in vivo functions. Thromb Res 1976; 9:345–57.

68. Scheffel U, Tsan MF, McIntyre PA. Labelling of human platelets with ^{111}In-8-hydroxy-quinoline. J Nucl Med 1979; 20:524.

69. Bunting RW, Callahan RJ, Finkelstein S, et al. A Modified method for labelling human platelets with indium-111 oxine using albumin density-gradient separation. Radiology 1982; 145:219.

70. Danpure HJ, Osman S, Brady F. The labelling of blood cells in plasma with ^{111}In-tropolonate. Br J Radiol 1982; 55:247.

71. Danpure HJ, Osman S. Cell labelling and cell damage with ^{111}In-acetylacetone—an alternative to indium-111 oxine. Br J Radiol 1981; 54:597.

72. Ezekowitz MD, Smith EO, Rankin R, Harrison LM, Krous HF. Left atrial mass: diagnostic value of transesophageal two-dimensional echocardiography and indium-111 platelet scintigraphy. Am J Cardiol 1983; 51:1563–64.

73. Thakur ML, McKenney SL, Park CH. Simplified and efficient labeling of human platelets in plasma using indium-111–2-mercaptopyridine-n-oxide: preparation and evaluation. J Nucl Med 1985; 26:510–7.

74. Becker W, Borner W, Borst U, et al. Tc-99m-HMPAO: a new platelet labelling compound. Eur J Nucl Med 1987; 13:267.

75. Dewanjee MK, Kapadvanjwala M, Dewanjee S, et al. New efficient cell labeling method with Tc-99m O_4 via neutral and lipid soluble Sn(II).

76. Harwig SSL, Harwig JF, Coleman RE, et al. In vivo behaviour of [99mTc]-fibrinogen and its potential as a thrombus-imaging agent (abstr). J Nucl Med 1976; 28:1930.

77. Higashi S, Kuniyasu Y. An experimental study of deep-vein thrombosis using [99mTc]-fibrinogen. Eur J Nucl Med 1984; 9:548.

78. Jeghers O, Abramovici I, Jonckheer M, et al. Chemical method for labeling of fibrinogen with [99mTc]. Eur J Nucl Med 1978; 3:95–100.

79. Jonckheer M, Abramovici I, Jeghers O, et al. The interpretation of phlebograms using fibrinogen labeled with [99mTc]. Eur J Nucl Med 1978; 3:233.

80. Vorne M, Leikas S, Sakki S, et al. Radionuclide venography and uptake imaging using [99mTc]-fibrinogen and its correlation with contrast venography. Nucl Med Commun 1987; 8:921.

81. Seigel ME, Malmud LS, Rhodes BA, Bell WS, Wagner HN. Scanning of Thromboemboli with ^{131}I-streptokinase. Radiology 1972; 103:695.

82. Som P, Rhodes BA, Bell WR. Radiolabeled streptokinase and urokinase and their comparative biodistribution. Thromb Res 1975; 6:247.

83. Weir GJ, Roberts RC, Wenzel F, et al. Visualization of thrombi with technetium-99m urokinase. Lancet 1976; 2:341.

84. Coller BS, Peerschke EI, Scudder LE. A murine monoclonal antibody that completely blocks the binding of fibrinogen to platelets produces a thrombasthenic like state in normal platelets and binds to glycoproteins IIb and/or IIIa. J Clin Invest 1983; 72:325–38.

85. Thakur ML, Thiagarajan P, White F III, et al. Monoclonal antibodies for specific cell labeling: consideration, preparations and preliminary investigation. Nucl Med Biol 1989; 14:51–8.

86. Som P, Oster ZH, Zamora PO, et al. Radioimmunoimaging of experimental thrombi in dogs using technetium-99m labeled monoclonal antibody fragments reactive with human platelets. J Nucl Med 1986; 27:1315–20.

87. Stuttle AWJ, Peters AM, Loutfi I, et al. Use of an antiplatelet monoclonal antibody F(ab')$_2$ fragment for imaging thrombus. J Nucl Med 1988; 27:1315–20.

88. Palabrica TM, Furie BC, Konstam MA, et al. Thrombus imaging in a primate model with antibodies specific for external membrane protein of activated platelets. Proc Natl Acad Sci USA 1989; 86:1036–40.

89. Ezekowitz MD, Coller B, Srivastava SC. Potential application of monoclonal antibodies for thrombus detection. Int J Nucl Med Biol 1986; 13:407–11.

90. Saito T, Powers J, Nossiff ND, et al. Radioimmuno-imaging of experimental thrombi in dogs using monoclonal antifibrin (AF) and antiplatelet (AP) antibodies: effect of heparin on uptake by pulmonary emboli (PE) and venous thrombosis (VT). J Nucl Med 1988; 29:825.

91. Rosebrough JG, McAfee JG, Grossman ZD. Thrombus imaging: a comparison study using T2G1s and GC4 fibrin-specific monoclonal antibodies (abstr). J Nucl Med 1988; 30:797.

92. Kudryk B, Rohoza A, Ahadi M, et al. Specificity of a monoclonal antibody for the NH_2 terminal region of fibrin. Mol Immunol 1984; 21:89–94.

93. Hui KY, Haber E, Matseuda GR. Monoclonal antibodies to a synthetic fibrin like peptide bind to human fibrin but not fibrinogen. Science 1983; 222:1120–32.

94. Rylatt DB, Blake AS, Cottis LE, et al. An immuno-assay for human D dimer using monoclonal antibodies. Thromb Res 1983; 31:767–78.

95. Gargan PE, Plopis VA, Scheu JD. A fibrin specific monoclonal antibody which interferes with the fibrinolytic effect of tissue plasminogen activator. Thromb Haemost 1988; 59:426–31.

96. Knight LC, Maurer AH, Kollmann M, et al. Imaging thrombi with improved formulation of I-123 fragment (abstr). Eur J Nucl Med 1989; 30:817.

97. Thakur ML, Thiagrajan P, White WF, et al. Monoclonal antibody as agents for specific cell labelling: concentration, preparation and preliminary evaluation. J Nucl Med 1987; 14:51.

98. Alavi A et al. Radiolabeled antifibrin antibody in the detection of venous thrombosis: preliminary results. Radiology 1990; 175:79–85.

99. Jung M et al. Deep vein thrombosis: scintigraphic diagnosis with In-111-labeled monoclonal antifibrin antibodies. Radiology 1989; 173:469.

100. Lusiani L, Zanco P, Visona A, et al. Immunoscintigraphic detection of venous thrombosis of lower extremities by means of human antifibrin monoclonal antibody labelling with In-111. Geology 1989; 40:671–677.

9

Magnetic Resonance Imaging

Gerald G. Blackwell
University of Alabama, Birmingham, Alabama

I. INTRODUCTION

This chapter will discuss the role of magnetic resonance imaging (MRI) methods in the diagnosis of intracardiac and intravascular masses and thrombi. In an attempt to better appreciate the contribution made by MRI, the discussion will begin by describing the basic principles of the technology together with the imaging sequences and special modifications required for successful cardiovascular applications. Finally, an attempt will be made to define the clinical role of MRI in detecting lesions of embolic potential.

It is important to appreciate that this exciting and evolving technology is in its infancy. High-resolution static and functional images of the heart have been available for just over 5 years, and dedicated software packages for cardiac applications have only recently been applied clinically. A limited number of sites worldwide have chosen to focus on cardiac imaging. Interest, however, seems to be expanding, and widespread use of this technology is anticipated.

II. OVERVIEW OF MAGNETIC RESONANCE METHODS

A. Basic Principles

The discipline of medical MRI exploits the magnetic properties of individual hydrogen nuclei to produce images of diagnostic quality (1). Magnetism is generally familiar at the macroscopic level. Its foundation is, however, at the level of atomic and subatomic particles (2). A magnetic field arises when charged particles are in motion. The hydrogen nucleus contains a single proton, which spins and possesses an electrical charge. Accordingly, each hydrogen nucleus produces a small, unopposed magnetic field and can be viewed as a tiny bar magnet (Fig. 1). The body does not have net magnetization, since nuclei are randomly oriented and opposing fields cancel each other. However, in the presence of a strong external magnetic field (i.e., a clinical MRI instrument) the body acquires a net magnetization vector since the field attracts these "magnetic" nuclei and causes them to align in a uniform fashion (3).

A magnetic resonance image is formed by the interaction of radiofrequency (RF) energy with hydrogen nuclei in the presence of the aforementioned external magnetic field. A fundamental principle of physics, the Larmor equation, states that a given nuclear species will precess (spin) at a specific frequency that is dependent on its gyromagnetic ratio and the strength of the external magnetic field. For hydrogen nuclei exposed to the field strength of commercial MRI instruments, the Larmor frequency, or resonance frequency, occurs in the radiofrequency range of the electromagnetic spectrum. Accordingly, we can influence atoms at low energy using apparently "safe" nonionizing radiation (1).

Fundamental to the understanding of MRI is the fact that all hydrogen nuclei exposed to the same magnetic field strength will spin at precisely the same frequency. An extension of this concept is the observation that varying the magnetic field strength will cause the hydrogen nuclei to spin at a different Larmor frequency (Fig. 2). The challenge of MRI is to transiently cause each group of hydrogen atoms, in a desired imaging plane, to experience a different magnetic field strength so they can be uniquely identified by their Larmor frequency. The bore of a commercial MRI unit has a very homogeneous, constant field strength. During imaging, however, the local field strength within the main magnet bore is transiently and rapidly altered so that each position in space is uniquely identified (Fig. 3). This is accomplished by a three-dimensional set of gradient coils that are wrapped around the main magnet. Gradient coils are simply electromagnets that are ramped-up in rapid succession. The order of application of these gradient coils determines the orientation of the imaging slice (1,4).

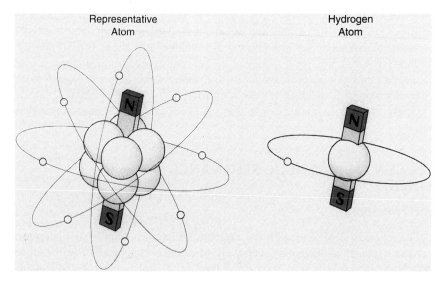

Figure 1   Schematic depiction of a hydrogen atom and a more complex atom. The unpaired, single proton of the hydrogen nucleus generates a small magnetic field as it spins and can be thought of as resembling a tiny bar magnet. (From Ref. 1.)

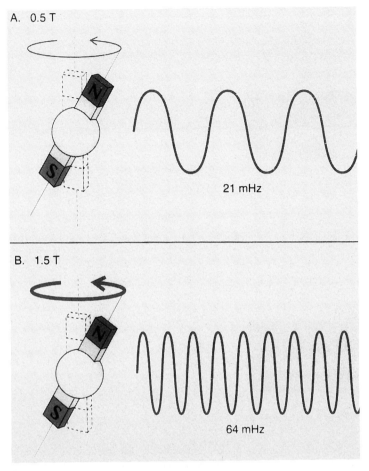

A. 0.5 T

21 mHz

B. 1.5 T

64 mHz

Figure 2 Graphic representation of the Larmor equation relating precession frequency to external magnetic field strength. At a field strength of 0.5 tesla all hydrogen nuclei precess with a frequency of approximately 21 MHz. At 1.5 tesla all hydrogen nuclei will precess at a frequency three times greater. (From Ref. 1.)

Specialized radiofrequency coils supply RF energy to the system. They are also used to detect the signal produced when the excited hydrogen nuclei return to equilibrium. A computer controls delivery of RF pulses and the timing of application of the gradient coils and transfers the resultant raw signal onto an image matrix. Complex mathematical manipulation of the data produces the image.

The terms relaxation times T1 and T2 require definition. When hydrogen nuclei are excited by RF energy, they dissipate the energy and return to equilibrium (relax) in a complex fashion that is influenced by the external applied field strength and the local environment, which includes adjacent nuclei, orbiting electrons, and molecular motion. T1 relaxation (spin-lattice or longitudinal relaxation) denotes the time required for the nuclei to reacquire net magnetization along the axis of the static magnetic field after being perturbed by applied RF energy. T2 relaxation (spin-spin or transverse relaxation) denotes

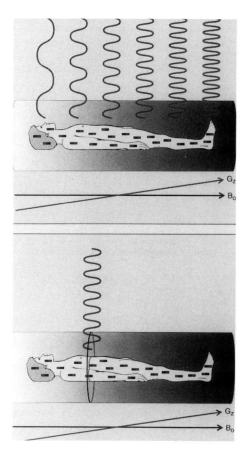

Figure 3 Top panel: In this cartoon hydrogen nuclei, represented as bar magnets, are precisely aligned in the presence of an external magnetic field (B_o). The precession frequency of the nuclei varies slightly from the patient's head to his feet, however, because a magnetic gradient (G_z) has been applied in this direction, superimposed on the main external magnetic field. Bottom panel: A specific slice is selected for imaging by applying radiofrequency (RF) energy at the precession frequency corresponding to the location desired. Supplying RF energy of a different frequency would be required to select a different slice for imaging. In clinical imaging, gradients are applied rapidly in three dimensions, and the unique position of each structure within the imaging plane is localized. See text for details. (From Ref. 1.)

the time required for the magnetization vector, in the transverse plane, to decay after nuclei are perturbed by applied RF energy. T1 and T2 relaxation times differ greatly and depend on the tissue composition. Thus, hydrogen nuclei contained within muscle, blood, fat, etc. all have unique T1 and T2 values (1).

B. Clinical Imaging Sequences

Magnetic resonance imaging permits flexibility not possible with other imaging modalities. Image production and contrast are influenced by multiple factors including tissue (hydrogen) density, magnetic relaxation properties of the specific tissue (T1 and T2), and blood flow. With appropriate manipulation of imaging parameters, images can be reconstructed to highlight each of these variables.

Two imaging sequences are currently used widely in cardiac imaging: spin-echo (black-blood images) and gradient-echo (white-blood images, cine MR) (Fig. 4). The standard imaging sequence used to produce high-resolution static images is referred to as the spin-echo sequence. In this sequence RF energy at the Larmor frequency is delivered to "flip" the hydrogen nuclei 90° from their equilibrium position. The spins are refocused by application of an additional radiofrequency pulse of 180°. Energy released by the spins as they return to equilibrium, referred to as an echo, is then sampled. First spin-echo images are typically acquired at 25–30 ms. A second 180° refocusing pulse can be applied and sampled, and these second spin-echo images are typically acquired at 60–120 ms (4).

Using the spin-echo technique, rapidly flowing blood does not generate a signal (black blood), because the spins originally excited by the RF pulse leave the imaging plane before the first echo signal is collected. The first spin-echo images of static tissues contain a great deal of MR signal and highlight anatomy. The later second echo images generate less image intensity. Areas of slowly moving blood and tissues with long T2 relaxation times, however, may appear brighter on these second spin-echo images, which thus may provide useful information. Changing the location of excitation permits acquisition in multiple tomographic planes (slices). An individual slice can be excited only once per cardiac cycle during an electrocardiogram (ECG)-gated spin-echo study (see below). To produce a high-resolution image, sampling of from 128 to 512 cardiac cycles is required. Thus, acquisition time of ECG-gated MR images is dependent on the patient's heart rate. In general, longer imaging times are required to produce images of higher resolution (4).

A second type of imaging sequence, the gradient-echo sequence, is used to evaluate cardiac function and blood flow (4,5). Images are acquired by repeatedly sampling a tomographic plane using limited RF "flip angles" (i.e., <90°). An echo signal is generated by rapid gradient-coil reversal rather than by application of an additional RF pulse as

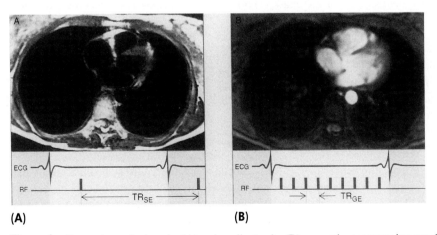

(A)   **(B)**

Figure 4   Comparison of spin-echo (A) and gradient-echo (B) magnetic resonance images. Conventional spin-echo imaging produces high-resolution, multislice, static images of a single cardiac phase in which the normal blood pool appears black. The gradient-echo sequence produces multiphase images that can be displayed in a cine format and in which the normal blood pool appears white. RF = radiofrequency pulse. TR = repetition time. See text for details. (From Ref. 4.)

is the case with the spin-echo sequences. Short echo times (TE) (3–12 ms) and short repetition times (TR) can be achieved with this imaging sequence. The brightest signal emanates from flowing blood (white blood), because static tissue within the imaging plane becomes saturated by the continuous, rapid pulses and has a low-intensity signal. In contrast, flowing spins (i.e., blood) entering the imaging plane have not been previously exposed to the pulses. Flowing blood, therefore, is capable of releasing more signal and appears brighter. Gradient-echo images can be produced with a high temporal resolution and are usually displayed in an endless-loop cine format, analogous to radionuclide ventriculo-grams. A multislice format can be used, but as the number of slices imaged per cardiac cycle increases, there is a significant reduction in temporal resolution (i.e., doubling the number of slices lessens the temporal resolution by a factor of 2). In gradient-echo MR images, excessively turbulent blood flow causes regions of signal loss in the image (6). Accordingly, disordered flow patterns associated with valvular pathology or mass lesions are easily identified.

Gradient-echo images are most helpful in quantitating parameters such as cardiac volumes and estimating ejection fraction and are also used to define anatomy (5). The spatial resolution, wide field of view, and ability to alter image contrast confers significant advantages on MRI in comparison with other imaging modalities for the purpose of defining anatomy. The cine format is useful for evaluating global and regional ventricular function as well as valvular pathology.

Several new pulse sequences are currently being developed. Echo-planar strategies, for example, permit image acquisition in a matter of milliseconds. In the next few years modifications that both reduce acquisition times and improve image quality for cardiovascular applications are likely.

C. Cardiac Gating

Magnetic resonance images of static organs such as the brain are accomplished with exquisite resolution. Unfortunately, imaging of the beating heart is considerably more difficult. To compensate for continuous motion, cardiovascular MR scans must be gated to an appropriate trigger, most commonly the ECG (7,8). When the heart rate is regular and the patient is cooperative, images of the heart of very high resolution can be obtained. If the heart rate is irregular or there is difficulty in obtaining a stable ECG trigger, considerable artifact is introduced into the image. Figure 5 illustrates this point by demonstrating the effect of atrial fibrillation, with a fast ventricular response, on image quality. Arrhythmia-rejection software and the development of ultrafast imaging sequences serve to reduce image degradation (4).

D. Safety

Because the magnetic field is always "on," special precautions must be taken to ensure that extraneous ferromagnetic materials are not inadvertently allowed into the field of the MRI instrument. These objects can become high-speed projectiles and cause serious injury to the patient and equipment. Most implantable materials have been tested for safety during MRI. In general, the most important absolute contraindications to MRI are intracerebral surgical clips and cardiac pacemakers. Sternal wires used in cardiovascular surgery present no safety risk, and almost all prosthetic valves can be imaged safely (9). Safety questions are addressed in detail in a number of texts (10–12).

The remainder of the chapter will focus on the clinical role of cardiovascular MRI methods in detecting lesions of embolic potential.

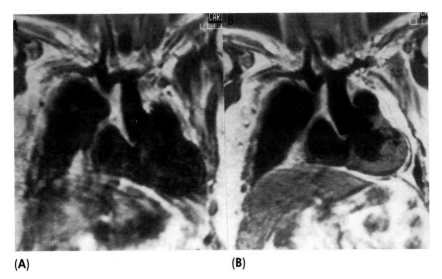

(A)   **(B)**

Figure 5 Coronal spin-echo images highlighting the importance of a regular cardiac trigger. Panel A is from a patient imaged during atrial fibrillation with a rapid, very irregular ventricular response. Panel B is the same imaging plane, in the same patient after conversion to normal sinus rhythm. Note the dramatic improvement in image quality. (From Ref. 4.)

III. DETECTION OF INTRACARDIAC LESIONS BY MAGNETIC RESONANCE METHODS

Transthoracic echocardiography is recognized as the imaging modality of first choice in the assessment of patients with known or suspected cardiac masses or thrombi. It is real-time, portable, and noninvasive and is quite accurate for the initial assessment of patients with these lesions. Before the development of echocardiographic techniques, the diagnosis of cardiac masses was seldom made ante mortem. There are well-known limitations of transthoracic echocardiography (see Chap. 7). With the development of transesophageal echocardiography and MRI techniques, many of these limitations can be obviated (13).

There are many case reports and larger studies demonstrating that MRI is useful for diagnosing mass lesions in any of the four cardiac chambers. Studies by several authors, notably Freedberg et al. (14) and Lund et al. (15), have suggested that MRI provides important additional information in assessing masses identified by transthoracic echocardiography and can be used to resolve equivocal ultrasound studies (16). Further, it may provide valuable additional information regarding the relationship of known lesions to adjacent structures.

It was originally hoped that MRI would be able not only to provide anatomic definition of mass lesions but also to reveal an etiology on the basis of tissue classification. Unfortunately, apart from identifying cystic lesions and lipomatous tissue, there is considerable overlap in signal intensity of different tissues. Thus, it is seldom possible to confidently diagnose the etiology of a mass solely on the basis of the MR signal intensity (17).

From a practical standpoint, MRI assumes a supplementary role in the diagnosis, being most helpful in the design of invasive and therapeutic strategies (18). There are no studies to date comparing the relative value of transesophageal echocardiography and MRI in the diagnosis of cardiac masses.

The following sections will describe specific lesions for which MRI may be clinically useful.

A. Left-Sided Lesions

1. Atrial Lesions

Primary cardiac tumors are unusual (19,20). The most common primary cardiac tumors are myxomas, which are histologically benign and most frequently arise in the left atrium. Usually occurring as solitary lesions, they present clinically by causing either obstructive symptoms or unexplained systemic emboli. Not infrequently, patients have a poorly defined clinical syndrome highlighted by general malaise and fever of undetermined origin. Classically, myxomas are attached by a stalk to the interatrial septum. They occasionally produce a "tumor plop" by prolapse of the tumor into the ventricle during diastole.

The diagnosis of a myxoma by MRI is suggested by the identification of tumor attachment to the interatrial septum (21). The signal intensity of myxomas on either spin-echo or gradient-echo MR images is not specific. The value of MRI resides in its ability to visualize the lesion in three-dimensional space. Figure 6 shows images from a patient with a surgically confirmed myxoma in close proximity to the mitral valve.

The body of the left atrium and the left atrial appendage are common locations for intracardiac thrombi. These thrombi are especially prevalent in patients with rheumatic

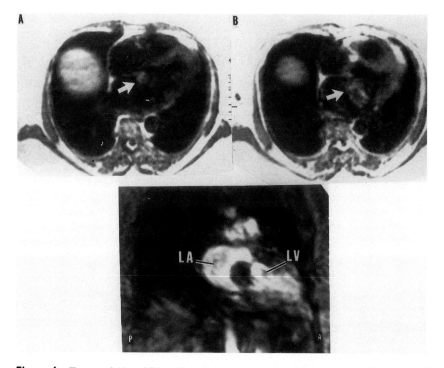

Figure 6 Top panel (A and B): Adjacent spin-echo images from a patient with a left atrial myxoma (arrow) intimately associated with the mitral valve. Bottom panel: Diastolic frame from a gradient-echo image acquired in the right anterior oblique equivalent projection. The signal void associated with the myxoma is well seen. LV = left ventricle; LA = left atrium.

mitral valve disease and in patients with atrial fibrillation unrelated to valvular pathology. The diagnostic accuracy of MRI is better than that of transthoracic echocardiography. The specificity of spin-echo MR images in identifying small atrial thrombi is reduced by artifact caused by slow-flowing blood. Gradient-echo images may be difficult to interpret. Recent experience suggests that transesophageal echocardiography may prove superior to both transthoracic echocardiography and MRI in identifying left atrial lesions, especially small thrombi confined to the left atrial appendage.

2. Ventricular Lesions

Tumors arising in the left ventricle are exceedingly rare in adults. Most intraventricular lesions are thrombi. Regional left ventricular dysfunction, such as occurs commonly in postinfarction patients, and global left ventricular dysfunction such as occurs in patients with cardiomyopathy both predispose to intraventricular thrombus formation. Sechtem and colleagues have compared spin-echo MRI with angiocardiography, transthoracic echocardiography, and computed tomography scanning in the diagnosis of left ventricular thrombi in patients referred for surgical aneurysmectomy (22). Spin-echo MRI methods had sensitivities and specificities that compared favorably with these of the best of the alternative techniques.

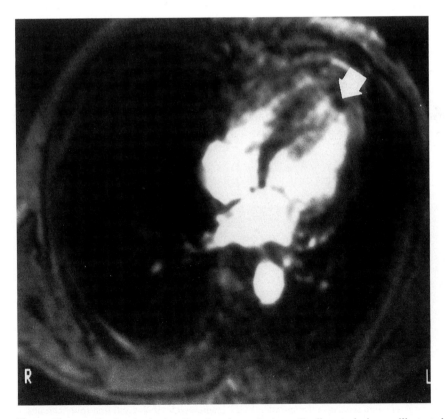

Figure 7   Apical left ventricular thrombus (arrow). A small, discrete lesion as illustrated in this figure is generally best seen using the gradient-echo technique.

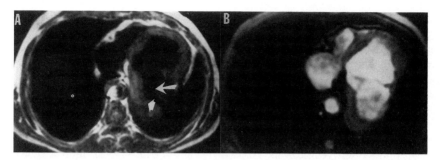

Figure 8   Companion transverse spin-echo (A) and gradient-echo (B) images from a patient with a large posterobasal left ventricular aneurysm filled with thrombus. Curved arrow = aneurysm cavity; arrowhead = thrombus.

A recent study compared the newer gradient-echo MRI technique with conventional spin-echo imaging in identifying left ventricular thrombi (23). Gradient-echo images permit greater discrimination between the lesion and surrounding blood pool/myocardium and were, therefore, diagnostically superior. Figure 7 shows a gradient-echo image from a patient with an apical left ventricular thrombus.

Maximum diagnostic information is obtained in most patients by a combination of dual spin-echo and a gradient-echo techniques. Spin-echo images obtained with a short echo time have the best anatomic resolution, while images with a long echo time are used to distinguish between slow blood flow and thrombus. As noted above, a companion gradient-echo image permits maximum differentiation of the lesion. Figures 8 and 9 show mural thrombi as they appear in companion spin-echo and gradient-echo images.

The comprehensive assessment of the entire left ventricle using transesophageal echocardiography, especially the apex, is often not possible. Theoretically, MRI may be more accurate in these patients, but comparisons with transesophageal echocardiography have not been undertaken.

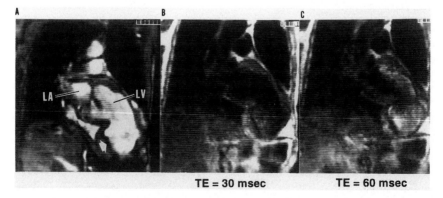

Figure 9   Gradient-echo image (A), first spin-echo (B), and second spin-echo (C) images demonstrating thrombus in a massive apical aneurysm. In the gradient-echo image and first spin-echo image the thrombus can be clearly seen (arrowhead). On the second spin-echo image there is marked signal enhancement of the blood pool within the aneurysm consistent with very slow flow. LV = left ventricle; LA = left atrium; TE = echo time.

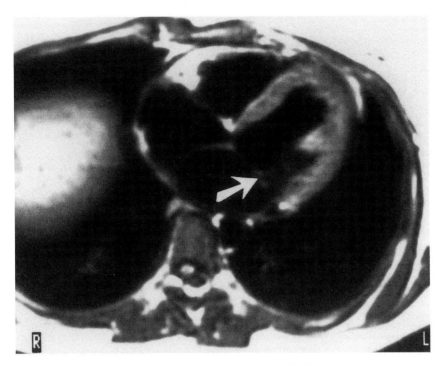

Figure 10   Mitral valve vegetation (arrow). Although echocardiography is clearly superior, large vegetations can be seen on high-resolution spin-echo images. The finding in this patient was confirmed at surgery.

3.   Valvular Lesions

Echocardiography-based techniques are superior to MRI in the assessment of valvular pathology. Magnetic resonance imaging is useful in identifying large lesions and excluding involvement of contiguous cardiac structures. The MR image in Figure 10 is from a patient in whom a bulky, poorly defined lesion related to the mitral valve had been identified by transthoracic echocardiography. The differential diagnosis included a lesion involving the atrial wall or an atypical myxoma. By MRI, the lesion was clearly seen and was limited to the mitral valve. At surgery the young patient was found to have endocarditis on an otherwise structurally normal valve.

B.   Right-Sided Lesions

Masses and thrombi within the right heart have been less frequently described using MRI. Atrial masses can traverse the interatrial septum, either through an atrial septal defect or via a patent foramen ovale, and produce systemic embolization. Alternatively, atrial lesions may embolize the pulmonary vasculature.

1.   Atrial Lesions

Right atrial lesions usually pose a diagnostic dilemma for both echocardiography and MRI. Mirowitz and Gutierrez recently described spin-echo MR images of the fibromuscular elements of the right atrium (24). These structures, which include the crista terminalis, Chiari network, and eustachian valve, are largely posterior in origin and can be misinterpreted as masses.

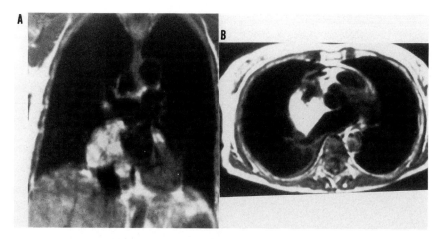

Figure 11 Right atrial lipoma. The distinctive high-signal-intensity lipomatous tissue is clearly seen on both the coronal (A) and the transverse (B) spin-echo images. Magnetic resonance imaging is well suited for determining the extent of bulky lesions, as illustrated in this patient. (From Ref. 13.)

Right atrial lipomas (25) and lipomatous hypertrophy of the interatrial septum (26) are well seen by MRI using standard spin-echo images (27,28) (Fig. 11).

A variety of other tumors, as well as thrombi and emboli in transit, have been identified within the right atrium by MRI (Fig. 12).

2. Ventricular Lesions

Mass lesions rarely occupy the right ventricle. Primary benign cardiac tumors, notably rhabdomyomas, fibromas, and myxomas, may involve the right ventricle, particularly in children (29,30). Malignant cardiac sarcomas and metastatic tumors can also involve the right ventricle (31). A prominent moderator band sometimes leads to diagnostic confusion.

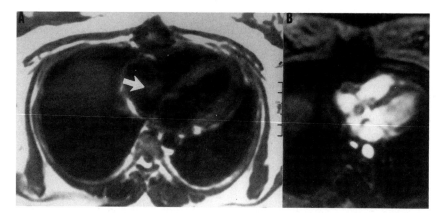

Figure 12 Companion transverse spin-echo (A) and gradient-echo (B) images from a patient with a presumed right atrial thrombus (arrowhead) related to a long-standing central venous catheter. (From Ref. 13.)

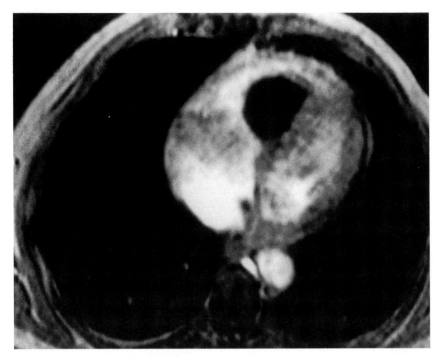

Figure 13 Calcified right ventricular mass. A well-circumscribed signal void is seen occupying a large portion of the right ventricle on this transverse gradient-echo image. This lesion of unknown etiology was surgically removed and contained calcium.

Magnetic resonance imaging is useful in the assessment of these tumors as well as right ventricular thrombi (32). Figure 13 is an image from a patient with a calcified right ventricular mass of undefined etiology.

IV. DETECTION OF INTRAVASCULAR THROMBOSIS BY MAGNETIC RESONANCE METHODS

The MR signal is inherently sensitive to motion, and considerable efforts are being directed at developing MR techniques that reliably describe normal and abnormal intravascular blood flow (33). Standard spin-echo and gradient-echo techniques have been applied in an attempt to visualize intravascular thrombus. More recently, phase velocity mapping (PVM) techniques have been used (34). By means of postprocessing algorithms, images can be constructed that define flow velocity throughout the vessel or chamber of interest. Thrombus is depicted as a region of zero velocity within the vessel lumen.

Arterial thrombi have been described in the thoracic and abdominal aorta (35–37). Several investigators have evaluated MRI for detecting venous thrombosis (36,38–42). Thrombi in major abdominal veins and the jugular vein have been identified (35,41). A recent report from Spritzer et al. describes a sensitivity of 100% and specificity of 92.9% for gradient-echo MRI in the detection of lower extremity deep venous thrombosis in a group of patients undergoing venography (42).

Table 1 Magnetic Resonance Imaging of Cardiac Tumors and Thrombi

Advantages	Disadvantages
Noninvasive	Cost
High resolution	Image quality degraded by patient motion or irregular cardiac rhythms
Not limited by acoustic windows	Less effective for small tumors and thrombi, especially those associated with cardiac valves
Intrinsically three-dimensional	Poor discrimination in region of atrial appendages
Wide field of view	
Good visualization of left ventricular apex	
Some tissue discrimination possible, especially fat-containing tumors	

Magnetic resonance angiography is being developed and may ultimately permit non-invasive visualization of lesions of embolic potential in either the arterial or venous circulation. Widespread clinical applicability awaits the development of improved imaging sequences and large-scale studies that compare MR with conventional modalities.

V. SUMMARY

Although in its infancy, MRI has expanded our diagnostic armamentarium in the detection of intracardiac and intravascular masses of embolic potential (Table 1). It is best considered as a complementary modality to echocardiography. The well-rounded clinician must have some familiarity with the technology, because in certain circumstances it provides diagnostically unique information. This information may be important in designing appropriate medical or surgical therapy.

REFERENCES

1. Doyle M, Blackwell, GG. Basic principles of MRI. In Blackwell GG, Cranney GB, Pohost GM, eds. MRI: cardiovascular system. New York: Gower Medical Publishing, 1992.
2. Saini S, Frankel RB, Stark DD, Ferrucci JT. Magnetism: a primer and review. Am J Roentgenol 1988; 150:735–44.
3. Doyle M, Cranney GC, Pohost GM. Basic principles of magnetic resonance. In: Pohost GM, O'Rourke RA, eds. Principles and practice of cardiovascular imaging. Boston: Little, Brown, 1991.
4. Blackwell GG, Doyle M, Cranney GB. Cardiovascular MRI Techniques. In Blackwell GG, Cranney GB, Pohost GM, eds. MRI: cardiovascular system. New York: Gower Medical Publishing, 1992.
5. Pettigrew RI. Dynamic cardiac MR imaging: techniques and applications. Radiol Clin 1989; 27: 1183–1203.
6. Mirowitz SA, Lee JKT, Gutierrez FR, Brown JJ, Eilenberg SSS. Normal signal-void patterns in cardiac cine MR images. Radiology 1990; 176:49–55.
7. Wendt RE, Rokey R, Vick GW, Johnston DL. Electrocardiographic gating and monitoring in NMR imaging. Magn Reson Imag 1988; 6:89–95.
8. Dimick RN, Hedlund LW, Herfkens RJ, Fram EK, Utz J. Optimizing electrocardiograph electrode placement for cardiac-gated magnetic resonance imaging. Invest Radiol 1987; 22:17–22.

9. Soulen RL, Budinger TF, Higgins CB. Magnetic resonance imaging of prosthetic heart valves. Radiology 1985; 154:705–7.

10. Shellock FG, Curtis JS. MR imaging and biomedical implants, materials and devices: an updated review. Radiology 1991; 180:541–50.

11. Kanal E, Shellock FG, Talagala L. Safety considerations in MR imaging. Radiology 1990; 176: 593–606.

12. Pohost GM, Blackwell GG. Safety of patients with medical devices during application of magnetic resonance methods. Ann NY Acad Sci 1992; 649:302–12.

13. Blackwell GG, Cranney GB. Cardiac and paracardiac masses. In Blackwell GG, Cranney GB, Pohost GM, eds. MRI: cardiovascular system. New York: Gower Medical Publishing, 1992.

14. Freedberg RS, Kronzon I, Rumancik WM, Liebeskind D. The contribution of magnetic resonance imaging to the evaluation of intracardiac tumors diagnosed by echocardiography. Circulation 1988; 77:96–103.

15. Lund JT, Ehman RL, Julsrud PR, Sinak LJ, Tajik AJ. Cardiac masses: assessment by MR imaging. Am J Radiol 1988; 152:469–73.

16. Gomes AS, Lois JF, Child JS, Brown K, Batra P. Cardiac tumors and thrombus: evaluation with MR imaging. Am J Radiol 1987; 149:895–9.

17. Brown JJ, Barakos JA, Higgins CB. Magnetic resonance imaging of cardiac and paracardiac masses. J Thorac Imag 1989; 4:58–64.

18. Winkler M, Higgins CB. Suspected intracardiac masses: evaluation with MR imaging. Radiology 1987; 165:117–22.

19. Salcedo EE, Cohen GI, White RD, Davison MB. Cardiac tumors: diagnosis and management. Curr Prob Cardiol 1992; 17:75–137.

20. Braunwald E. Heart disease. Philadelphia: W.B. Saunders, 1992.

21. Conces DJ, Vix VA, Klatte EC. Gated MR imaging of left atrial myxomas. Radiology 1985; 156: 445–7.

22. Sechtem U, Theissen P, Heindel W, Hungerberg K, Deutsch HJ, Welslau R, Curtius JM, Hugel W, Hopp HW, Schicha H. Diagnosis of left ventricular thrombi by magnetic resonance imaging and comparison with angiocardiography, computed tomography and echocardiography. Am J Cardiol 1989; 64:1195–1200.

23. Jungehulsing M, Sechtem U, Theissen P, Hilger HH, Schicha H. Left ventricle thrombi: evaluation with spin-echo and gradient-echo MR imaging. Radiology 1992; 182:225–9.

24. Mirowitz SA, Gutierrez FR. Fibromuscular elements of the right atrium: pseudomass at MR imaging. Radiology 1992; 182:231–3.

25. Tuna IC, Julsrud PR, Click RL, Tazelaar HD, Bresnahan DR, Danielson GK. Tissue characterization of an unusual right atrial mass by magnetic resonance imaging. Mayo Clinic Proc 1991; 66:498–501.

26. Levine RA, Weyman AE, Dinsmore RE, Southern J, Rosen BR, Guyer DE, Brady TJ, Okada RD. Noninvasive tissue characterization: diagnosis of lipomatous hypertrophy of the atrial septum by nuclear magnetic resonance imaging. J Am Coll Cardiol 1985; 7:688–92.

27. Rokey R, Mulvagn SL, Cheirif J, Mattox KL, Johnston DL. Lipomatous encasement and compression of the heart: antemortem diagnosis by cardiac nuclear magnetic resonance imaging and catheterization. Am Heart J 1989; 117:952–3.

28. Hananouchi GI, Goff WB. Cardiac lipoma: six-year follow-up with MRI characteristics, and a review of the literature. Magn Reson Imag 1990; 8:825–8.

29. Rienmuller R, Lloret JL, Tiling R, Groh J, Manert W, Muller KD, Seifert K. MR imaging of pediatric cardiac tumors previously diagnosed by echocardiography. J Comput Assist Tomogr 1989; 13:621–6.

30. Camesas AM, Lichstein E, Kramer J, Liebeskind D, Kronzon I, Tyras D, Bodenheimer M. Complementary use of two dimensional echocardiography and magnetic resonance imaging in the diagnosis of ventricular myxoma. Am Heart J 1987; 114:440–2.

31. Kim EE, Wallace S, Abello R, Coan JD, Ewer MS, Salem PA, Ali MK. Malignant cardiac

fibrous histiocytomas and angiosarcomas: MR features. J Comput Assist Tomogr 1989; 13: 627–632.

32.   Johnson DE, Vacek J, Gollub SB, Wilson DB, Dunn M. Comparison of gated cardiac magnetic resonance imaging and two-dimensional echocardiography for the evaluation of right ventricular thrombi: a case report with autopsy correlation. Cathet Cardiovasc Diagn 1988; 14:266–8.

33.   Von Schulthess GHK, Higgins CB. Blood flowing imaging with MR: spin phase phenomenon. Radiology 1985; 157:687.

34.   Underwood SR, Firmin DN, Klipstein RH, Rees RSO, Longmore DB. Magnetic resonance velocity mapping: clinical application of a new technique. Br Heart J 1987; 57:404–12.

35.   Higgins CB. The vascular system. In: Higgins CB, Hricak H, Helms CA, eds. Magnetic Resonance Imaging of the Body. New York: Raven Press, 1992.

36.   Tavares NJ, Auffermann W, Brown JJ, et al. Detection of thrombus by using phase-image MR scans: ROC curve analysis. Am J Radiol 1989; 153:173–8.

37.   Pan X, Rapp JP, Harris HW, Krupski WC, Hale JD, Sheldon P, Kaufman L. Identification of aortic thrombus by magnetic resonance imaging. J Vasc Surg 1989; 9:801–5.

38.   Rapoport S, Sostman HD, Pope C, Camputaro CM, Holcomb W, Gore JC. Venous clots: evaluation with MR imaging. Radiology 1987; 162:527–30.

39.   Pope CF, Dietz MJ, Ezekowitz MD, Gore JC: Technical variables influencing the detection of acute deep vein thrombosis by magnetic resonance imaging. Magn Reson Imag 1991; 9:379–388.

40.   Erdman WA, Weinreb JC, Cohen JM, Buja LM, Chaney C, Peshock RM. Venous thrombosis: clinical and experimental MR imaging. Radiology 1986; 161:233–8.

41.   Braun I, Hoffman J Jr, Malko J, Pettigrew R, Dannels W, Davis P. Jugular venous thrombosis: MR imaging. Radiology 1985; 157:357–60.

42.   Spritzer CE, Sostman HD, Wilkes DC, Coleman RE. Deep venous thrombosis: experience with gradient-echo MR imaging in 66 patients. Radiology 1990; 177:235–41.

10

Comprehensive Cardiac Evaluation with Cine Computed Tomography

Robert M. Weiss and William Stanford
University of Iowa College of Medicine, Iowa City, Iowa

I. INTRODUCTION

Stroke is caused by abrupt interruption of perfusion to a region of brain. Derangements in cardiac structure and function such as arrhythmia or acute pump dysfunction may act as contributing factors in the presence of compromised cerebral circulation. The heart may also directly precipitate stroke by acting as a source of systemic embolus. The precise cardiac and vascular events that cause stroke are rarely observed. Therefore, delineation of the role of the heart in the events leading up to a stroke is usually circumstantial. The role of cardiac imaging in this setting is to provide information about the structure and function of the heart that will enable the clinician and clinical researcher to determine prospectively the likelihood of a cardiac etiology for stroke.

Cine computed tomography is one of a newer generation of advanced cardiac-imaging modalities. This technique has been shown to provide reliable tomographic images of the heart and great vessels with very high temporal and spatial resolution. This technique has several unique attributes that make it a valuable tool for comprehensive cardiac assessment. Two approaches have been employed to obtain cine tomographic images of the heart through detection of x-rays. The first was the dynamic spatial reconstructor, which employs computer integration of information obtained by multiple image intensifiers (1). This technique, which provides excellent temporal and spatial resolution, has been employed on a research basis only and is not commercially available. The second approach uses the Imatron C-100 ultrafast computed tomography scanner. This device became commercially available in the 1980s. Detailed descriptions have been previously published (2). This technique uses gun-generated electron beams that are magnetically focused onto semicircular x-ray–emitting tungsten targets. The emitted x-rays are collimated and vertically directed at a semicircular array of 210 photodiode detectors. Information from the detector array is then converted by a computer to tomographic images. These data are then transferred to an off-line image-analysis computer for further study. In the multislice mode, image acquisition requires 50 ms per tomogram. This minimizes the effects of cardiac motion and allows dynamic visualization of the heart in the cine format. The technique requires only a single 50-ms acquisition period for each final image, thus eliminating the necessity of electrocardiographic "gating." This minimizes the effects of patient and respiratory motion. The whole heart can be interrogated with an imaging time of less than 10 s, the entire procedure usually lasting less than 10 min. The technique yields slices 8 mm thick with in-plane resolution of approximately 1.5 mm.

II. PREVIOUS STUDIES OF CARDIAC STRUCTURE AND FUNCTION WITH CINE COMPUTED TOMOGRAPHY

From the outset, this technique has demonstrated the ability to provide precise quantitative assessment of cardiac anatomy and function. Left ventricular mass can be quantitated with less than 5% error (3) (Fig. 1). Similar accuracy can be obtained in the assessment of right ventricular mass (4). This technique offers advantages over conventional techniques because mass calculations do not rely on geometrical assumptions about cardiac shape. This is a particular advantage under conditions where cardiac geometry is distorted, as after acute myocardial infarction. Cardiac chamber volumes can be quantitated with a high degree of accuracy (5). Figure 2 shows the excellent correlation between stroke volume measurements made with cine computed tomography and those obtained with thermodilution or electromagnetic flow probe as the reference standard. These studies were conducted in laboratory animals. More recently, a similar degree of accuracy was demonstrated in human subjects (6). Reliable evaluation of global left ventricular volumes and contractile function is useful in the identification of important thromboembolic "substrates," e.g., dilated cardiomyopathy. Regional ventricular function can be quantified using an off-line interactive

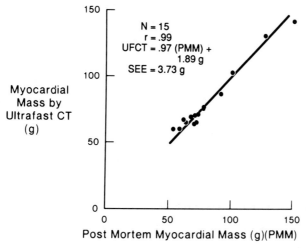

Figure 1 Correlation between cine computed tomography (Ultrafast CT) measurements of left ventricular mass and the actual postmortem mass in 15 experimental animals. (From Ref. 3.) (Ultrafast CT is a registered trademark of the Imatron Corporation, South San Francisco, CA.)

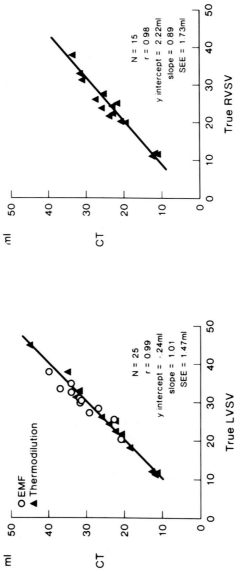

Figure 2 Correlation between cine computed tomography (CT) measurements of stroke volume and those made by either electromagnetic flow probe (EMF) or thermodilution. LVSV = left ventricular stroke volume; RVSV = right ventricular stroke volume. (From Ref. 5.)

image-analysis program (7). The ability to clearly identify endo- and epicardial borders is a particular advantage in this setting. This method has been used to serially assess the size and location of myocardial infarction—a key risk factor for systemic embolization (8,9). The entire left and right atria are reliably imaged in virtually 100% of patients with cine computed tomography. In addition, both atrial appendages are clearly visualized, a distinct advantage over transthoracic echocardiography. The latter point is important because of the predilection for clot formation in the left atrial appendage (see below). Preliminary studies have been conducted that demonstrate superior accuracy of this method in the quantitation of left and right atrial volumes (10). This capability can thus identify the "substrate" for future thrombus formation, even when no clot is present at the time of the study.

The clinical importance of this high degree of quantitative precision has not been sufficiently established. However, one preliminary study by Grenadier et al. demonstrated the superiority of cine computed tomography over conventional techniques (including transthoracic echocardiography and contrast ventriculography) in the diagnosis of left ventricular aneurysm—an important risk factor for stroke (11). A study by Hopson et al. demonstrated gross abnormalities of cardiac chamber size or function in a majority of patients in whom conventional assessment (including two-dimensional echocardiography) previously yielded a diagnosis of "lone atrial fibrillation" (12). These preliminary studies suggest that quantitatively accurate volumetric cardiac assessment can uncover abnormalities not seen by routine evaluation.

A second method of cardiac function analysis employs indicator dilution analysis of contrast medium. This technique has been shown to provide precise assessment of cardiac output as well. This technique can be utilized to identify and quantify hemodynamically significant intracardiac shunts (13)—a condition predisposing to "paradoxical" systemic embolization. The presence of a patent foramen ovale has been incidentally noted with cine computed tomography. However, no studies of the sensitivity and specificity of this finding have been performed.

III. ASSESSMENT OF VALVULAR DYSFUNCTION

The superior spatial resolution of cine computed tomography affords visualization of abnormalities of all four cardiac valves. However, to date no studies have prospectively demonstrated superiority over other methods such as conventional echocardiography. Valvular regurgitation can be identified and precisely quantitated by this technique (14).

IV. IDENTIFICATION OF CARDIAC MURAL THROMBUS

The very high resolution of this technique makes it well suited for detection of cardiac mural thrombi. Figure 3 shows a short-axis tomogram at the level of the left atrium. A thrombus is present in and adjacent to the left atrial appendage and is identified as a "filling defect." This region is not reliably imaged with conventional techniques such as transthoracic echocardiography. Figure 4 shows a tomogram in the apical region of the left ventricle. Once again a thrombus is identified as a filling defect.

Rooholamini et al. evaluated 260 consecutive patients with unexplained stroke or systemic embolization (15). They demonstrated cardiac mural thrombi in 30 and main pulmonary artery thrombus in an additional 5 (total = 13%). A second study by Love et al. compared cine computed tomography with two-dimensional echocardiography in 37 pa-

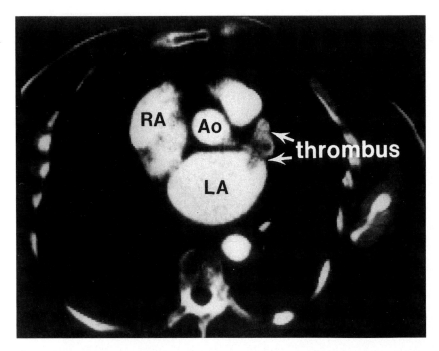

Figure 3   Short-axis tomogram at the cardiac base. Ao = proximal aorta. LA = left atrium. RA = right atrium. A thrombus is present in the left atrial appendage. This was not seen by transthoracic echocardiography.

tients with previously unexplained stroke or transient ischemic attack (16). The results were concordant in only 78% of these patients. A "gold standard" (autopsy) was available in only 2 of 8 discordant cases—both concurring with cine computed tomographic findings. The ultimate clinical importance of the presence or absence of cardiac mural thrombus in this setting has not been prognostically evaluated at this time. Of particular importance was that 32% of the echocardiographic studies in this unselected clinical population were of insufficient quality, whereas only 5% of cine computed tomography studies were technically inadequate. Poor cine tomographic images are usually due to mistakes in timing of contrast injection or to erroneous electrocardiographic triggering as a result of arrhythmia. Repeat studies in those patients usually provide acceptable images.

V.   CARDIAC TUMORS

The presence of cardiac tumors is a predisposing factor for systemic embolus. A number of reports have demonstrated the ability of cine computed tomography to visualize both primary and metastatic cardiac tumors (17–19).

VI.   ADVANTAGES OF CINE COMPUTED TOMOGRAPHY

The chief advantage of cine computed tomography is its consistency in obtaining excellent high-resolution images of the whole heart and surrounding structures (Table 1). The

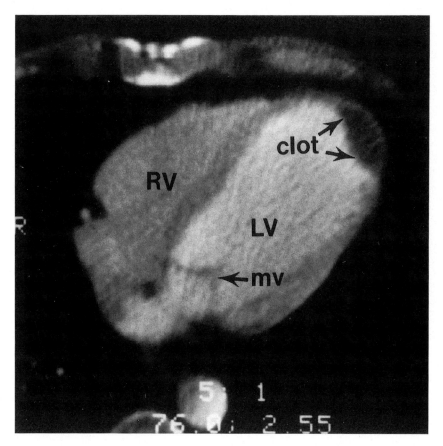

Figure 4 Tomogram taken at the midventricular level. RV = right ventricle; LV = left ventricle; MV = mitral valve.

quantitatively accurate measurements of chamber structure and function are an added advantage. The technique is minimally invasive, requiring only peripheral intravenous access. The technique requires only about 10 min to perform and is suitable for study in critically ill patients. Finally, the technique can provide insight into unsuspected disease processes such as pulmonary embolus (15), pericardial disease (20), aortic dissection (21),

Table 1 Characteristics of Cine Computed Tomography

Advantages	Disadvantages
Consistent images	Limited availability
Superior spatial resolution	Radiation exposure
Rapid image acquisition	Iodinated contrast required
Precise quantitation	Immobile
Minimally invasive	

Table 2 Relative Costs of Imaging Techniques[a]

Imaging techniques	Relative cost
Transthoracic echocardiography	1.0
Transesophageal echocardiography	1.4
Cine computed tomography	1.1
Cine magnetic resonance imaging	1.8
Platelet scan[b]	1.0

[a]Total cost to patients of the University of Iowa Hospitals and Clinics.
[b]Indium-labeled platelet scintigraphy.

and coronary atherosclerosis (22). Future developments may include the ability to quantify regional myocardial and cerebral perfusion.

VII. DISADVANTAGES OF CINE COMPUTED TOMOGRAPHY

The main disadvantage of this technique is its limited availability; currently only 24 referral centers in the United States have scanners in operation (Table 1). A corollary to this shortcoming is the limited clinical and prognostic data that are available with this new modality; few studies are available that compare its usefulness with that of other methods in the setting of stroke. The technique exposes the patient to ionizing radiation. A complete volumetric study of the heart yields about 2.5 rad to the target organ. It also requires administration of iodinated contrast medium, with its attendant risks (23). The apparatus requires a sizable initial investment. Fortunately, the cost per procedure is approximately the same as for transthoracic echocardiographic examination (Table 2). Finally, the imaging apparatus is immobile and thus requires that the patient be transported to the facility.

VIII. SUMMARY

Cine computed tomography is one of a new generation of cardiac imaging techniques with the potential to be highly useful in the evaluation of patients who are at risk for stroke. Early experience suggests that this modality can provide highly accurate, comprehensive cardiac assessment with consistently excellent image quality.

REFERENCES

1. Iwasaki T, Sinak LJ, Hoffman EA, et al. Mass of left ventricular myocardium estimated with dynamic spatial reconstructor. Am J Physiol 1984; 246:H138.
2. Boyd DB. Computerized transmission tomography of the heart using scanning electron beams. In: Higgins CH, ed. Computed tomography of the heart and great vessels. New York: Futura, 1983.
3. Feiring AJ, Rumberger JA, Reiter SJ, et al. Determination of left ventricular mass in dogs with rapid-acquisition cardiac computed tomographic scanning. Circulation 1985; 72:1355.
4. Hajduczok ZD, Weiss RM, Stanford W, Marcus ML. Determination of right ventricular mass in humans and dogs with ultrafast cardiac computed tomography. Circulation 1990; 82:202.

5. Reiter SJ, Rumberger JA, Feiring AJ, et al. Precision of measurements of right and left ventricular volume by cine computed tomography. Circulation 1986; 74:890.

6. Oren RM, Schobel HP, Hill GA, Stanford W, Ferguson DW, Weiss RM. Precise assessment of ventricular stroke volume with cine computed tomography utilizing the long axis in humans. Circulation 1992; 86:II165.

7. Feiring AJ, Rumberger JA, Reiter SJ, et al. Sectional and segmental variability of left ventricular function: experimental and clinical studies using ultrafast computed tomography. J Am Coll Cardiol 1988; 12:415.

8. Stark CA, Rumberger JA, Marcus ML. Determination of myocardial risk area following coronary occlusion with cine computed tomography. J Am Coll Cardiol 1987; 9:158A.

9. Hajduczok ZD, Stanford W, Weiss RM. Effects of acute loading changes on the extent and severity of left ventricular dysfunction after acute myocardial infarction. J Am Coll Cardiol 1991; 17:229A.

10. Vandenberg BR, Weiss RM, Kinzey JE, Marcus ML. Left atrial volume measurements: cine computed tomography and echocardiography. J Am Coll Cardiol 1988; 11:217A.

11. Grenadier E, Weiss RM, Lemmer JH, et al. Surgically resectable left ventricular aneurysm: specific characteristics by ultrafast computed tomography. J Am Coll Cardiol 1989; 13:47A.

12. Hopson JR, Weiss RM, Stanford W, Kienzle MG. Cine computed tomographic abnormalities in "lone" atrial fibrillation. Circulation 1990; 82:III58.

13. Reiter SJ, Feiring AJ, Stanford W, et al. Precise measurements of contrast clearance curve cardiac outputs using cine computed tomography. J Am Coll Cardiol 1987; 9:161A.

14. Reiter SJ, Rumberger JA, Stanford W, Marcus ML. Quantitation of aortic regurgitant volumes in dogs by ultrafast computed tomography. Circulation 1987; 76:758.

15. Rooholamini SA, Galvin JR, Stanford W. Ultrafast CT for the detection of intracardiac and proximal pulmonary artery thromboembolism. Radiology 1989; 173(P):489.

16. Love BB, Struck LK, Stanford W, Biller J, Kerber RE, Marcus ML. Comparison of two-dimensional echocardiography and ultrafast cardiac computed tomography for evaluating intracardiac thrombi in cerebral ischemia. Stroke 1990; 21:1033.

17. Stanford W, Rooholomini SA, Galvin JR. Assessment of intracardiac masses and extracardiac abnormalities by ultrafast computed tomography. In: Marcus ML, Schelbert HR, Skorton DJ, Wolf GL, eds. Cardiac imaging. Philadelphia: W.B. Saunders, 1991:703–13.

18. Scholtz TD, Boskis M, Roust L. Noninvasive diagnosis of recurrent familial left atrial myxoma. Am J Cardiac Imag 1989; 3:142.

19. Stanford W, Galvin JR. The radiology of right heart dysfunction: chest roentgenogram and computed tomography. J Thorac Imag 1989; 4(3):7–19.

20. Oren RM, Stanford W, Weiss RM. Accurate pre-operative diagnosis of pericardial constriction using cine computed tomography. J Am Coll Cardiol 1993 (in press).

21. Stanford W, Rooholamini SA, Galvin JR. Ultrafast computed tomography in the diagnosis of aortic aneurysms and dissections. J Thorac Imag 1990; 5(4):32–9.

22. Janowitz WR, Agatston AS, Zusmer NR, et al. Comparison of ultrafast computed tomography and fluoroscopy in detecting coronary artery calcification. Circulation 1989; 80:II108.

23. Hessel SJ, Adams DF, Abrams HL. Complications of angiography. Radiology 1981; 138:273.

Miscellaneous Techniques

Patrick H. McNulty

Yale University School of Medicine, New Haven, Connecticut

Michael D. Ezekowitz

*Yale University School of Medicine, West Haven Veterans Affairs,
and Cardiovascular Thrombosis Research Laboratory,
New Haven, Connecticut*

I. INTRODUCTION

Since dos Santos et al. first reported examination of the abdominal aorta by direct needle puncture in 1929 (1), angiography has become a safe and accurate procedure for obtaining images of the cardiovascular system. Despite equally dramatic progress in the development of noninvasive imaging techniques, angiography remains a uniquely valuable tool in the evaluation of many patients with suspected thromboembolic disease.

Angiographic examinations are generally performed first to confirm an anatomic abnormality suggested by a noninvasive imaging test, and second, as a primary imaging technique when detailed anatomic information about a small vascular structure is required.

Because angiographic procedures pose greater risks than noninvasive imaging techniques, careful consideration must be given to the type of angiographic procedure required and the risk-benefit ratio of the anticipated procedure for individual patients.

II. FUNDAMENTALS OF ANGIOGRAPHIC TECHNOLOGY

Contrast angiography depends on the relative impenetrance of iodine-containing solutions to x-rays. Such solutions, termed radiocontrast materials, are water-soluble and can be introduced by injection either directly into, or proximally to, a vascular structure of interest. Simultaneous irradiation and collection of x-rays traversing the area of interest results in a transmission image in which vascular structures containing radiocontrast are opacified and therefore are readily distinguished from surrounding soft tissue. These images provide excellent anatomical and functional information and thus can identify congenital and acquired diseases of the thoracic and abdominal aorta and the pulmonary, carotid, and intracerebral arteries. They can also demonstrate the presence of intravascular thrombus (which appears as a filling defect within the contrast-filled lumen of an artery or vein, or a contrast-stained area) or embolic occlusion of distal arteries. They are, in addition, useful in identifying conditions that may predispose to thromboembolism (such as dissection, aneurysmal dilation, or flow-limiting stenoses of the aorta and its major branches) as well as arteriovenous communications that may predispose to paradoxical arterial embolization.

A. Radiographic Equipment

Several more-detailed reviews of the radiographic equipment used for contrast angiography are available (2–4). Contrast angiography utilizes the same ionizing radiation used to make traditional x-ray images. The equipment required for angiographic studies is represented schematically in Figure 1. Briefly, within the x-ray generator tube a metal filament (the cathode) is heated to produce electrons. These electrons impact on a metal target within the generator (the anode), which releases some of the energy thus generated as x-rays. One of the limitations of this process is that only a small fraction (typically 1–2%) of the energy generated by the anode is in the form of x-rays, while the remainder is released as heat. Angiographic procedures generally require a generator tube capable of producing rapid, high-energy x-ray pulses. Accumulation of heat within the anode places an upper limit on the duration and power of the x-ray stream that can be produced by the tube.

X-rays pass from the generator tube through the anatomic area to be examined. These x-rays may be absorbed by tissue, deflected (scattered), or transmitted unimpeded. Only those x-rays transmitted directly without absorption or scatter are collected by an image intensifier mounted coaxially with the x-ray generator tube on the opposite side of the patient. Interposed between the image intensifier and the patient is a scatter-reduction grid, which is composed of lead filters oriented to pass linearly transmitted x-rays to the image intensifier, while absorbing scattered radiation.

Image intensifiers are composed of an input surface coated with a phosphor (typically cesium iodide) that emits photons upon absorbing electromagnetic energy; an electronic focusing system; and a recording system to which the photon stream is directed. Three types of recording systems may be used: plain film is used to record static x-ray transmission images; a 35-mm film camera may be used for cineangiography; or a video camera may be used and the image information converted to digital form and stored on videotape.

Each image-recording technique has advantages in particular cases. Plain film allows x-ray images to be recorded over large fields and is commonly used to produce static images of the thoracic aorta or pulmonary artery and their branches. Cineangiography allows the

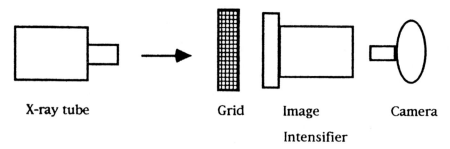

X-ray tube   Grid   Image   Camera

Intensifier

Figure 1 Components of a cineangiographic imaging system.

capture of images on film at 30 to 60 frames per second, permitting such physiologically relevant phenomena as regional cardiac left ventricular contraction and cardiac valvular regurgitation to be examined. Both plain film and cineangiography generally produce images of higher spatial resolution than video recordings, and have therefore traditionally been favored for recording images of small structures such as coronary and intracerebral arteries. Video recording techniques allow x-ray images to be stored and recalled easily, simplify computer-aided quantification of vessel size, and when used with digital subtraction systems are sufficiently sensitive to changes in transmitted x-ray intensity to allow arterial structures to be imaged with very small amounts of selectively injected radiocontrast material, or even radiocontrast injected intravenously (for example, images of the cardiac left ventricle can be made after radiocontrast injection into a peripheral vein).

Diagnostic angiographic examinations result in exposure of both patient and operators to ionizing radiation. While the radiation exposure to each patient during a single examination is small, the potential cumulative exposure for operating personnel is more significant. The principal source of x-ray exposure during angiographic examinations is scatter produced when the incident x-ray beam passes through the examining table and the patient. Exposure requires both passive surveillance and active protection on the part of angiographic personnel. Protection includes minimizing the duration of x-ray exposure for each examination, maximizing the distance between operating personnel and the x-ray generator tube, and wearing lead-lined garments over bone marrow (pelvis and sternum), gonads, and thyroid. Surveillance includes the use of film badges worn both outside and inside lead-lined garments. These badges serve the dual purpose of monitoring x-ray generating equipment for the infrequent problem of excessive leakage and quantifying cumulative personal x-ray exposure. Current regulatory agency guidelines permit radiologic personnel a cumulative exposure of not more than 5 rem (roentgen equivalent man) per year.

B. Technical Considerations in the Performance of Vascular Catheterization

Radiocontrast angiographic studies carry perhaps the greatest potential for patient discomfort and risk of all the imaging modalities used in the evaluation of thromboembolic problems. Nevertheless, the use of modern equipment and careful technique has made these studies generally safe and routine. Most angiographic studies performed to evaluate thromboembolic events—including carotid and cerebral angiography, aortography, and cardiac ventriculography—employ the technique of selective arterial catheterization with intra-arterial contrast injection. It may be illustrative, therefore, to review some common features of this procedure.

In selective arterial contrast angiography, the operator must accomplish four related tasks: (1) obtaining access to the arterial blood stream; (2) positioning an angiographic catheter appropriately for the desired examination; (3) opacifying the vessels of interest and recording the result; and (4) using appropriate pharmacologic measures to prevent and treat potential complications.

While in special circumstances arterial access may still be gained by direct surgical cutdown, the safer and faster Seldinger technique (5), using percutaneous needle puncture followed by guidewire placement, has become the universal standard.

In this procedure, the skin over the artery to be entered is prepared with antiseptic solution and sterile drapes. After infiltration of the surrounding tissues with a local anesthetic (e.g., 2% lidocaine), an angiographic needle is used to puncture the artery. While a variety of needles are in use, the most common are thin-walled, size 18 or 20 gauge, and 6–8 cm in length. Following successful needle puncture, a 0.032- to 0.035-inch-diameter stainless steel guidewire is introduced through the needle and advanced retrograde into the aorta under fluoroscopic guidance. The guidewires commonly used for this purpose have soft, deformable tips curved into a "J" shape, to avoid traumatizing diseased arteries during retrograde advancement of the wire and subsequent catheters.

Following guidewire placement, the needle is removed from the artery and replaced with the desired angiographic catheter. The catheter is then advanced into position in the aorta or one of its branches over the guidewire. The needle/guidewire/catheter procedure thus has the advantages of allowing a relatively large catheter (which may also have a preformed distal end) to be introduced into a peripheral artery through a relatively small needle puncture, and of allowing the catheter to be directed through the arterial system atraumatically as it tracks the flexible guidewire.

The site from which arterial access is most commonly obtained is the right common femoral artery. This artery has the advantages of being large enough to accommodate angiographic catheters without compromising distal blood flow, superficial enough to be readily identified in most persons, and easily compressed against the bony pelvis in the femoral canal to control bleeding after removal of the angiographic catheters.

Other arterial entry sites, in approximate order of suitability, are the left common femoral artery, the right or left axillary artery, and the right or left brachial artery. The axillary or brachial artery is frequently used when atherosclerotic obstruction of the iliac or femoral arteries prevents safe passage of a catheter from the common femoral artery into the aorta. Entry into the aorta, followed by selective angiography of the aortic root, aortic arch, descending aorta, cardiac left ventricle, and carotid arteries may be accomplished from any of these sites.

Carotid angiography by direct needle puncture of the common carotid artery, while still practiced (particularly in children), is less common than angiography via the femoral route. Similarly, direct translumbar aortic puncture for aortography is now of mostly historic interest.

For the common femoral artery, needle puncture is performed two fingers' breadth below the inguinal ligament, where the artery crosses the floor of the bony pelvis. This position assures hemostasis after removal of catheters from the vessel by allowing the puncture site to be compressed against the pelvic floor, while preventing puncture distally in the superficial femoral branch of the common femoral artery, which is small enough to be occluded and thrombosed by large catheters. The axillary artery is correctly punctured over the head of the humerus lateral to the axillary fold, with the patient's arm abducted to 90°; some operators prefer to secure the ipsilateral hand behind the head as well. The brachial artery is quite superficial and easily entered just proximal to the elbow skin crease with the arm abducted and supinated.

A variety of catheters can be used to perform selective contrast angiography. Angiographic catheters were originally made of woven Dacron, but now are more frequently of either polyurethane or polyethylene impregnated with heavy metal salts to make the catheters radiopaque. Adult angiographic catheters range in length from 60 to 125 cm and in diameter from 5 to 8 French gauge.

Catheters used to opacify large arteries (e.g., in aortography) typically have multiple side holes, arranged several centimeters proximal to the distal tip of the catheter, through which contrast can be ejected at high rates. The distal ends of these catheters are either straight or more commonly pig-tailed in shape; the spiral curve of the distal end of a pig-tail catheter allows contrast to exit the catheter in multiple directions, producing rapid opacification and preventing the catheter from recoiling. Selective cannulation of smaller arteries (e.g., the common carotid) requires catheters with tips shaped to enter the desired artery from the aorta. Catheters with many different distal curves are available commercially; some operators prefer to shape a straight catheter into the form required during a particular examination.

Once a catheter has been selected and advanced into the aorta from the arterial entry site, it can be directed into the left cardiac ventricle or any aortic branch through a process of gentle manipulation, and selective angiography can then be performed.

Successful angiographic examination depends on fully opacifying the vascular structure of interest during the time that radiographic images are obtained. This requires that the operator choose a radiocontrast injection rate and volume appropriate to the examination being performed. For small arteries (e.g., the coronary arteries), radiocontrast may be injected by hand through a syringe attached to the hub of the angiographic catheter. Most examinations, however, are better performed using an automated power injector. This device consists of a calibrated glass or plastic syringe in which the plunger is advanced hydraulically, allowing flow rate and injection volume to be programmed with greater precision than is possible with a hand injection. In addition, the power injector is capable of delivering radiocontrast at higher flow rates than can be achieved by hand, and is therefore necessary in the angiographic examination of large vessels.

Finally, several pharmacologic agents may be used during contrast angiography. While the practice is not universal, many laboratories administer heparin intravenously, at the start of arterial catheterization studies, to prevent thrombus formation in catheters and at the arterial entry site. Similarly, it is common to premedicate patients with a mild sedative. Antihistamines may also be given in the hope of minimizing allergic reactions due to radiocontrast-induced mast cell degranulation. Injection of high-osmolarity radiocontrast into the coronary circulation may cause bradycardia requiring treatment with atropine.

Of great importance is the availability of equipment, drugs, and personnel to treat anaphylaxis and other serious adverse reactions to contrast injection. These include a defibrillator, a medication cart with epinephrine, lidocaine, and corticosteroids, and equipment for endotracheal intubation.

C. Properties of Radiocontrast Materials

Radiocontrast materials are used in the performance of well over one million angiographic procedures yearly in the United States. A number of water-soluble contrast materials are currently available; all contain between 30% and 40% iodine and a variable concentration of osmotically active particles. Radiocontrast agents are conveniently classified on the basis of their relative osmolalities: traditional high-osmolality or "ionic" types contain sodium or meglumine salts and have osmolalities of 1400–1700 mOsm/L (i.e., more than five times that of plasma), while newer low-osmolality or "nonionic" types contain instead organic monomers and have osmolalities of 600–800 mOsm/L.

Injection of radiocontrast into the blood stream during angiographic examination may cause several types of adverse response. The most significant of these is anaphylactic reaction to iodine, which occurs with an incidence of approximately 1 in 20,000. Anaphylaxis may occur following the injection of even small amounts of radiocontrast intravenously, and is usually manifested within minutes. In such patients, there is occasionally a remote history of previous contrast allergy, which should be carefully sought before the procedure. If an allergic history is suggested, premedication with a corticosteroid and the antihistamine diphenhydramine for 12 h before contrast exposure has been shown to significantly reduce this risk.

Other effects of radiocontrast injection are dependent on the volume of material injected, the rate of injection, the route of administration, and the type of agent used.

Rapid intra-arterial injection of significant amounts of high-osmolality radiocontrast (as is done in the performance of aortography or cardiac ventriculography) expands intravascular volume within a few seconds; in patients with elevated pulmonary venous pressure due to cardiac left ventricular dysfunction this may produce pulmonary edema. Shortly after this volume expansion, blood pressure may fall as a result of the direct vasodilatory action of radiocontrast. Heart rate may increase secondary to the fall in blood pressure, or may slow if radiocontrast enters the coronary circulation (for example, after aortic root angiography), where it directly inhibits sinoatrial and A-V nodal function. In addition, selective injection of radiocontrast into small arteries may be painful. Finally, occasional patients develop nausea or vomiting after intra-arterial contrast injection.

A number of studies (6–8) have documented that the newer low-osmolality radiocontrast agents cause less discomfort and fewer hemodynamic and electrocardiographic effects than traditional high-osmolality agents. However, two recent randomized, prospective comparisons of high- and low-osmolality radiocontrast agents in cardiac angiography have suggested that the incidence of life-threatening side effects is little different (9,10). Because the unit cost of low-osmolality agents is 10–20 times higher than that of traditional radiocontrast, the appropriate uses for each type are currently being debated. Low-osmolality agents have, however, become the standard for use in procedures requiring selective injection into distal arteries (e.g., carotid arteriography) and in patients expected to be poorly tolerant of the hemodynamic effects of high-osmolality agents.

III. PATIENT SELECTION, PREPARATION, AND COMPLICATIONS

A. Patient Selection

While of primary diagnostic importance in certain situations, angiographic examinations are frequently used to supplement data readily available from noninvasive studies. Thus, one needs to consider carefully their incremental value in the evaluation of suspected thromboembolic disease in very ill patients.

Several absolute and relative contraindications to selective arterial angiographic studies have been suggested.

First, most operators recognize the need to discuss the potential risks and benefits of elective angiographic procedures with patients beforehand, and to obtain written consent. This is both a legal and a practical necessity, since most examinations require the patient's cooperation in breath holding, swallowing, or other tasks. Thus, the inability to give fully informed consent or to cooperate with the examination should usually exclude patients from elective studies. Contrast arteriography, like all studies using ionizing radiation, should be avoided in early pregnancy. Uncorrected bleeding diathesis is a relative contraindication to arterial catheterization, because of the risk of bleeding complications following catheter removal.

Anuric renal failure or severe renal insufficiency increases the risk of hemodynamic compromise during the plasma volume expansion that follows contrast injection. In addition, because radiocontrast may precipitate renal failure in patients with reduced glomerular filtration rates, this risk should be weighed against the information to be gained from the study in patients with renal insufficiency.

Poorly compensated congestive heart failure is a strong relative contraindication to elective angiography because of the risk of pulmonary edema during acute plasma volume expansion, compounded by the negative inotropic effect of radiocontrast agents on the myocardium. Dehydration predisposes to contrast-mediated renal injury, and both it and congestive heart failure should be corrected before the performance of elective angiographic studies. Severe hypertension (diastolic blood pressure over 110–120 mm Hg) is a relative contraindication to arterial catheterization.

Previous severe allergic reaction to contrast is a relative contraindication only, since the risk of recurrence is probably less than 25% (11) and because effective prophylaxis can be given by pretreatment with corticosteriods and antihistamines.

B. Preparation of the Patient

Patient care and procedural success in angiography are improved when the operator visits the patient before the study. This enables the operator to determine the adequacy of the femoral or other arterial pulse, obtain informed consent, and examine relevant laboratory data. These data should include at a minimum blood hemoglobin and urea nitrogen measurements, platelet count, and clotting studies (prothrombin time in all patients, and partial thromboplastin time in patients receiving heparin).

Patients should be instructed to discontinue oral anticoagulants 3–4 days before elective angiographic studies. Food and liquids should be withheld for 8 h before the study. The anticipated arterial entry site should be shaved and scrubbed with antiseptic soap the night before the procedure. Finally, it is common practice to premedicate the patient with a benzodiazepine and an antihistamine (e.g., diazepam 5 mg and diphenhydramine 25 mg orally). Care must be taken with elderly patients not to oversedate, which may render the patient unable to cooperate with the operator during the procedure.

C. Complications of Angiographic Procedures

Adverse events occurring during angiography can be divided into those resulting from radiocontrast, and mechanical complications of vascular catheterization.

In the former category are hypersensitivity reactions to radiocontrast, hemodynamic complications of rapid contrast injection, and nephrotoxicity. Allergy of any degree to radiocontrast is estimated to occur in 2–3% of patients (12), is mediated by mast cell degranulation with histamine release, and is usually limited to pruritus or urticaria. These manifestations are usually self-limited and may be managed with antihistamines. Major allergic reactions occur with an incidence of approximately 0.05–0.01% (13,14), may include bronchospasm and circulatory collapse, and require treatment with adrenergic agonists and corticosteroids. These reactions can occur following either intravenous or intraarterial contrast injection.

The major hemodynamic complication of angiography is pulmonary edema; this occurs most commonly in patients with poorly compensated congestive heart failure and is attributable to the high osmolality of traditional agents (15). This complication is less common when low-osmolality contrast agents are used. Hypotension following contrast injection is also more common with high-osmolality agents, and it can be exacerbated by dehydration. It usually responds promptly to volume expansion.

Acute tubular necrosis following contrast injection is a dose-dependent phenomenon, but nevertheless it is uncommon except in patients with preexisting renal impairment (16). Diabetic nephropathy is a particular risk factor for contrast renal injury. Patients with acute tubular necrosis usually develop oliguria but usually not anuria, and renal function usually returns to baseline from a few days to several weeks following the contrast study. Management is conservative, consisting of expanding extracellular fluid volume and judicious use of diuretic agents.

Mechanical complications due to needle, guidewire, or catheter advancement may be minor or severe, depending on location. Arterial injury at the vascular entry site (including thrombosis, hematoma, bleeding, or pseudoaneurysm formation) occurs with an incidence of approximately 1% after arterial angiography (17). When the common femoral artery is used with careful technique, distal thrombosis or embolization is uncommon; more serious is the risk of retroperitoneal hemorrhage following vascular catheter removal when the arterial puncture has inadvertently been made too proximal, although this also is uncommon.

While hemostasis is more easily achieved after brachial or axillary artery procedures, the incidence of thrombosis is somewhat higher in the smaller brachial and axillary arteries than in the femoral artery. Hematoma formation is potentially more serious at these sites than in the femoral canal, because of the risk of compartment syndrome or brachial plexus compression and neuropathy with an expanding hematoma. Most authors note that local complications following arterial angiography are more common in women (whose arteries may be small) and in elderly patients with atherosclerotic vascular disease.

Other potential mechanical complications include subintimal dissection, arterial or cardiac perforation, and embolization of cholesterol particles or atheromatous debris to the extremities or the renal or splanchnic circulation. The severity of these problems depends largely on the site at which they occur. Cerebral embolization, the greatest potential risk in studies requiring catheter manipulation in the aortic arch, has a reported incidence of 0.1–0.2% (18,19).

IV. SPECIFIC ANGIOGRAPHIC PROCEDURES USEFUL IN THE EVALUATION OF THROMBOEMBOLIC DISEASES

A. Cardiac Left Ventriculography

Angiography of the left cardiac ventricle is performed to assess global and regional myocardial contractility in patients with a variety of cardiovascular diseases. In patients with cerebral or systemic arterial thromboembolism, this procedure may disclose thrombus within the ventricle, suggesting an embolic source, but is neither sensitive nor specific (see Chap. 12). Most thrombi occur in large ventricles, which are difficult to opacify fully; thus false-positive studies are common. Conversely, thrombi that do not project into the cavity of the left ventricle are often not identified on the ventriculogram. Ventriculography may also identify prolapse of the mitral valve (20) or areas of regional contractile dysfunction or aneurysm, both potential sites of thrombus formation.

Cardiac ventriculography is most commonly performed by direct injection of contrast into the left ventricular cavity. This procedure entails advancing a 5- to 8-French gauge pigtailed catheter from the right or left femoral artery into the aortic root, and across the aortic valve into the left ventricle with gentle manipulation; if the aortic valve is calcified or stenotic, it may be necessary to enter the ventricle with a straight guidewire, over which the pig-tail catheter is then advanced.

The angiographic catheter is best positioned with its distal end either centrally in the body of the ventricle or in the left ventricular inflow tract near the mitral valve. In these positions the catheter tip will not come into contact with the endocardium, producing premature beats and distorting the pattern of ventricular contraction while angiographic images are being recorded. The tip should appear to move freely on fluoroscopy; a catheter "trapped" in trabeculations on the floor of the ventricle, or the submitral apparatus, may inject contrast into the myocardium ("staining"), producing ventricular dysrhythmias, or into the left atrium.

Contrast injections in the left ventricle are usually made at a rate of 10–15 ml/s, and cardiac images are most commonly recorded on cineangiography film at 30 or 60 frames per second with the image intensifier positioned in the 30° right anterior oblique projection. If biplane recording equipment is available, orthogonal images may be simultaneously recorded in the 60° left anterior oblique projection. Biplane imaging improves the sensitivity of ventriculography for detecting hypokinetic myocardial segments, potential sites of thrombus formation.

The potential risks of cardiac left ventriculography are dysrhythmia, intramyocardial injection (more common with straight than with pig-tailed catheters), and embolization of air or thrombus during contrast injection. Left ventricular angiography would logically seem more hazardous in ventricles harboring mural thrombi, although firm evidence in support of this is difficult to find. Nevertheless, care should be taken to avoid disturbing a known ventricular thrombus with the angiographic catheter, and one may in fact want to review carefully the indications for ventriculography in such patients, particularly if the history suggests recent embolization.

Cardiac left ventriculography can also be performed using digital subtraction angiography (DSA) (2,21,22) after injection of radiocontrast into a central vein. This procedure has the advantage of not requiring arterial cannulation, avoiding many potential complications and allowing it to be performed on an outpatient basis. In addition, since the angiographic catheter does not enter the ventricle, image quality is not distorted by premature beats during the period when the ventricle is opacified. With this technique, a "mask" x-ray image is obtained over the area of interest just before contrast injection. The video recording screen is then divided into pixels, and the image information within each pixel is digitized by assigning numbers proportional to the intensity of transmitted photons. Subsequent images are obtained after contrast injection, and the "mask" is electronically subtracted from each. Alternatively, DSA may be used after left ventricular contrast injection. The superior sensitivity afforded by DSA in this situation allows the injection of smaller contrast volumes than are used for cineangiographic ventriculography.

B. Aortography

Arch aortography is commonly performed to determine the degree of atherosclerotic stenosis at the origins of the carotid and vertebral arteries in patients with clinical evidence of stroke or transient ischemic attack. Arch aortography may also reveal other anatomic lesions occasionally responsible for thromboembolic events, including aortic aneurysm, dissection, aortitis, and aortic trauma.

This procedure is performed with a thin-walled 5-French pig-tail catheter, inserted via the femoral artery and positioned in the ascending aorta just proximal to the origin of the innominate artery. The axillary artery may be used for vascular access in patients with iliofemoral atherosclerosis or obstruction of the descending aorta (e.g., by aortic coarctation).

For arch aortography the image intensifier is usually positioned in the 45° left anterior oblique position (i.e., with the x-ray tube 45° right posterior oblique), and contrast is injected at 20–22 ml/s. Plain film or video exposures are obtained three times per second for 3 s, then once per second for an additional 3 s. When video image recording is chosen, DSA allows the use of somewhat smaller injection volumes. In cases where aortic valvular regurgitation is suspected (for example, in a type A aortic dissection with disruption of the aortic valve ring), images may be recorded on cineangiography film, which allows better visual interpretation of the degree of regurgitant flow into the left ventricle.

As with cardiac ventriculography, the primary risk is embolization of air, atheroma, or thrombus during contrast injection.

The images obtained with arch aortography in patients with suspected arterial thromboembolism are generally complementary to those available using contrast computed tomography scanning or magnetic resonance imaging, with the exception that aortography provides more useful information regarding aortic insufficiency.

C. Carotid and Cerebral Angiography

Carotid angiography is the definitive imaging technique in the evaluation of patients with cerebral ischemia and evidence suggesting carotid atherosclerosis. Such evidence may consist of an audible bruit over one or both carotid arteries on examination, Doppler evidence of acceleration of blood flow through a carotid stenosis, or evidence of asymmetric hemispheric perfusion (e.g., by ocular plethysmography or radionuclide perfusion scanning) in the patient with stroke or transient ischemic attack.

The procedure usually begins with performance of arch aortography, which allows the proximal vertebral and carotid arteries to be examined and identifies their origins and course for subsequent selective angiography. While it is possible to record images of the aorta and the carotid and cerebral arteries using DSA after large-volume intravenous contrast injection, selective arterial studies are performed more commonly and produce superior images.

Selective carotid angiography is most commonly performed via the right or left common femoral artery. The arteries are cannulated individually using a small (4 or 5 French) endhole catheter; a catheter with a short hook (e.g., Berenson) or more complex distal curves (e.g., "headhunter") may be manipulated in the aortic arch to point into the origin of the common carotid artery, after which it is advanced to several centimeters below the artery's bifurcation. Selective cannulation of the vertebral arteries is similarly possible.

Low-osmolality radiocontrast is generally used for carotid and cerebral angiography, as it is less painful and less toxic to the central nervous system than high-osmolality agents. For selective carotid angiography, 10–12 ml of contrast is injected with an automated injector, and images are obtained in oblique and lateral projections. Digital subtraction imaging, using electronic subtraction of a previously obtained mask from angiographic video images, aids in visualization of carotid lesions with lower volumes of contrast and is now commonly practiced. This procedure requires that the patient cooperate to the extent of avoiding swallowing or head movement while subtraction masks are being acquired.

Potential complications of selective carotid angiography include cerebral embolization of atheroma, thrombus, or air, and central nervous system toxicity (transient visual loss, seizure) attributed to the interaction of radiocontrast with the blood-brain barrier. In experienced hands using low-osmolality contrast, the serious complication rate should not exceed 0.5–1.0%.

D. Lower Extremity Phlebography

Lower limb ascending contrast phlebography is the most accurate means of detecting the presence and extent of deep venous thrombosis in patients with pulmonary embolism or suspected paradoxical arterial embolism. The sensitivity of this procedure for venous thrombosis approaches 100%, although it is not always possible to distinguish between acute and chronic venous obstruction. The test is most commonly used to confirm a diagnosis of proximal (i.e., above the knee) lower extremity deep venous thrombosis suggested by physical examination or by a noninvasive test, such as impedance plethysmography or Doppler flow interrogation.

Ascending phlebography is usually performed with the patient secured to a tilting radiographic table. A small-gauge butterfly needle is inserted into a vein on the dorsum of the foot and connected to a syringe filled with low-osmolality radiocontrast. With a tourniquet occluding venous flow at the level of the knee, contrast is injected into the dorsal vein, and the table is slowly tilted until contrast can be seen to fill the calf veins on fluoroscopy; images of these veins are then recorded on plain x-ray film. The tourniquet at the knee is then removed and the table is tilted further to allow contrast to fill the deep veins of the thigh and the groin. Elevation of the leg and compression of the calf often allows adequate opacification of the femoral and iliac veins and the distal inferior vena cava. At the end of the examination, contrast is cleared from the leg veins by injecting saline through the angiographic needle.

If the iliac veins and inferior vena cava fail to opacify during ascending phlebography (as is the case in approximately 50% of examinations), direct pelvic venography may be necessary. This procedure involves needle puncture of the common femoral vein in the femoral canal, under local anesthesia. Contrast is injected through the needle by hand, and antero-posterior radiographs are taken to demonstrate the femoral and iliac veins and the vena cava.

The potential risks of lower extremity phlebography include those detailed above for exposure to radiocontrast material. The indications for phlebography should be considered with particular care in patients with a previous severe reaction to contrast media. Other potential complications include chemical cellulitis from extravasation of contrast, local pain during injection, and the potential for thrombosis in veins filled with radiocontrast. These complications occur very infrequently when low-osmolality contrast agents are used.

The major limitation of ascending phlebography is technical. About 10% of studies are technically inadequate, precluding a definitive interpretation. The interpretation of technically adequate studies is variable. Thus, although this technique remains the standard, important limitations exist.

V. VASCULAR CATHETERIZATION IN THE EVALUATION OF PARADOXICAL EMBOLIZATION

Paradoxical embolization is embolization of a thrombus or other material from the venous into the arterial system (see Chap. 15). This logically requires that a communication exist between the venous and arterial circulations proximal to the lungs; the most common such communications in adults are patent foramen ovale and atrial septal defect. Less common examples include ventricular septal defect, patent ductus arteriosus, and tetralogy of Fallot.

While paradoxical embolization accounts for only a small fraction of arterial occlusive events (e.g., stroke) in adults overall, it is proportionally more important as a cause of stroke in young patients without atherosclerotic vascular disease.

In addition to the presence of an arteriovenous communication, paradoxical embolization requires that right-sided cardiac pressures be equal to or higher than left-sided pressures across the communication at the time of embolization. Cyanotic congenital cardiac anomalies, including tetralogy of Fallot, transposition of the great arteries, and the "Eisenmenger complex" resulting from chronic left-to-right shunting across a large ventricular septal defect, are examples of intracardiac communications with chronic equalization of right and left heart pressures. In the patient with suspected paradoxical embolization, these conditions should be considered if (1) resting arterial hypoxemia is present without an apparent explanation, and (2) hypoxemia is not fully corrected (i.e., 99–100% arterial oxygen saturation) with administration of oxygen.

By far the more common cause of paradoxical embolization is reversal of flow in a communication that normally shunts blood left to right (e.g., atrial septal defect), or the opening of a patent foramen ovale as a consequence of sudden evaluation in thoracic venous pressure. This can occur with a Valsalva maneuver, during parturition or positive pressure mechanical ventilation, or as a consequence of acute pulmonary hypertension (e.g., following a pulmonary embolism).

Although the presence of an atrial septal defect or patent foramen ovale can be suggested by Doppler or contrast echocardiography, intracardiac catheterization is usually required to confirm the finding and to assess the magnitude of shunting. Confirmation of atrial septal defect or patent foramen ovale is obtained when an angiographic catheter can be advanced under fluoroscopic guidance from the right to the left atrium. The presence, location, and magnitude of an intracardiac communication associated with left-to-right shunting of blood can also be determined by sequential measurement of blood oxygen saturation during passage of a sampling catheter through the right cardiac chambers (23). Blood oxygen saturations in the superior vena cava, right atrium, right ventricle, and pulmonary arteries are normally between 50% and 75%, and differ by no more than 7%. An increase ("step-up") in oxygen saturation between the vena cavae and the pulmonary artery indicates entry of oxygenated blood from the left heart into the right heart. The level of the step-up (right atrial, right ventricular, etc.) localizes the intracardiac communication, which may be considered a potential route of paradoxical embolization. When a right-to-left intracardiac shunt has been confirmed its magnitude can be determined by subtracting measured pulmonary blood flow (comprising net cardiac output plus left-to-right shunt flow) from systemic blood flow (24).

VI. IMPEDANCE PLETHYSMOGRAPHY

Impedance plethysmography is a technique that measures changes in blood volume. Its major application relates to the diagnosis of deep vein thrombosis. When there is obstruction to venous flow, the decline in blood volume following deflation of a pneumatic cuff is reduced and delayed (25–27). Commercially available units (IPG-200; Codman) use the occlusion-cuff technique described by Wheeler et al. (25,26). Patients are examined while they are lying supine with their legs elevated 15–30°. A pneumatic cuff is applied to the mid-thigh and inflated to occlude venous return; it is then deflated. Changes in blood volume produce changes in electrical impedance that are recorded on a strip chart recorder. The rise in blood volume and the changes in impedance after cuff occlusion are plotted against the fall in blood volume during the first 3 s after deflation. The ratio of the rise over the fall, called the venous function index, is plotted on a graph with a discriminant line. Patients whose venous function index values fall below the discriminant line are called abnormal. If an abnormal result is obtained up to four repeat examinations are performed (27). If, on repeat examination, the venous function index value falls into the normal range, the examination is interpreted as normal. If the venous function index value remains in the abnormal range at the end of four repeat examinations, the final result is interpreted as abnormal. This technique is totally noninvasive and is cheap, costing approximately $100.

False-negative plethysmographic studies occur in patients with good venous collaterals and in patients with nonocclusive thrombi. Thrombi located in the calf have a low detection rate.

False-positive studies occur in patients with heart failure or in those with nonthrombotic proximal occlusions. In addition, studies may be falsely positive if the patient is tense or positioned incorrectly or has severe arterial disease reducing in-flow.

REFERENCES

1. Dos Santos R, Lamas AC, Pereira-Caldas J. Arteriografia da aorta e dos vasas abdominales. Med Contemp 1929; 43:93.
2. Collins DA, Skorton DJ, eds. Cardiac imaging and image processing. New York: McGraw-Hill, 1986.
3. Grossman W, ed. Cardiac catheterization and angiography. 3d ed. Philadelphia: Lea & Febiger, 1986.
4. Whitehouse GH, Worthington BS, eds. Techniques in diagnostic imaging. 2d ed. Oxford: Blackwell Scientific Publications, 1990.
5. Seldinger S. Catheter replacement of needle in percutaneous arteriography: a new technique. Acta Radiol 1953; 39:368–76.
6. Hirshfeld JW. Cardiovascular effects of iodinated contrast agents. Am J Cardiol 1990; 66: 9F–17F.
7. Hirshfeld JW, Laskey WK, Martin JL, Groh WC, Untereker W, Wolf GL. Hemodynamic changes induced by cardiac angiography with ioglaxate: comparison with diatrizoate. J Am Coll Cardiol 1983; 2:954–7.
8. Mancini GBJ, Bloomquist V, Bhargava V. Hemodynamic and electrocardiographic effects in man of a new nonionic contrast agent (iohexol): advantages over standard ionic agents. Am J Cardiol 1983; 51:1218–22.
9. Barrett BJ, Parfrey PS, Vavasour HM, O'Dea F, Kent G, Stone E. A comparison of nonionic, low osmolality radiocontrast agents with ionic, high-osmolality agents during cardiac catheterization. N Engl J Med 1992; 326:431–6.
10. Steinberg EP, Moore RD, Powe NR, Gopalan R, Davidoff AJ, Litt M, Graziano S, Brinker JA. Safety and cost effectiveness of high-osmolality as compared with low-osmolality contrast materials in patients undergoing cardiac angiography. N Engl J Med 1992; 326:425–30.
11. Shehadi WH. Contrast media adverse reactions: occurrence, recurrence and distribution patterns. Radiology 1982; 143:11–7.
12. Goldberg M. Systemic reactions to intravascular contrast media: a guide for the anesthesiologist. Anaesthesiology 1984; 60:46.
13. Mills SR, Jackson DC, Older RA, Heaston DK, Moore AV. The incidence, etiologies, and avoidance of complications of pulmonary angiography in a large series. Radiology 1980; 136:295.

14. Hessel SJ, Adams DF, Abrahams HL. Complications of angiography. Radiology 1982; 138: 273–81.

15. Iseri LT, Kaplan MA, Evans MJ, Nickel ED. Effect of concentrated contrast media during angiography on plasma volume and plasma osmolality. Am Heart J 1965; 69:154.

16. D'Elia JA, Gleason RE, Alsay M, Malarick C, Godley K, Warram J, Kaldany A, Weinruch LA. Nephrotoxicity from angiographic contrast material: a prospective study. Am J Med 1982; 72:719.

17. Adams DF, Fraser DB, Abrams HL. The complications of coronary angiography. Circulation 1973; 48:609–15.

18. Kennedy JW. Complications associated with cardiac catheterization and angiography. Cathet Cardiovasc Diagn 1982; 8:5–11.

19. Braunwald E, Swan HCJ, eds. Cooperative study on cardiac catheterization. Circulation 1968; 37(suppl III):1.

20. Criley JM, Lewis KB, Humphries JO, Ross RS. Prolapse of the mitral valve: clinical and cineangiographic findings. Br Heart J 1966; 28:488.

21. Kruger RA, Riederer SJ. Digital subtraction angiography. Boston: G.K. Hall, 1984.

22. Levin DC, Shapiro RM, Baxt LM, Dunham L, Harrington DP, Ergun DL. Digital subtraction angiography: principles and pitfalls of image improvement techniques. Am J Roentgenol 1984; 143:447.

23. Antman EM, Marsh JD, Green LH, Grossman W. Blood oxygen measurements in the assessment of intracardiac left to right shunts: a critical appraisal of methodology. Am J Cardiol 1980; 46:265–70.

24. Flamm MD, Cohn KE, Hancock EW. Measurement of systemic cardiac output at rest and exercise in patients with atrial septal defect. Am J Cardiol 1969; 23:258.

25. Hull RD, Van Aken WG, Hirsh J, Gallus AS, Hoicka G, et al. Impedance plethysmography using the occlusive cuff technique in the diagnosis of venous thrombosis. Circulation 1976; 53: 696–700.

26. Wheeler HB, Pearson D, O'Connell D, Mullick SC. Impedance plethysmography. Arch Surg 1972; 104:164–9.

27. Hull R, Taylor DW, Hirsh J, Sackett DL, Powers P, Turpie AGG, Walker I. Impedance plethysmography: the relationship between venous filling and sensitivity and specificity for proximal vein thrombosis. Circulation 1978; 58:898–902.

III

MANAGEMENT CONSIDERATIONS

12

The Left Ventricle

Michael D. Ezekowitz

Yale University School of Medicine, West Haven Veterans Affairs, and Cardiovascular Thrombosis Research Laboratory, New Haven, Connecticut

I. INTRODUCTION

With the demonstration of reliable techniques for the identification of left ventricular thrombi (1–10), important questions have emerged concerning the value of these tests not only for diagnosis, but also for stratifying risk for embolization and identifying patients who would benefit most from treatment. This chapter will critically review each technique and attempt to define a rational approach to the diagnosis of left ventricular thrombi in the settings of acute myocardial infarction, chronic left ventricular aneurysms, and poor ventricular function. Each of these entities is marked by either global or regional left ventricular dysfunction, a prerequisite for the development of a ventricular thrombi. Tumors are much rarer causes of intraventricular masses that might embolize. Following the discussion of the diagnostic approaches, strategies for treatment will be developed.

II. TECHNIQUES FOR DIAGNOSIS OF LEFT VENTRICULAR THROMBI

A. Echocardiography

Echocardiography (see Chap. 7) is the most widely used technique for the diagnosis of left ventricular clot. It is the least expensive of the available imaging techniques and is the most widely available, and it is totally noninvasive, without known danger. Most present-day two-dimensional echocardiographic instruments are compact and portable, enabling evaluation at the patient's bedside in the intensive care unit. Echocardiography also provides important additional information in patients with myocardial infarction. While echocardiography is mostly superfluous for diagnosis of acute infarction (11), it often provides important prognostic information. Several studies have shown an important relationship between the extent of left ventricular dysfunction and serious complications such as death, shock, heart failure, and arrhythmias (12–15). It has been shown that patients with detectable anatomical impairment have a much higher risk for major in-hospital complications (13,14). A baseline study also serves as a frame of reference for complications that may occur later.

In general, for the evaluation of the left ventricle a 2- or 2.25-MHz transducer is used. This choice represents a good compromise between penetration of the ultrasonic beam into the tissue and resolution of the image. Generally, the higher the frequency the better the resolution of the image and the poorer the penetration. For the evaluation of the left ventricle, it is critical to evaluate the anteroapical segment, the most important site of thrombus formation. The apical two- and four-chamber views are those that are most commonly utilized. To acquire this view, the transducer is placed over the cardiac apex with the patient lying supine in the left lateral position. Two imaging planes are usually recorded. The first, in the cross-sectional view, provides an image of all four cardiac chambers, and the second, in a longitudinal fashion, provides an image of the left ventricle and the left atrium.

1. Accuracy of Echocardiography

Studies performed over the past decade have defined the accuracy of echocardiography in identifying thrombi in the left ventricle of the heart. In early studies that used M-mode echocardiography the technique was neither sensitive nor specific for identifying left ventricular thrombus, since with this method it is seldom possible to examine the cardiac apex, where over 90% of these thrombi occur (16–19). The modality of choice is therefore two-dimensional echocardiography, which offers spatial resolution enabling examination of the cardiac apex from either the apical or the subxyphoid transducer position. To distinguish thrombus from artifact it is important to use strict criteria for thrombus diagnosis (10). The thrombus should (1) be adjacent to (but distinct from) abnormally contracting myocardium, (2) be seen in at least two transducer positions, and (3) be distinguished by a clear thrombus-blood interface. The echogenicity of the interior of the thrombus can vary; it may be highly echogenic, or if the thrombus is homogeneous, the interior may be relatively echo-free (Fig. 1). Thrombi may be classified according to spatial characteristics as mural, protuberant, or highly mobile (20–22). The accuracy of two-dimensional echocardiography in diagnosing thrombus has been assessed in five studies (Table 1). In one of the largest prospective studies, Visser et al. in 1983 (23) found that echocardiography had a sensitivity of 92% and a specificity of 88% in a series of 67 patients. The reference standard was either aneurysmectomy or autopsy. Fifty-one patients underwent left ventricular aneurysmectomy, and an additional 16 patients were studied before death during the acute phase of myocardial infarction. A second study by Ezekowitz et al. (10) of 53 patients studied prospectively before aneurysmectomy (n = 50) or death (n = 3) found the sensitivity and specificity of echocardiography to be 77% and 96%, respectively. A third study by Stratton et al. (24), in which aneurysmectomy and platelet scintigraphy were used as the reference standard, found a sensitivity of 95% and a specificity of 86% in a series of 78 patients. The study by Starling et al. (25), which included 21 patients undergoing echocardiography before aneurysmectomy, reported a sensitivity of 77% and a specificity of 100%. In the most recent study, Sheiban et al. (26) reported a sensitivity of 100% (14/14) and a specificity of 97% (57/59) in a series of 73 patients with surgical validation. The four earlier studies were performed almost 5 years before Sheiban's study. As reflected in the Sheiban study, the technology of echocardiography has improved significantly. In addition, color Doppler promises to provide further information (27) by demonstrating flow patterns that might predict the development of thrombi or emboli. Thus, for the vast majority of patients,

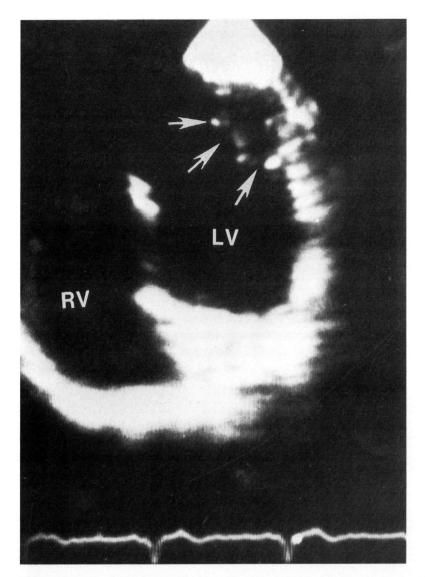

Figure 1 Left ventricular thrombus (arrowed). LV = left ventricle; RV = right ventricle.

Table 1 Accuracy of Echocardiography for the Diagnosis of Left Ventricular Thrombus

	Sensitivity[a]	Specificity[b]	Validation
Ezekowitz et al., 1982 (10)	10/13 = 77%	26/27 = 96%	Surgery
Stratton et al., 1982 (24)	21/22 = 95%	48/56 = 86%	Surgery/autopsy/platelet scan
Visser et al., 1983 (23)	24/26 ± 92%	36/41 = 88%	Surgery/autopsy
Starling et al., 1983 (25)	10/13 = 77%	8/8 = 100%	Surgery/autopsy
Sheiban et al., 1987 (26)	14/14 = 100%	57/59 = 97%	Surgery

[a]Sensitivity = true positive/(true positive + false negative).
[b]Specificity = true negative/(true negative + false positive).

echocardiography is a very accurate technique for the identification of left ventricular thrombus.

2.   The Optimal Timing for Imaging in Patients After Myocardial Infarction

The optimal time to acquire an echocardiogram in the acute phase of myocardial infarction depends not only on when thrombi can be best visualized, but also on when emboli occur and on the expected effect of therapy. It has long been recognized that most mural thrombi occur very early after myocardial infarction (6,28–31). Asinger et al. (5) found that thrombi occurred a mean of 5 ± 3 (mean ± 1 SD) days after the acute event. Gueret et al. (32) found, in a series of 21 patients with thrombi, that these occurred a mean of 4.3 ± 3 days after infarction, with 10 seen by day 2 and 20 of 21 by day 4. Davis et al. (29) reported that 23 of 29 patients had thrombi by the third day after acute infarction, and Spirito et al. (30) found that approximately half of their patients had thrombi by 48 h. Domenicucci et al. (31) found in 59 nonanticoagulated patients, when serial echocardiograms were performed following acute myocardial infarction, that thrombi developed 12 ± 47 (mean ± 1 SD) days after infarction, with a range of 1 to 362 days. Eighty-three percent of the thrombi were seen in the first week, with 5% in weeks 1–2 and 12% after week 2. Thus most left ventricular clots are imaged in the first week after acute myocardial infarction; however, over 15% of thrombi developed after the first week. It is also important to recognize that very early studies, i.e., within the first 48 to 72 h after the infarction, may fail to identify thrombi that presumably have not yet formed. In the study of Asinger et al. (5), only one of 12 thrombi was seen at less than 72 h, and similarly, in three other studies (29,30,32) only about 50% of thrombi were iden-

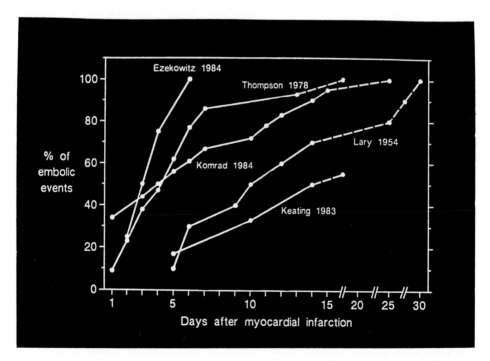

Figure 2   Maximum time for the thrombus to become apparent after acute myocardial infarction. (Ezekowitz MD, Azrin MA. Should patients with large anterior wall myocardial infarction have echocardiography to identify left ventricular thrombus and should they be anticoagulated? In: *Dilemmas in Clinical Cardiology*, Melvin D. Cheitlin (guest editor), pp. 105–121 (1990).

tified by 48 h. Therefore, evaluation in the first few days after infarction will fail to detect a large proportion of thrombi, whereas by the end of the first week almost all thrombi can be visualized.

In patients with acute myocardial infarction the risk of embolization is highest in the first few days (Fig. 2) and decreases over time, with approximately two-thirds of systemic emboli occurring within the first week after the index infarction (20–22,33–43). In a retrospective study, Stratton and Resnick (34) demonstrated that increased embolic risk was not restricted to the immediate postinfarction period. Patients with left ventricular thrombi continue to be at risk of embolization for as long as 5 years after myocardial infarction. Thus, the risk of embolization is highest immediately after infarction, and emboli may occur as early as the first day, but the presence of thrombus is a marker of an increased risk at any time.

3. Stratification of Risk

Because the overall incidence of embolization following myocardial infarction is low, it is important to identify subgroups of patients who are at higher risk. A number of investigators have identified anterior transmural myocardial infarction as the major predisposing factor to the formation of intracardiac thrombi and subsequent systemic embolization (6,9,32, 33,43–47). The incidence of systemic embolization in patients with inferior myocardial infarction and subendocardial myocardial infarction is low (6,9,42,43,45,46). Large inferior myocardial infarctions with involvement of the anteroapical segment present a risk of thromboembolism similar to that associated with transmural anterior myocardial infarction.

The presence of thrombus alone is a marker of significant risk for subsequent embolization (34,44,47,48). The morphology and mobility of the thrombus both can predict added risk for embolization. Several studies have shown a positive correlation between the mobility of the clot, its protuberance into the ventricular cavity, and the risk of subsequent embolization (20–22,34,47,49). The more mobile and protuberant the thrombus, the more likely it is to embolize. Domenicucci et al. (31) reported considerable spontaneous variation in the characteristics of a thrombus at different times, confirming an earlier case report by Johannessen (47). Domenicucci et al. (31) found that five of eight mobile thrombi later became nonmobile, while 12 originally nonmobile thrombi subsequently became mobile, and that 41% of thrombi changed from mural to protuberant or vice versa. They also noted that these changes occurred over widely disparate times. Thus, the analysis of the morphologic features of thrombi may have limitations. Recently Johannessen et al. (49) studied a large group of patients with anterior myocardial infarction and noted that in addition to thrombus mobility and protuberance, patient age (>68 years) was also a significant predictor of subsequent embolization, although this finding is at variance with a previous report (34).

4. Competing and Complementary Technology

There are several techniques that compete with or complement echocardiography in the diagnosis of intracardiac clot. These are indium-111 (^{111}In) platelet scintigraphy (see Chap. 8), magnetic resonance imaging (see Chap. 9), x-ray tomography (see Chap. 10), and contrast ventriculography (see Chap. 11).

B. Platelet Imaging

Working at Hammersmith Hospital in London, Thakur and associates (50) first chelated indium 111, a gamma-emitting radioisotope, with 8-hydroxyquinoline, a molecule that permitted passage of an imageable isotope into the cell without altering the physiologic function of the cell (50). Thus, it was theoretically possible to inject labeled platelets into patients and image clots in any location in the body. This radionuclide-based technique depends on the active exchange of platelets between the blood and the thrombus surface, and it not only allows identification of the thrombus but also reflects its activity (51,52). In patients with left ventricular aneurysms this technique has been found to be highly specific, approaching 100% (10). Its sensitivity, however, was lower, at 72% (10). The lower sensitivity reflects the relative inactivity of the clot. Although comparative studies have not been performed in patients with acute infarction, it is anticipated that sensitivity would be higher because of the active formation of clot.

1. Interpretation of Images

The interpretation of platelet images is usually decisive. Thrombi are most often represented as a single "hot spot" (Fig. 3). Multiple hot spots may be seen but are less common (Fig. 4). A thrombus may be imaged tangentially, in which case a linear area of increased activity is depicted (Fig. 5). Occasionally, when the clot is laminated against the wall of an aneurysm, a doughnut-shaped image is seen. In patients with elevated left hemidiaphragms (Fig. 6), the spleen may cause difficulty with interpretation of the anterior and right anterior oblique images. The main point of differentiation between splenic activity and that due to thrombus is that the activity due to the spleen characteristically accumulates early, within minutes of injection. Increased activity due to a thrombus tends to be maximal 3 to 4 days after injection of the platelet suspension (Fig. 7). This is contrasted with a series of negative images (Fig. 8). Occasionally, cardiac myxomas may accumulate platelets on their surface and be mistaken for thrombi (53) (Fig. 9). With attention to these details, errors in interpretation are unusual.

In a retrospective analysis of 662 images obtained from 64 patients read on two separate occasions by three blinded observers, the intra- and interobserver agreement was 91% and 88%, respectively (54). The optimal time for imaging was in the 3- to 4-day period following the injection of the platelet suspension. The left anterior oblique view was the optimal view (Fig. 10). For best diagnostic accuracy, images acquired on the first and third or

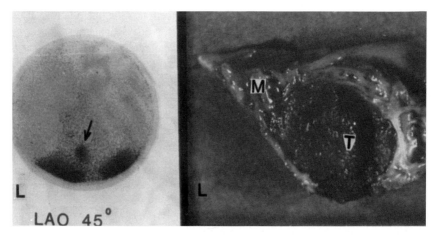

Figure 3 An area of increased activity representing a left ventricular thrombus. This image was acquired 72 h after the injection of labeled platelets suspension. The corresponding surgical specimen from or after an aneurysectomy is shown adjacent. T = thrombus, M = muscle.

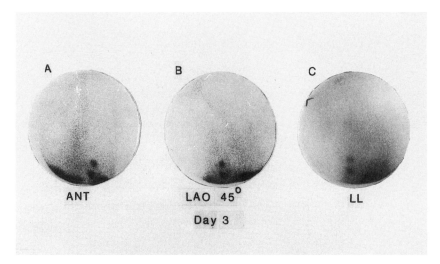

Figure 4 Images in the anterior, left anterior oblique, and left lateral views demonstrating two large thrombi in the apex of the left ventricle. This image was obtained 3 days after the injection of labeled platelet suspension.

fourth days after injection of the isotope in the left anterior oblique view are usually adequate. In patients imaged during the acute phase of myocardial infarction, multiple imaging views are often used for localization of the thrombus to a particular chamber. These patients are prone to have thrombi in multiple sites, and it is important to distinguish thrombi in the coronaries, right ventricle, or in the atria from those in the left ventricle (55–57) (Figs. 11 and 12). Tomographic imaging may be useful (Fig. 13).

Platelets interact in a dynamic manner at the blood thrombus interface. Therefore, platelet scintigraphy might be used as a direct index of thrombus activity. The effect of aspirin on the incorporation of ^{111}In-labeled platelets into cardiac thrombi has been studied (52,55). Stratton and Ritchie (52) noted that one of six positive platelet scans became negative in patients treated with aspirin and dipyridamole, and that sulfinpyrazone and warfarin administration converted three of seven and two of three positive platelet scans, respectively. In another study, by Ezekowitz et al., the in vitro and in vivo behavior of platelets was compared in 11 patients with aneurysms and mural thrombi (55). In all patients, platelet images were positive, whether the patients were treated with aspirin or not. Thus, although in vitro platelets from patients receiving aspirin aggregated abnormally (Fig. 14), they nevertheless took part in thrombosis in vivo. This study by Ezekowitz et al. suggests a disparity between the in vivo behavior of platelets and their in vitro function (55).

2. *Quantification of Images*
Quantification of intracardiac imaging is difficult. The quantity of radioactivity detected depends on the size, shape, and orientation of the object in the area of interest as well as the distance of the object from the detector and the characteristics of the imaging system (57). Since platelets circulate in the blood and provide a dark background differentiation of circulating platelets from those accumulating on a thrombogenic surface can be difficult. Attempts to obviate these problems have been made by developing a dual-isotope blood pool subtraction technique (57). This technique assumes that labeled red cells are not taken up by

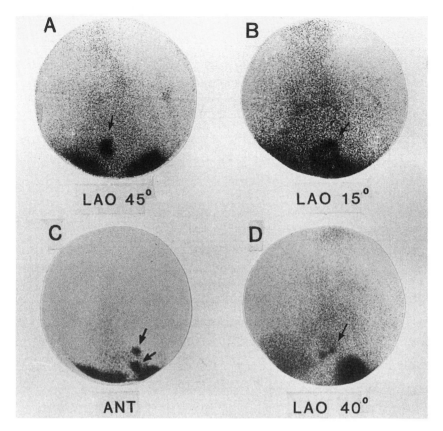

Figure 5 Scintiphotos obtained 72 h after injection of the platelet suspension. Images are oriented with the top of the illustration cephalad. The increased activity in the lower left quadrant in each panel is from the liver. The arrows point to areas of increased activity within the left ventricle and represent typical active thrombi within large anteroapical left ventricular aneurysms. These images were obtained from four different patients.

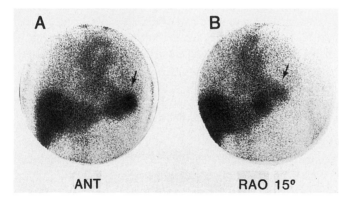

Figure 6 Image of a patient with a raised left hemidiaphragm. The arrow points to areas of increased activity which superficially resembles a thrombus in the apex of the ventricle. This patient had normal ventricular function and on chest x-ray had a left raised hemidiaphragm. The arrow reflects activity from the spleen. (From Ezekowitz MD, et al. Diagnostic accuracy of indium-111 platelet scintigraphy in identifying left ventricular thrombi. Am J Cardiol 51:1712–1716, 1983.)

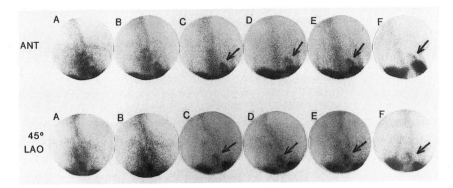

Figure 7 Series of images obtained on the day of injection of the labeled platelet suspension (Panel A) and daily thereafter. The arrows point to an area of increased activity representing a thrombus in the left ventricle. (Heynes AP, Badenhorst PN, Lotter MG (eds). Platelet Kinetics and Imaging, CRC, Boca Raton, 1985.)

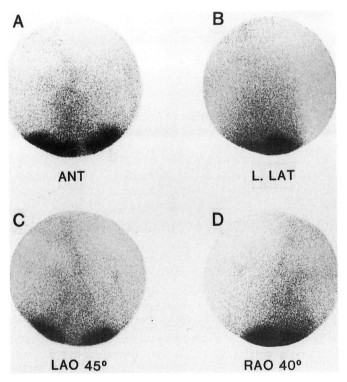

Figure 8 The area of increased activity in panels A and C in the right lower zone is due to the spleen and that in the left lower zone is due to the liver. In panels B and D there is superimposition of liver and splenic activity in the lower portions of both panels. This figure represents a typical series of negative images obtained 72 h after injection of the platelet suspension. ANT = anterior; LAO = left anterior oblique; LLAT = left lateral; RAO = right anterior oblique. (From Ezekowitz, MD et al. Diagnostic accuracy of indium-111 platelet scintigraphy. Am J Cardiol 51: 1712–1716, 1983.)

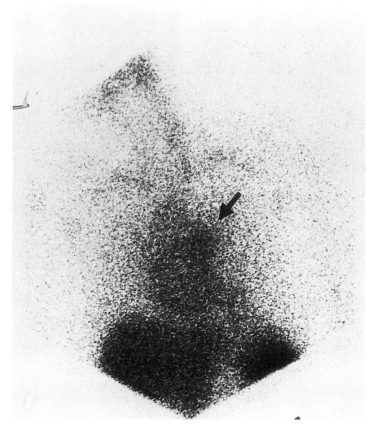

Figure 9 Image obtained in the anterior projection 48 h after injection of the platelet suspension. The top of the image is cephalad. Arrow = area of increased activity due to the left atrial myxoma. This activity was maximally positive at 24 to 48 h after injection of the platelet suspension. The area of increased activity in the right lower zone is caused by the spleen; that seen in the left lower zone is caused by the liver. (From Ezekowitz, MD, et al. Left atrial mass: diagnostic value of transesophageal two-dimensional echocardiography and indium-111 platelet scintigraphy. Am J Cardiol 51: 1583–1584, 1983.)

the thrombus, whereas the activity due to the ^{111}In-labeled platelets is found both within the thrombus and in the blood. The ratio of activity from technetium 99m–labeled red cells and ^{111}In platelets is determined by quantitative imaging of a remote vascular zone or by direct analysis of a blood sample. The ratio is used for subtraction of the blood pool from the cardiac images. The indium excess represents the clot. Potential problems with this technique are the nonspecific uptake of red cells by the thrombus, the statistical significance of data derived by subtraction involving two large numbers with a small difference from each other, and patient movement during acquisition of the images. Stratton (51) recently demonstrated that ^{111}In platelet scintigraphy is a good predictor of embolic risk and serves to further enhance the stratification of high- and low-risk patients and the selection of patients for therapy.

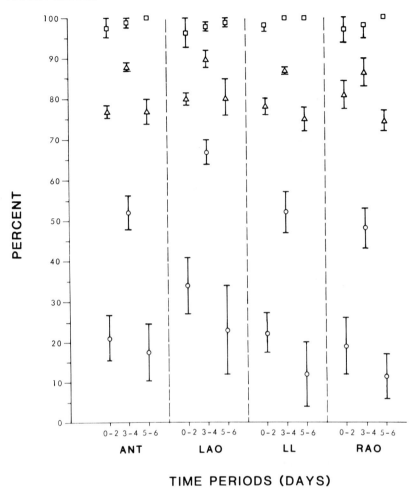

Figure 10 Percent sensitivity, specificity, and diagnostic accuracy in the anterior (ANT), left anterior oblique (LAO), left lateral (LL), and right anterior oblique (RAO) views for all images in time periods 0 to 2, 3 to 4, 5 to 6 days. The data excludes patients with inactive thrombi. These were defined as thrombi in which the surface indium-111 activity was <6 times the activity in the blood normalized by mass. (From Ezekowitz, MD, et al. Diagnostic accuracy of indium-111 platelet scintigraphy in identifying left ventricular thrombi. Am J Cardiol 51: 1712–1716, 1983.)

C. Magnetic Resonance Imaging/X-Ray Computed Tomography

Magnetic resonance imaging systems generate high-resolution images of the cardiovascular system. Thus, theoretically it is possible to noninvasively image thrombi in the left ventricle. Studies have demonstrated the feasibility of this technique in identifying left ventricular masses (58–62). However, systematic studies during the acute phase of myocardial infarction have not been performed. The technique is costly and cumbersome, and it is not usually feasible to transport sick patients to the imaging facilities. The same applies to computed tomography, which can accurately identify intraventricular masses or thrombi (63–68).

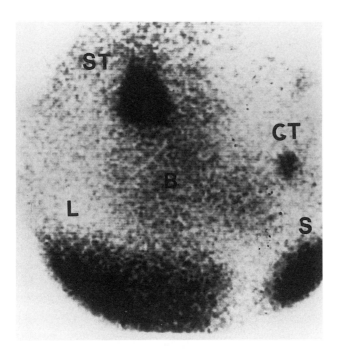

Figure 11 Right anterior oblique indium-111 scintiphoto obtained 24 h after injection of platelet suspension. Top of the image is cephalad. L = liver; S = spleen; CT = presumed coronary thrombus. The intense area of activity in the sternal area was a subcutaneous hematoma (ST). (From *Radiolabeled Cellular Blood Elements*. ML Thakur, ed. Plenum Publishing Corporation, 1985.)

D. Contrast Ventriculography

Contrast ventriculography (70–72) was first used for the diagnosis of left ventricular clot. In general, it lacks both sensitivity and specificity. It is insensitive because clots are often laminated against the wall of the ventricle and cannot be seen. It is nonspecific because thrombi form in large-volume ventricles that are incompletely opacified with contrast material, and therefore apparent filling defects due to incomplete mixing often are seen, leading to overdiagnosis.

E. Radionuclide Angiography

Stratton and his colleagues evaluated radionuclide angiography as a means of identifying left ventricular thrombi (73). The diagnosis of a left ventricular thrombus should be considered if a discrete filling defect or a squared ventricular apex was identified on routine images. The technique, however, has proved insensitive to small thrombi. The low sensitivity of this technique precludes its use as a routine clinical test. However, the specificity of the technique for detecting thrombi is quite high.

F. Conclusion

Echocardiography is the technique of choice for the diagnosis of left ventricular thrombi. Platelet imaging plays a complementary role. Echocardiography reflects thrombus mass, whereas platelet scintigraphy reflects the activity on the thrombus surface. In general,

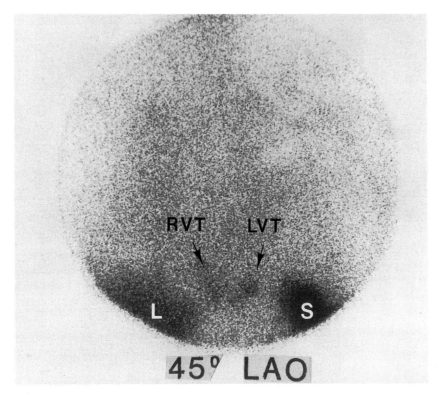

Figure 12 Indium-111 platelet scintiphoto obtained 72 h following injection of platelet suspension. Top is cephalad. LVT = left ventricular thrombus; RVT = right ventricular thrombus; S = spleen; L = liver. Both thrombi were confirmed at autopsy. (From Ezekowitz, MD et al. Detection of active left thrombosis during acute myocardial infarction using indium-111 platelet scintigraphy. Chest 86: 35–39, 1984.)

echocardiography is the less cumbersome technique, but in those cases where technical considerations preclude the acquisition of a technically satisfactory study, platelet scintigraphy may be useful in identifying clot and directing therapy by predicting the risk of subsequent embolization. Magnetic resonance imaging and x-ray computed tomography are expensive alternatives to echocardiography. Contrast ventriculography and radionuclide angiography should not be routinely employed, because of their low sensitivity.

III. TREATMENT

This section will separate the treatment approach for patients in the acute phase of myocardial infarction from that for patients with poor ventricular function, and those with left ventricular aneurysms.

A. Acute Myocardial Infarction

Systemic embolization is one of the rarer complications of acute myocardial infarction. With greater preservation of myocardial function in patients experiencing an acute myocardial infarction, this complication is likely to decrease further. Nonetheless, stroke or embolization following acute myocardial infarction, when it does occur, can be devastating. Treat-

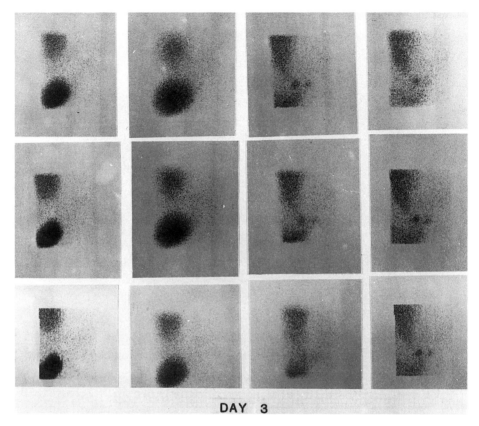

Figure 13 Intracardiac thrombus identification by tomographic imaging. Series of tomographic slices obtained from a Pho/Con 192 gamma scintillation camera. Image 1 is the most anterior image and image 12 is the most posterior image. Tops of the images are cephalad. The arrows point to two mural left ventricular thrombi seen in the most anterior images and not seen posteriorly. These images were obtained on the fifth day after injection of the labeled platelet suspension. (From *Diagnostic Nuclear Medicine*, 2nd Edition. A Gottschalk, PB Hoffer, EJ Potchen and Assoc. Ed. HJ Berger, eds. Williams and Wilkins, 1988.)

ment options for stroke prevention fall into four categories. The first is anticoagulation, which is the most widely employed. Anticoagulation involves a combination of heparin followed by the chronic use of either subcutaneous heparin or warfarin. Heparin followed by warfarin constitutes the cornerstone of therapy. Fibrinolytic agents and antiplatelet agents, as well as surgery, have also been employed and will be discussed.

1. Anticoagulation

The possibility of using anticoagulants to prevent the development of mural thrombi in patients during the acute phase of myocardial infarction was first entertained by Solandt et al., in 1938 (74). While the prevention of thrombus formation using anticoagulants has not been consistently demonstrated, there is considerable evidence supporting a role for anticoagulation in the prevention of embolization (7,9,32,42,43,75,76). Early trials of anticoagulation in a large number of patients with acute myocardial infarction provide the

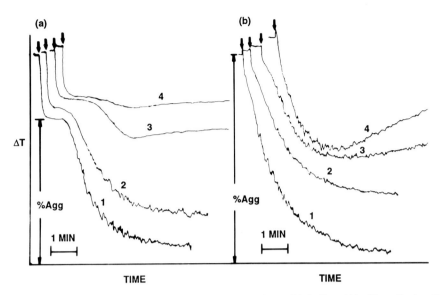

Figure 14 Platelet aggregation before and after labeling with indium-111. (From Ezekowitz, MD et al. Failure of aspirin to prevent incorporation of indium-111 labeled platelets into cardiac thrombi in man. Lancet, August 29, 1981.)

strongest evidence for the prevention of embolic events. Wright et al. in 1948 (77) treated 800 patients with acute myocardial infarction with heparin followed by dicumarol to maintain the prothrombin time at twice the normal value. They compared this group with an untreated group and found that 3.4% in the untreated group had cerebrovascular accidents versus only 1.4% in the treated group. There was also a decrease in peripheral embolization from 3% in the control group to 1% in the treated group. Similar results were found in a British study (78) that showed a reduction in the frequency of clinically evident systemic embolic complications from 3.4% to 1.3% among 1427 patients randomized to either 36 h of heparin administration with phenindione to maintain the thrombotest at 15% (mean dose 72 mg/day) or low dose phenindione (1 mg/day) without heparin. Another study by Harvald et al. (79) published in 1962 found a reduction in strokes. One of 45 patients treated with long-term dicumarol (2%) and 11 of 170 patients not given anticoagulation (6%) suffered cerebrovascular accidents. Drapkin and Merskey's study (35) complicated the field by reporting that among more than 1000 patients randomized to heparin and phenindione (prothrombin time at 2–2½ times control), a reduction in the number of cerebrovascular accidents was seen only among women (1.5% vs. 3.9% among controls) and not among men (1.5% vs. 1.8% among controls). However, the event rate in each subgroup was small. In the VA Cooperative Study of 999 patients (80), there was a decrease in the number of emboli among patients treated with heparin followed by warfarin (prothrombin time at twice normal), with a reduction in the occurrence of emboli from 3.8% in the placebo group to 0.8% in the treated group. In the VA study, anticoagulated patients had a decreased prevalence of mural thrombi at autopsy as compared with controls, a finding also reported by Hilden et al. (87); this suggests that the decreased incidence of emboli with anticoagulation might in part be due to a reduced incidence of ventricular clot. More recently, two small echocardiographic studies found a decreased incidence of left ventricular thrombus in patients treated with anticoagulant therapy (44,45). However, there are several other studies (6,9,42,43,75,82) in which no significant reduction in thrombus was seen with anticoagulation. Interestingly, in three of these studies (9,42,43), in spite of failure to show a reduction in the incidence of ventricular clot, embolic complications were nevertheless reduced. In the study by Friedman et al. (9), left ventricular thrombi occurred in 9 of 45 patients who were anticoagulated (20%), an incidence that was not different from that of the control group (two of eight, 25%). A trend toward reduction of emboli was found. In the study by Weinreich et al. (42), mural thrombi were noted in 44 of 130 patients with anterior myocardial infarction (34%). A follow-up study of survivors at 6 months found no significant difference in the incidence of thrombus; thrombi occurred in 11 of 19 patients (58%) receiving anticoagulation and six of ten patients (60%) not being treated (p = NS). Nevertheless, there was significant difference in embolic complications ($p < 0.05$), with no emboli among the 25 anticoagulated patients and 7 emboli among the 18 control patients. A similar finding was reported by Keating et al. (43). Of 54 patients with anterior myocardial infarction, 17 had mural thrombi; 10 (18%) were receiving anticoagulation and 7 (13%) were not (p = NS). There were no emboli in the anticoagulated group, and 6 (86%) in the group that did not receive anticoagulation ($p < 0.001$). In spite of the absence of a clear-cut effect on thrombi, these studies, in general, support the conclusion that anticoagulation prevents emboli in patients with left ventricular clot.

Stratton and Resnick (34) and Tramarin et al. (45) studied patients with chronic left ventricular thrombi and found a reduction of both emboli and clot among anticoagulated patients. Tramarin et al. (45) compared 19 anticoagulated patients with 19 controls. There was a significant reduction in the dimensions of mural thrombi at 15 days, at 3 months, and at 1 year. At the final follow-up evaluation at 1 year, 15 of 17 patients in the treated group (88%) had resolution of thrombus, whereas only 4 of 17 patients in the untreated group (24%) had resolution. Stratton and Resnick (34) studied 85 patients with ventricular thrombi by echocardiography. The presence of thrombus was associated with an increased risk of emboli, which occurred in 11 of 85 patients with thrombi (13%). There were 11 emboli in 62 nonanticoagulated patients (18%) and no emboli in the 23 patients who were fully anticoagulated. These two studies demonstrate the efficacy of long-term anticoagulation both in the resolution of thrombi and in the prevention of emboli.

The timing of anticoagulation may influence the benefit seen. The earlier the anticoagulation is administered, the greater the benefit. An animal study by Solandt et al. (74) as well as investigations in patients support this idea (47). When heparin was given early, 4.6 ± 2.5 (mean $\pm$ 1 SD) h after the myocardial infarction (47), there was a decreased incidence of thrombi as compared to heparin given later, at 6.5 ± 3.3 and 5.2 ± 4.6 h in two other studies, where a decrease was not observed (76,82). As discussed in the next section, early thrombolytic therapy, as opposed to later therapy, also reduced the frequency of ventricular thrombi. No difference was found in the incidence of left ventricular thrombi in patients given intravenous full-dose heparin as compared with those receiving subcutaneous low-dose heparin therapy (82).

2. Thrombolytic Therapy

Thrombolytic therapy is standard treatment in the hyperacute phase of acute myocardial infarction. The studies that have specifically evaluated the effect of thrombolysis on the formation, resolution, or embolization of ventricular thrombi have not been consistent (Table 2). Stratton et al. (83), in 1985, compared 45 patients treated with streptokinase and 38 concurrent controls receiving heparin. Only four patients had left ventricular thrombi on

Table 2 Thrombolytic Therapy and Left Ventricular Thrombus

Study	Anterior MI	Incidence of LVT		p Value	Therapy used
		Treated	Controls		
Eigler et al., 1984 (87)	22	1/12 = 8%[a]	7/10 = 70%	<.005	Streptokinase 750,000 U < 3 h after MI, then full anticoagulation with adjusted-dose intravenous heparin, then warfarin[b]
Stratton et al., 1985 (83)	29	5/19 = 26%[c]	0/10 = 0%	NS	IC streptokinase 1000 U/min up to 300,000 U, total 4.7 ± 2.5 h after MI, then full anticoagulation with adjusted-dose intraenous heparin, followed by warfarin[d]
Sharma et al., 1985 (84)	30	8/30 = 27%[e]	No controls		IC streptokinase 10,000 (1985) U/min up to 750,000 U 3.7 ± 2.0 h after MI, then full anticoagulation with intravenous heparin[f]
Natarajan et al., 1988 (88)	40	0/22 = 0%[g]	8/18 = 44%	<.05	Streptokinase 750,000 U < 6 h after MI, then full anticoagulation with adjusted-dose intravenous heparin for 3–4 days, followed by unspecified antiplatelet therapy[b]
Held et al., 1988 (85)	43	1/92 = 1.1%[h]	6/14 = 43%	NS	Streptokinase 1,500,000 U <7 h after MI, then full anticoagulation with adjusted-dose intraenous heparin[i]
		7/20 = 35%[h]	6/14 = 43%	NS	t-PA 80mg over 3 h, <7 hr after MI, then full anticoagulation with adjusted dose intravenous heparin[i]

[a]Echocardiography performed <36 h and 9 ± 2 days after infarction.
[b]Controls received no anticoagulation.
[c]Echocardiogram performed at 8 ± 3 weeks after infarction.
[d]Controls received adjusted dose heparin followed by oral coumadin.
[e]Echocardiography performed <24 h and 10 days after infarction.
[f]No Control group.
[g]Echocardiography performed at 8–10 days after infarction.
[h]Echocardiography performed at 48–72 h.
[i]Controls received heparin 5000 U subcutaneously bid.
Anterior MI = number of patients in the study with anterior myocardial infarction; LVT = left ventricular thrombus as determined echocardiographically; IC streptokinase = intracoronary streptokinase; t-PA = tissue plasminogen activator.

serial echocardiography, and all four were in the streptokinase-treated group. Although this difference did not reach statistical significance, it suggested that the incidence of left ventricular thrombi was not reduced by thrombolysis. Sharma et al. (84) reported a 27% incidence of left ventricular thrombi after intracoronary streptokinase. They similarly concluded that the incidence of thrombi was not reduced by thrombolysis, although their study lacked a control group. Most recently, Held et al. (85) failed to find a statistically significant decrease in the incidence of left ventricular thrombi after thrombolytic therapy with either tissue plasminogen activator or streptokinase (Thrombolysis in Myocardial Infarction Study), although there was a trend toward reduction, especially with streptokinase (86). Eigler et al. (87) in one of the earliest studies and Natarajan et al. (88) in a larger series of 40 patients with anterior myocardial infarction found a statistically significant decrement in the incidence of left ventricular thrombi in patients treated early with thrombolytic therapy. In addition Keren et al. (89) and Kremer et al. (90) have demonstrated efficacy in lysis of ventricular thrombi present in the postinfarction period.

The effects of thrombolysis on mural thrombi may include the direct lysis of the thrombus or result from a decrease in infarct size, with less substrate for thrombus formation, because of preserved wall motion and overall function. There is also the theoretical possibility, supported by isolated clinical observations (personal communication, Funke-Kupper), that embolization may actually result from thrombolytic therapy. Patients receiving thrombolytic therapy for a second myocardial infarction, with a history of a prior anterior myocardial infarction and existing left ventricular thrombi, may have fragmentation of clot and subsequent embolization. In a large series of patients receiving thrombolytic therapy during the hyperacute phase of myocardial infarction, the low incidence of stroke is outweighed by the beneficial effects on mortality (91). Thus, in the absence of consistent and strong evidence the use of thrombolytic agents to treat ventricular thrombi is of questionable benefit and may actually cause stroke by fragmenting the clot. In the setting of an acute myocardial infarction thrombolytic therapy is indicated primarily for myocardial preservation, not thrombus prevention. Because of the danger of inducing an embolus, thrombolysis may be contraindicated in situations where a thrombus is demonstrated.

3. *Thrombectomy/Aneurysmectomy/Infarctectomy*

Left ventricular aneurysmectomy may be indicated for recurrent thromboembolism (92). Surgical removal of thrombus in the setting of acute myocardial infarction has only rarely been undertaken (93,94). Resection of myocardial tissue (infarctectomy) is difficult and inexact because of the lack of definite margins, and the absence of scar early after infarction adds to the technical difficulty of the operation. Nevertheless, if patients can be identified who are at sufficiently high risk of embolization, operative removal may very occasionally be considered.

4. *Antiplatelet Drugs*

Antiplatelet drugs have not been systematically studied. While Ezekowitz et al. (95) demonstrated the lack of effect of aspirin on platelet scintigraphy, Stratton and Ritchie (52) found that platelet deposition as measured by indium-111 labeled platelets was inhibited by sulfinpyrazone as well as by aspirin and dipyridamole given together. However, thrombus size as determined by echocardiography was not significantly affected. Thus, while antiplatelet therapy may alter platelet activity or uptake by thrombus, there is no evidence of a clinically important effect.

5. *Warfarin and Aspirin for Secondary Prevention of Acute Myocardial Infarction*

The need to prevent recurrent myocardial infarction with anticoagulation may supersede the rarer indication for preventing systemic embolization after acute myocardial infarction. It is generally agreed that the majority of acute myocardial infarctions result from obstruction due to an intracoronary thrombus (96). The first paper to suggest that agents which modify blood coagulation could prevent myocardial infarction was published in 1947 by Nicol and Fasset (97). Since then, scores of clinical trials have been undertaken to assess the efficacy of anticoagulants and antiplatelet agents in preventing death and reinfarction in survivors of acute myocardial infarction (Tables 3 and 4). The failure of most of these trials to enroll a sufficient number of patients to demonstrate a survival benefit has resulted in the lack of agreement concerning the efficacy of these agents. In recent years, the pendulum of opinion has turned toward the reevaluation and reutilization of these agents for secondary prevention of myocardial infarction. The motivation for this change has been the resolution of the debate concerning the role of thrombosis in causing acute myocardial infarction, and the demonstrated efficacy of thrombolytic agents in the hyperacute phase of infarction, further supporting the contention of a central role for thrombosis in acute coronary syndromes.

Thus, recommendations concerning the use of anticoagulant drugs in preventing systemic embolization will probably be overshadowed by the need to use either antiplatelet or anticoagulant agents to prevent reinfarction and death. It is therefore relevant in any discussion concerning the prevention of systemic embolization following acute infarction to

Table 3 Anticoagulants in Secondary Prevention of Myocardial Infarction (MI)

	MRC (100)	VA COOP (105)	GAMIS (104)	WARIS (108)
Study accrual	1955–60	1957–60	1970–77	1983–86
Delay after MI to entry	4–6 weeks	3 weeks	4–7 weeks	4 weeks
Target INR	2–2.5	2–2.5	2.5–5.0	2.8–4.8
% of visits with PT range	60	82	62–75	75
Years on treatment	4	5	2	5
# randomized	383	739	626	1214
Mean age (yr)	55–60	53	45–70	61
% with >1 previous MI	ND	20	20	20
% with a transmural index MI	ND	ND	ND	69
% withdrawals	20	22	17	18
% mortality				
Control	21	33	10	20
Treated	15	31	12	15
% CV mortality				
Control	21	24	7	?
Treated	14	20	8	?
% tot mort rel risk reduction	30	4.3	−18	24
% Reinfarction				
Control	46	21	8	20.4
Treated	16	16	5	13.5

Table 4 Antiplatelet Agents in Secondary Prevention of Myocardial Infarction

	CARDIFF I (MRC I) (000)	CARDIFF II (MRC II) (100)	PARIS I (102)	PARIS II (103)	GAMIS (104)
Study accrual	1971–72	1974–77	1975–76	1980–83	1970–77
Delay after MI to entry	0–6 months	0–1 month	2–60 months	1–4 months	1–2 months
Active drug	ASA 300 mg qd	ASA 900 mg qd	ASA 972 mg qd	ASA mg 972 + DIP 225 mg qd	ASA mg 1500 qd
% complaint at 1 yr	70	70	70	70	80
Years on treatment	1.0	1.0	3.0–4.0	2.0	2.0
# randomized	1239	1682	2026	3128	1340
Mean age (yr)	55	56	56	57	ND
% with a transmural index MI	ND	ND	54	70	ND
% mortality					
Control	10.9	14.8	12.8	7.3	10.3
Treated	8.3	12.3	10.5	7.1	8.5
% CV mortality					
Control	ND	ND	11.1	6.6	7.1
Treated	ND	ND	9.1	6.1	4.1
% tot mort rel risk reduction	22 (NS)	17 (NS)	18 (NS)	9 (NS)	18 (NS)
% reinfarction					
Control	ND	7.4	15.6	5.2	4.8
Treated		3.4	9.4	4.9	3.5

	CDP-A (98)	AMIS (101)	ARIS (140)	ART (141)
Study accrual	72–74	75–76	76–79	75–77
Delay after MI to entry	>60	2–60	0–1	1
Active drug	ASA 972 mg qd	ASA 1000 mg qd	SULPHINP 800 mg qd	SULPHINP 800 mg qd
% complaint at 1 yr	80	90	80	80
Years on treatment	2	3	1.7	1.3
# Randomized	1529	4524	727	1620
Mean age (yr)	?	53	55	57
% with > 1 previous MI	24	13	10	21
% with a transmural index MI	53	ND	80	ND
% mortality				
Control	8.3	9.7	7.4	7.9
Treated	5.8	10.8	7.9	5.6
% CV mortality				
Control	6.4	8.0	4.9	7.9
Treated	4.6	8.7	5.2	5.5
% tot mort rel risk reduction	30 (NS)	−11 (NS)	−6 (NS)	29 (?)
% reinfarct				
Control	4.2	11.6	9.4	?
Treated	3.7	9.5	4.1	?

ASA = acetylsalicylic acid; DIP = dipyridamole; SULPHINP = sulphinpyrazone; ND = no data.

discuss the value of using aspirin and warfarin as agents for secondary prevention of myocardial infarction.

Aspirin and Secondary Prevention.   The practice of prescribing aspirin for secondary prevention is based on the findings of several large clinical trials comparing aspirin, in a variety of doses, with placebo among patients discharged following acute myocardial infarction (98–103). Using mortality as the major end point, five of the six prospective, randomized trials found a nonsignificant survival benefit for aspirin. A pooled analysis of these trials showed that the differences were statistically significant for death ($p < 0.01$) and for re-infarction ($p < 0.001$) (104). The latter figure included both fatal and nonfatal myocardial infarction.

Warfarin in Secondary Prevention.   The use of warfarin always entails an educated evaluation of the benefit of the medication against the danger of hemorrhage. Thus, despite evidence suggesting that warfarin may be superior to aspirin in secondary prevention following acute myocardial infarction, long-term oral anticoagulation has not generally been prescribed. Two trials published before 1980 were able to demonstrate a survival advantage at 1 and 3 years after the first event that was not seen at 5 years after infarction (105,106). The third study showed no benefit at all (100). The International Anticoagulant Review Group pooled the data from nine prospective trials involving over 2400 subjects and concluded that long-term anticoagulant administration reduced mortality by 20% (107). The 60+ Reinfarction Study revived the question of long-term anticoagulation after acute myocardial infarction (108). In this study all patients were initially given warfarin; half were withdrawn, while the remainder were allowed to continue medication. In patients randomized to continue warfarin there was a 55% reduction in the reinfarction rate as compared with the patients who were randomized to discontinue therapy. More recently, the Warfarin Reinfarction Study demonstrated a 24% reduction in death and a 34% reduction in reinfarction rate among patients randomized to receive warfarin following acute myocardial infarction (109). Differences between treated patients and controls for both these end points were statistically significant. The authors cite the increased intensity of anticoagulation in this trial (international normalized ratio [INR] = 2.8 to 4.8) and the large sample size to account for their highly statistically significant result. This study was well designed and provides compelling support for the routine use of anticoagulation after acute myocardial infarction. If generally accepted, this use would supersede the indications of warfarin to prevent systemic embolization, a much rarer complication. A limitation of the Warfarin Reinfarction Study is that patients were not stratified by risk (110,111).

Combination of Warfarin and Aspirin in Secondary Prevention (Combined Hemotherapy). Currently there are no data concerning the efficacy of combination therapy in secondary prevention of ischemic heart disease. The simultaneous inhibition of platelet function by aspirin and reduction of circulating procoagulants by warfarin would produce a significantly greater antithrombotic effect than either agent used alone. The danger of this combination is bleeding. However, the Thrombosis Prevention Trial showed no increase in gastric bleeding above the very low level attributable to aspirin alone (35,112). A second study, which will be conducted by the Veterans Administration Cooperative Studies Program, has the goal of randomizing patients who have undergone peripheral artery bypass grafting to either aspirin alone at a dose of 325 mg/day or aspirin at that dose combined with warfarin, with a target INR of 1.5. The primary end point will be graft patency. Another study, with Fiori and Ezekowitz as co-principal investigators, will test the value of low-dose warfarin and aspirin in a secondary-prevention trial in acute myocardial infarction (The Champ Study).

6. Summary

Systemic emboli occur in only a small percentage of patients (35,52,77–79) after myocardial infarction. However, the reported incidence of emboli is markedly increased in certain subgroups. Approximately one-third of patients with anterior myocardial infarctions will have left ventricular thrombi (9,72,80,98–102). The reported incidence of emboli among patients with left ventricular thrombus varies widely; in patients not treated with anticoagulants the incidence varies from only a few per hundred in one large study (103) to 27% in another large study and as high as 86% (9). Improved selection of patients at risk may be enhanced by the finding of thrombus protrusion, thrombus mobility, positive platelet scintigraphy, advanced age, or Doppler evidence of low flow adjacent to poorly contracting myocardium. The best data to support the use of anticoagulation in acute infarction are found in the older literature. More recent studies have not been completely consistent, but they support the beneficial effect of anticoagulation. The role of thrombolytic agents is in the process of evolution. In the acute setting, the importance of myocardial salvage overshadows consideration of embolic risk. The role of delayed thrombolysis, for example, for high-risk mobile thrombi has not been clarified; it remains experimental and is probably dangerous. Antiplatelet agents are not useful. Surgery has been undertaken only rarely. Thrombectomy remains primarily an incidental procedure during surgery for other indications. The standard of therapy, therefore, remains anticoagulation. There is evidence to guide the optimal timing of therapy. The occurrence of emboli soon after infarction supports a role for early anticoagulation. The optimal timing of echocardiography depends on the peak occurrence of thrombus formation and the most cost-effective time to perform the study. In the case of anterior infarction, echocardiography is not necessary before starting anticoagulation. It is likely, however, that the indication of warfarin and/or aspirin to prevent reinfarction and death will supersede the indications for prophylaxis against systemic embolization.

B. Cardiomyopathy and Systemic Embolization

The association between systemic embolization and left ventricular dysfunction has long been recognized (6,113–117) and is independent of the cause of the ventricular myopathy (115). In a retrospective study of 104 patients with the diagnosis of idiopathic dilated cardiomyopathy based on clinical and angiographic criteria, identified between 1960 and 1973 and followed for 6 to 20 years (116), it was found that systemic emboli occurred in 18% of those who were not treated with anticoagulant therapy and in none of the patients who received anticoagulant therapy. While this study made an important contribution, it was limited because it represented a retrospective analysis. Also, no attempt was made to quantify left ventricular function. However, it has formed the basis for the recommendation that patients with left ventricular dysfunction should be treated with warfarin. Gottdiener et al. provided important supplemental information in a later study using two-dimensional echocardiography to identify thrombi in patients with chronic dilated cardiomyopathies (118). They found thrombi in 36% of patients. Events compatible with systemic embolization occurred in 11% of these patients but were not more frequent in patients in whom thrombi were not detected. That report suggests that in patients with poor ventricular function, echocardiographic identification of thrombus is not useful in segregating risk with respect to embolic complications. Studies in Africa among the indigenous population provide one of the most convincing sources of evidence that cardiomyopathies and embolic stroke are connected (117). Cardiomyopathies are common at a young age and atherosclerotic vascular disease is uncommon. Thus, the usual competing causes of stroke are absent, although hypertension is a common disorder among black Africans. At the present time there are no prospective, controlled trials evaluating the effect of warfarin in patients with poor ventricular function.

C. Left Ventricular Aneurysms and Systemic Embolization

Left ventricular aneurysms, both pseudoaneurysms and true aneurysms, represent a paradox. Thrombi frequently complicate aneurysms, yet it appears that systemic embolization is relatively uncommon. This appears to be so for true aneurysms as well as pseudoaneurysms (119). Both true and false aneurysms most commonly complicate acute transmural myocardial infarction. It is generally accepted that false aneurysms often contain thrombi (120–123). Reports of cerebrovascular events in patients with pseudoaneurysms have appeared sporadically in the literature (122–124).

The general approach to patients with true aneurysms with thrombi is to use anticoagulation therapy unless there is a contraindication. Pseudoaneurysms should be treated surgically unless there is a compelling reason to contraindicate the procedure. Occasionally, thrombi within aneurysms may become infected, and theoretically this may lead to embolization.

IV. CARDIAC TUMORS

Cardiac tumors are less common than thrombi but may present with an embolic event. The triad of valve obstruction, embolization, and constitutional symptoms characterizes intracavitary tumors, especially myxomas. Tumors of the heart may be primary or secondary. The most common benign primary cardiac tumors are myxomas, which are described in detail in Chapter 14. While 75% of these tumors are located in the left atrium, myxomas are also found in the right atrium, the right ventricle, and, in 2.5% of cases, the left ventricle (125). Systemic embolization occurs in about half of patients with left atrial myxomas and in about two-thirds of patients with left ventricular myxomas. Characteristically, these patients suffer episodes of syncope, have symptoms of short duration, and may have a mass on echocardiography that appears to obstruct the aortic valve (125,126). Rhabdomyomas are the most frequent cardiac tumors in infants and children (127,128) and most often involve the ventricular myocardium. Fibromas are usually ventricular and intramural and also occur most commonly in infants and children (127,129,130). Lipomas may occur throughout the heart.

Primary malignant tumors are almost always sarcomas and most frequently angiosarcomas (131). In general, the prognosis of patients with malignant tumors of the heart is poor and their survival is short (127,132–135). Secondary tumors of the heart gain access by direct continuous growth from an adjacent structure, by hematogenous or lymphatic spread, or by direct growth along the vena cava or pulmonary veins (136–138). Cardiac metastasis occurs with all types of tumors but is more frequent with bronchogenic carcinoma and carcinoma of the breast. Metastatic cardiac tumors are 16 to 40 times more common than primary cardiac tumors. They may occasionally lead to systemic or pulmonary emboli, but this complication is less common than with primary tumors. Carcinoid tumors occur more commonly in the right side of the heart and are hardly ever seen in the left ventricle.

In general, cardiac tumors are easily diagnosed by ultrasound. Further definition of the extent of the mass can be obtained with magnetic resonance imaging or angiography.

REFERENCES

1. Ports TA, Cogan J, Schiller NB, Rapaport E. Echocardiography of left ventricular masses. Circulation 1978, 58:528–36.
2. DeMaria AN, Bommer W, Neumann A, et al. Left ventricular thrombi identified by cross-sectional echocardiography. Ann Intern Med 1978; 90:14–8.
3. Meltzer RS, Guthaner D, Rakowski M, Popp RL, Martin R. Br Heart J 1979; 42:261–5.
4. Come PC, Mankis JE, Vine HS, Sacks B, McArdle C, Raminez A. Echocardiographic diagnosis of left ventricular thrombus. Am Heart J 1980; 100:523–30.
5. Asinger RW, Mikell FL, Elsperger J, Hodges M. Incidence of left ventricular thrombosis after acute transmural myocardial infarction: serial evaluation by two-dimensional echocardiography. N Engl J Med 1981; 305:297–302.
6. Reeder GS, Tajik AJ, Seward JB. Left ventricular mural thrombus: two dimensional echocardiographic diagnosis: Mayo Clin Proc 1981; 56:82–6.
7. Stratton JR, Ritchie JL, Hamilton GW, Hammermeister KE, Harker LA. Left ventricular thrombi: in vivo detection by indium-111 platelet imaging and two dimensional echocardiography. Am J Cardiol 1981; 47:874–81.
8. Ostfelt AM: A review of stroke epidemiology. Epidemiol Rev 1980; 2:136–52.
9. Friedman MJ, Carlson K, Marcus FI, Woolfenden JM. Clinical correlations in patients with acute myocardial infarction and left ventricular thrombus detected by two-dimensional echocardiography. Am J Med 1982; 72:894–8.
10. Ezekowitz MD, Wilson DA, Smith EO, Burow RD, Harrison LH Jr, Parker DE, et al. Comparison of indium-111 platelet scintigraphy and two-dimensional echocardiography in the diagnosis of left ventricular thrombi. N Engl J Med 1982; 306:1509–13.
11. Kloner RA, Parisi AS. Acute myocardial infarction: diagnostic and prognostic applications of two-dimensional echocardiography. Circulation 1987; 75:521–4.
12. Horowitz RS, Morganroth J, Parrotto C, Cher CC, Soffer J, Pauletto FJ. Immediate diagnosis of acute myocardial infarction by two dimensional echocardiography. Circulation 1982; 65:323.
13. Gibson RS, Bishop HL, Stamm RB, Crampton RS, Beller GA, Martin RP. Value of early two dimensional echocardiography in patients with acute MI. Am J Cardiol 1982; 49:1110.
14. Nishimura RA, Tajik AJ, Shub C, Miller FA, Ilstrup DM, Harrison CE. Role of two-dimensional echocardiography in the prediction of in hospital complications after myocardial infarction. J Am Coll Cardiol 1984; 4:1080.
15. Horowitz RS, Morganroth J. Immediate detection of early high risk patients with acute myocardial infarction using two-dimensional echocardiographic evaluation of left ventricular regional wall motion abnormalities. Am Heart J 1982; 103:814.
16. Horgan JH, O'M Shiel F, Goodman AC. Demonstration of left ventricular thrombus by conventional echocardiography. J Clin Ultrasound 1976; 4:287.
17. Kramer NE, Rathod R, Chawla KK, Patel R, Towne WD. Echocardiographic diagnosis of left ventricular mural thrombi occurring in cardiomyopathy. Am Heart J 1978; 96:381.
18. Dejoseph RL, Shiroff FA, Levenson LW, Martin CE, Zelis RF. Echocardiographic diagnosis of intraventricular clot. Chest 1977; 71:417.
19. Van den Bos AA, Bletter WB, Hagemeijer F. Progressive development of a left ventricular thrombus. Detection and evolution studied with echocardiographic techniques. Chest 1978; 74:307.
20. Meltzer RS, Visser CA, Kan G, Roelandt J. Two-dimensional echocardiographic appearance of left ventricular thrombi with systemic emboli after myocardial infarction. Am J Cardiol 1984; 53:1511.

21. Haugland JM, Asinger RW, Mikell FL, Elsperger J, Hodges M. Embolic potential of left ventricular thrombi detected by two-dimensional echocardiography. Circulation 1984; 70:588.

22. Visser CA, Kan G, Meltzer RS, Dunning AJ, Roelandt J, Van Corler M, de Koning H. Embolic potential of left ventricular thrombus after myocardial infarction: a two dimensional echocardiographic study of 119 patients. J Am Coll Cardiol 1985; 5:1276.

23. Visser CA, et al. Two-dimensional echocardiography in the diagnosis of left ventricular thrombus. Chest 1983; 83:228–32.

24. Stratton JR, Lighty GW, Pearlman AS, Ritchie JL. Detection of left ventricular thrombus by two dimensional echocardiography: sensitivity specificity, and causes of uncertainty. Circulation 1982; 66:156–66.

25. Starling MR, Crawford MM, Sorenson SG, Grover FL. Comparative value of invasive and noninvasive techniques for identifying left ventricular mural thrombi. Am Heart J 1983; 106: 1143–9.

26. Sheiban I, Casarotto D, Trevi G, et al. Two dimensional echocardiography in the diagnosis of intracardiac masses: a prospective study with anatomic validation. Cardiovasc Intervent Radiol 1987; 10:157–61.

27. Maze SS, Kotler MA, Pavy WR. The contribution of color Doppler flow imaging to the assessment of left ventricular thrombus. Am Heart J 1988; 115:479–82.

28. Jordan RA, Miller RD, Edwards JE, Parker RL. Thromboembolism in acute and in healed myocardial infarction. I. Intracardiac mural thrombosis. Circulation 1952; 6:1–6.

29. Davis MJE, Ireland MA. Effect of early anticoagulation on the frequency of left ventricular thrombi after anterior wall acute myocardial infarction. Am J Cardiol 1986; 57:1244–7.

30. Spirito P, Bellotti P, Chairella F, Domenicucci S, Sementa A, Vecchio C. Prognostic significance and natural history of left ventricular thrombi in patients with acute anterior myocardial infarction: a 2D echocardiographic study. Circulation 1985; 72:774–80.

31. Domenicucci S, Bellotti P, Chiarella F, Lupi G, Vecchio C. Spontaneous morphologic changes in left ventricular thrombi: a prospective two-dimensional echocardiographic study. Circulation 1987; 75:737–43.

32. Gueret P, Duborg O, Ferrier A, Farcot JC, Rigand M, Courdarias J. Effects of full-dose heparin anticoagulation on the development of left ventricular thrombosis in acute transmural myocardial infarction. J Am Coll Cardiol 1986; 8:419–26.

33. Komrad MS, Coffey CE, Coffey KS, McKinnis R, Massey EW, Califf RM: Myocardial infarction and stroke. Neurology 1984; 34:1403–9.

34. Stratton JR, Resnick AD. Increased emboli risk in patients with left ventricular thrombi. Circulation 1987; 75:1004–11.

35. Drapkin A, Merskey C. Anticoagulant therapy after acute myocardial infarction: relation of therapeutic benefit to patient's age, sex, and severity of infarction. JAMA 1972; 222:541.

36. Resnekov L, Chediak, Hirsh J, Lewis D. Antithrombotic agents in coronary artery disease. Chest 1986; 89:54S.

37. Thompson JE, Weston AS, Signler L, Raut PS, Austin DJ, Patman RD. Arterial embolectomy after myocardial infarction: a study of 31 patients. Ann Surg 1970; 171:979.

38. Darling RC, Austen G, Linton RR. Arterial embolism. Surg Gynecol Obstet 1967; 124:106.

39. Lary BG, de Takats G. Peripheral arterial embolism after myocardial infarction: occurrence in unsuspected cases and ambulatory patients. JAMA 1954; 155:10.

40. Thompson PL, Robinson JS: Stroke after myocardial infarction: relation to infarct size. Br Med J 1978; 2:457.

41. Bean WB. Infarction of the heart: III. Clinical course and morphological findings. Ann Intern Med 1938; 12:71.

42. Weinreich DJ, Burke JF, Pauletto FJ. Left ventricular mural thrombi complicating acute myocardial infarction: long-term follow-up with serial echocardiography. Ann Intern Med 1984; 100:789.

43. Keating EC, Gross SA, Schlamowitz RA, Glassman J, Mazur JH, Pitt WA, Miller D. Mural thrombi in myocardial infarctions: prospective evaluation by two-dimensional echocardiography. Am J Med 1983; 74:989.
44. Johannessen KA, Nordrehaug JE, Lippe G. Left ventricular thrombosis and cerebrovascular accident in acute myocardial infarction. Br Heart J 1984; 51:553–6.
45. Tramarin R, Pozzoli M, Feko O, Opasich C, Columbo E, Cobelli F, Specchia G. Two-dimensional echocardiographic assessment of anticoagulant therapy in left ventricular thrombosis early after myocardial infarction. Eur Heart J 1986; 7:482–92.
46. Nordrehaug JE, Johannessen K, VonDerlippe G. Usefulness of high-dose anticoagulants in preventing left ventricular thrombus in acute myocardial infarction. Am J Cardiol 1985; 55: 1491–3.
47. Johannessen K. Peripheral emboli from left ventricular thrombi of different echocardiographic appearance in acute myocardial infarction. Arch Intern Med 1987; 147:641–4.
48. Kinney EL. The significance of left ventricular thrombi in patients with coronary heart disease: a retrospective analysis of pooled data. Am Heart J 1985; 109:191–4.
49. Johannessen KA, Nordrehaug JE, VonDerLippe G, Vollset SE. Risk factors for embolization in patients with left ventricular thrombi and acute myocardial infarction. Br Heart J 1988; 60:104–10.
50. Thakur ML, Welch MJ, Joist JM, Coleman RC. Indium-111 labeled platelets: studies on the preparation and evaluation of in vitro and in vivo functions. Thromb Res 1976; 9:345–57.
51. Stratton JR. Indium-111 platelet imaging of left ventricular thrombi: predictive value for systemic emboli. Presented at The International Meeting Left Ventricular Thrombosis After Myocardial Infarction. Genoa, Italy, October 21, 1988.
52. Stratton JR, Ritchie JL. The effects of antithrombotic drugs in patients with LV thrombi: assessment with indium-111 platelet imaging and two-dimensional echocardiography. Circulation 1984; 69:561–8.
53. Ezekowitz MD, Smith EO, Rankin R, Harrison LM, Krous HF. Left atrial mass: diagnostic value of transesophageal two-dimensional echocardiography and indium-111 platelet scintigraphy. Am J Cardiol 1983; 51:1563–4.
54. Ezekowitz MD, Smith EO, Streitz TM. Identifying patients at risk for systemic emboli during the hospital phase of acute myocardial infarction—study using indium-111 labeled platelets (abstr). J Am Coll Cardiol 1983; 1:648.
55. Ezekowitz MD, Smith EO, Cox AC, Taylor FB. Failure of aspirin to prevent incorporation of indium-111 labeled platelets into cardiac thrombi in man. Lancet 1981; 2:440–3.
56. Powers WJ, Siegel BA. Thrombus imaging with indium-111 platelets. Semin Thromb Hemost 1983; 9:115–31.
57. Bergman SR, Lerch RA, Mathias CJ, Sobel BE, Welch MJ. Noninvasive detection of coronary thrombi with indium-111 platelets: concise communication. J Nucl Med 1983; 24:130–5.
58. Choyke PL, Kressel HY, Rerchek N, Axel L, Gefter W, Mamourian AC, Thickman D. Nongated cardiac magnetic resonance imaging; preliminary experiences at 0.12T. Am J Radiol 1984; 143:1143–59.
59. Higgins CB, Lanzer P, Stark D, Botrimick E, Schilter NB, Crooks L, Kayman L, Lipton MJ. Imaging by nuclear magnetic resonance in patients with chronic ischemic heart disease. Circulation 1984; 69:523–31.
60. Dooms GC, Higgins CB. MR imaging of cardiac thrombi. J Comput Assist Tomog 1986; 10: 415–20.
61. Gomes AS, Lois JF, Child JS, Brown K, Batra P. Cardiac tumors and thrombus: evaluation with MR imaging. Am J Radiol 1987; 149:895–9.
62. Council on Scientific Affairs. Magnetic resonance imaging of the cardiovascular system. Present state of the art and future potential. JAMA 1988; 259:253–9.
63. Tomoda H, Hoshai M, Furuya M, Shotsu A, Ootaki M, Matsuyama S. Evaluation of left ventricular thrombus with computed tomography. Am J Cardiol 1981; 48:573–7.

64. Goldstein JA, Schiller NB, Lipton MJ, Ports TA, Brundage BM. Evaluation of left ventricular thrombi by contrast enhanced computed tomography and two-dimensional echocardiography. Am J Cardiol 1986; 57:757–60.

65. Nair CK, Sketch MM, Mahoney PD, Lynch JD, Moss AN, Kenney NP. Detection of left ventricular thrombi by computerized tomography: a preliminary report. Br Heart J 1981; 45: 535–41.

66. Goodwin JD, Herykens RJ, Skoldebrand CG, Brundage BM, Schiller NB, Lipton MJ. Detection of intraventricular thrombi by computed tomography. Radiology 1981; 138:717–21.

67. Tomora H, Hoshia M, Furuya H, Kurebayashi S, Ootaki M, Matsuyana S, Koide S, Kawada S, Shotsu A. Evaluation of intracardiac thrombus with computed tomography. Am J Cardiol 1983; 51:843–51.

68. Foster CJ, Sekiya T, Love MG, Broundee WC, Griffin JF, Isherwood I. Identification of intracardiac thrombus: comparison of computed tomography and cross sectional echocardiography. Br J Radiol 1987; 60:327–31.

69. Swan HJC. Aneurysm of the cardiac ventricle: its management by medical and surgical intervention. West J Med 1978; 129:26–40.

70. Raphael MJ, Steiner RC, Goodwin JF, Oakley CM. Cineangiography of left ventricular aneurysm. Clin Radiol 1972; 23:129–39.

71. Cooley. Surgical treatment of left ventricular aneurysm: experience with excision of post infarction lesions in 80 patients. Prog Cardiovasc Dis 1968; 11:222.

72. Takamato T, Kim D, Uric PM, Guthaner DF, Gordon MJ, Karen A, Popp RL. Comparative recognition of left ventricle thrombi by echocardiography and cineangiography. Br Heart J 1985; 53:36–42.

73. Stratton JR, Ritchie JL, Hammermeister KE, et al. Detection of left ventricular thrombi with radionuclide angiography. Am J Cardiol 1981; 48:565.

74. Solandt DY, Nassim R, Best CM. Production and prevention of cardiac mural thrombosis in dogs. Lancet 1938; 2:592.

75. Arvan S. Mural thrombi in coronary artery disease. Recent advances in pathogenesis, diagnosis, and approaches to treatment. Arch Intern Med 1984; 144:113–6.

76. Simpson MT, Oberman A, Kouchoukos NT, Rogers WJ. Prevalence of mural thrombi and systemic embolization with left ventricular aneurysm: effect of anticoagulation therapy. Chest 1980; 77:463–9.

77. Wright IS, Marple CD, Beck DF. Anticoagulant therapy of coronary thrombosis with myocardial infarction. JAMA 1948; 138: 1074–9.

78. Arnott WM, et al. Assessment of short-term anticoagulant administration after cardiac infarction. Br Med J 1969; 1:335–42.

79. Harvald B, Hilden T, Lund E. Long-term anticoagulant therapy after myocardial infarction. Lancet 1962; 2:626.

80. VA Hospital Investigators. Anticoagulants in acute myocardial infarction. JAMA 1973; 225: 724–9.

81. Hilden T, Iversen K, Raaschan F, Schwartz M. Anticoagulation in acute myocardial infarction. Lancet 1961; 2:327–31.

82. Davis MJE, Ireland MA. Effect of early anticoagulation on the frequency of left ventricular thrombi after anterior wall acute myocardial infarction. Am J Cardiol 1986; 57:1244.

83. Stratton JR, Speck SM, Caldwell JM, Stadius ML, Maynard C, Davis KB, Ritchie JL, Kennedy JW. Late effects of intracoronary streptokinase on regional wall motion, ventricular aneurysm and left ventricular thrombus in myocardial infarction: results from the Western Washington Randomized Trial. J Am Coll Cardiol 1985; 5:1023–8.

84. Sharma B, Carvalho A, Wyeth R, Franciosa JA. Left ventricular thrombi diagnosed by echo in patients with acute MI treated with intracoronary streptokinase followed by intravenous heparin. Am J Cardiol 1985; 56:422–5.

85. Held AC, Gore JM, Parasko J, Pape LA, Ball SP, Corrao JM, Alpert JS. Impact of thrombolytic

therapy on left ventricular mural thrombi in acute myocardial infarction. Am J Cardiol 1988; 62:310–1.

86. The TIMI Study Group. The Thrombolysis in Myocardial Infarction trial: phase I finding. N Engl J Med 1985; 312:932–6.

87. Eigler N, Maner G, Shah PK. Effects of early systemic thrombolytic therapy on left ventricular mural thrombus formation in acute anterior myocardial infarction. Am J Cardiol 1984; 54:261–3.

88. Natarajan D, Hotchandani RK, Nigan PD. Reduced incidence of left ventricular thrombi with intravenous streptokinase in acute anterior myocardial infarction: prospective evaluation by cross-sectional echocardiography. Int J Cardiol 1988; 20:201–7.

89. Keren A, Medina A, Gottleib S, Banai S, Stern S. Lysis of mobile left ventricular thrombi during acute myocardial infarction with urokinase. Am J Cardiol 1987; 60:1180–1.

90. Kremer P, Fiebig R, Tilsner V, Bleifeld W. Lysis of left ventricular thrombi with urokinase. Circulation 1985; 72:112–8.

91. ISIS-2 Collaborative Group. Randomized trial of intravenous streptokinase, oral aspirin, both or neither among 17,187 cases of suspected acute myocardial infarction: ISIS-1. Lancet 1988; 349–60.

92. Rutherford JD, Braunwald E, Cohn PF. In Braunwald E, ed. Heart disease. A textbook of cardiovascular medicine. Philadelphia: W.B. Saunders, 1988:1364–6.

93. Lew AS, Federman J, Harper RW, et al. Operative removal of mobile pedunculated left ventricular thrombus detected by 2-dimensional echocardiography. Am J Cardiol 1983; 52: 1148–9.

94. Fournial G, Glock Y, Berthoumieu F, Allibelli MJ, Desrez X, Marco J. Thrombus flottant du ventricle gauche après infarctus du myocarde récent traité chirurgicalement. Arch Mal Coeur 1980; 73:1415–20.

95. Ezekowitz MD, Smith EO, Cox AC, et al. Failure of aspirin to prevent incorporation of indium-111 labelled platelets into cardiac thrombi in man. Lancet 1981; 1:440.

96. Mizuno K, Satomura K, Miyamoto A, Arakawa K, Shibuya T, Arai T, Kurita A, Nakamura H, Ambrose J. Angioscopic evaluation of coronary-artery thrombi in acute coronary syndromes. N Engl J Med 1992; 326:287–91.

97. Nichol ES, Fassett DW. An attempt to forestall acute coronary thrombosis. South Med J 1947; 40:631–7.

98. Elwood PC, Cochrane AL, Burr ML, et al. A randomized controlled trial of acetylsalicylic acid in the secondary prevention of mortality from myocardial infarction. Br Med J 1974; 1:436–40.

99. The Coronary Drug Project Research Group. Aspirin in coronary heart disease. J Chronic Dis 1976; 29:625–42.

100. Breddin K, Loew D, Lechner K, et al. Secondary prevention of myocardial infarction: a comparison of acetylsalicylic acid, placebo and phenprocoumon. Hemostasis 1980; 9:325–44.

101. Elwood PC, Sweetnam PM. Aspirin and secondary mortality after myocardial infarction. Lancet 1979; 2:1313–5.

102. Aspirin Myocardial Infarction Research Group. A randomized controlled trial of aspirin in persons recovered from myocardial infarction. JAMA 1980; 243:661–9.

103. The Persantine-Aspirin Reinfarction Study Research Group. Persantine-aspirin reinfarction study. Circulation 1980; 62(Suppl 2):II1–22.

104. Peto R. Aspirin after myocardial infarction (editorial). Lancet 1980; 1:1172.

105. Second report of the Working Party on Anticoagulant Therapy in Coronary Thrombosis to the Medical Research Council. An assessment of long term anticoagulant administration after cardiac infarction. Br Med J 1964; 2:837–43.

106. Ebert RV, Borden CW, Hipp HR, Holzman D, Lyon AF, Schnaper H. Long term anticoagulant therapy after myocardial infarction: final report of the Veteran's Administration Cooperative Study. JAMA 1969; 207:2263–7.

107. International Anticoagulant Review Group. Collaborative analysis of long term anticoagulant administration after acute myocardial infarction. Lancet 1970; 1:203.

108. Report of the 60+ Reinfarction Study Research Group. A double-blind trial to assess long term anticoagulant therapy in elderly patients after myocardial infarction. Lancet 1980; 2:989–94.

109. Smith P, Arnesen H, Holme I. The effect of warfarin on mortality and reinfarction after myocardial infarction. N Engl J Med 1990; 323:147–52.

110. Laarman G, Wahberg P, Labib S, et al. Warfarin after myocardial infarction (editorial). N Engl J Med 1990; 323:1839–41.

111. Meade TW. Low dose warfarin and low dose aspirin in the primary prevention of ischemic heart disease. Am J Cardiol 1990; 65:7C–11C.

112. Prichard PJ, Kitchingman GK, Walt RP, et al. Human gastric mucosal bleeding induced by low dose aspirin but not warfarin. Br Med J 1989; 298:493–6.

113. Segal JP, Stapleton JF, McClellan JR, Waller BF, Harvey WP. Idiopathic cardiomyopathy: clinical features, prognosis and therapy. Curr Prob Cardiol 1978; 3:1–48.

114. Johnson RA, Palacios I. Dilated cardiomyopathies of the adult (part I). N Engl J Med 1982; 307:1051–8.

115. Roberts WC, Ferrans VJ. Pathologic anatomy of the cardiomyopathies: idiopathic dilated and hypertrophic types, infiltrative types, and endomyocardial disease with and without eosinophilia. Hum Pathol 1975; 6:287–342.

116. Fuster V, Gersh B, Giuliani E, Tajik A, Brandenburg R, Frye R. The natural history of idiopathic dilated cardiomyopathy. Am J Cardiol; 47:525–31.

117. Cosnett JE, Pudifin DJ. Embolic complications of cardiomyopathy. Br Heart J 1964; 26:544.

118. Gottdiener JS, Gay JA, Van Voorhees L, DiBianco R, Fletcher RD. Frequency and embolic potential of left ventricular thrombus in dilated cardiomyopathy: assessment by 2-dimensional echocardiography. Am J Cardiol 1983; 52:1281–5.

119. D'Cruz IA, Sinden JR, Sridharan MR, Kleinman D. Case report: thromboembolization complicating left ventricular pseudoaneurysm: serial two-dimensional and color-flow Doppler echocardiographic observations. Am J Med Sci 1989; 298:123–5.

120. Chesler E, Korns ME, Seruba T, Edwards JE. False aneurysms of the left ventricle following myocardial infarction. Am J Cardiol 1969; 23:76–82.

121. Catherwood E, Mintz GS, Kotler MN, Parry WR, Segal BL. Two-dimensional echocardiographic recognition of left ventricular pseudoaneurysm. Circulation 1980; 62:294–303.

122. Gatewood RP, Nanda NC. Differentiation of left ventricular pseudoaneurysm from true aneurysm with two dimensional echocardiography. Am J Cardiol 1980; 46:869–78.

123. Saner HE, Asinger RW, Daniel JA, Olson J. Two-dimensional echocardiographic identification of left ventricular pseudoaneurysm. Am Heart J 1986; 112:977–85.

124. Davidson KH, Parisi AF, Harrington JJ, Barsamian EM, Fishbein MC. Pseudoaneurysm of the left ventricle: an unusual echocardiographic presentation. Ann Intern Med 1977; 86:430–3.

125. Meller J, Teichholz LE, Pichard AD, Matta R, Litwak R, Herman MV, Massie KF. Left ventricular myxoma: echocardiographic diagnosis and review of the literature. Am J Med 1977; 63:816–7.

126. Mazer MS, Harrigan PR. Left ventricular myxoma: M-mode and two-dimensional echocardiographic features. Am Heart J 1982; 104:875.

127. McAllister HA Jr. Primary tumors and cysts of the heart and pericardium. Curr Prob Cardiol 1979; 4.

128. Mahoney L, Schieken RM, Doty D. Cardiac rhabdomyomas simulating pulmonic stenosis. Cathet Cardiovasc Diagn 1979; 5:385.

129. Hoen AG, Ellis EJ. Intramural fibroma of the heart. Am J Cardiol 1966; 17:579.

130. Reul GJ Jr, Howell JF, Rubio PA, Peterson PA. Successful partial excision of an intramural fibroma of the left ventricle. Am J Cardiol 1975; 36:262.

131. Panella JS, Paige ML, Victor TA, Sermerdjian RA, Heuter DC. Angiosarcoma of the heart, diagnosis by echocardiography. Chest 1979; 76:21.

132. Coe GC. Primary rhabdomyosarcoma of the heart. Am Heart J 1960; 52:1124.

133. Schwartz JE, Schwartz GP, Judson PL, Siebel JE, Trumbull HR. Complete resection of a

primary cardiac rhabdomyosarcoma: case report, review of the literature, and management recommendations. Cardiovasc Dis Bull Tex Heart Inst 1979; 6:413.

134. Baldelli P, De Angeli D, Dolora A, Diligenti LM, Marchi F, Salvatore L. Primary fibrosarcoma of the heart. Chest 1972; 62:234.

135. Gough JC, Connolly CE, Kennedy JD. Primary sarcoma of the heart: a light and electron microscopic study of two cases. J Clin Pathol 1979; 32:601.

136. Prichard RW. Tumors of the heart: review of the subject and report of one hundred and fifty cases. Arch Pathol 1951; 51:98.

137. Timmis AD, Smallpeice C, Davies AC, MacArthur AM, Grishen P, Jackson G. Intracardiac spread of intravenous leiomatosis with successful surgical excision. N Engl J Med 1980; 303:1043.

138. Kadir S, Coulan CM. Intracaval extension of renal cell carcinoma. Cardiovasc Intervent Radiol 1980; 3:180.

139. Paris II: J Am Coll Cardiol 1986; 7:251–69.

140. Anturane Reinfarction Italian Study. Lancet 1982; 1:237–42.

141. Anturane Reinfarction Trial. N Engl J Med 1980; 302:250–6.

13

Cardiac Valves: Native and Prosthetic

Ira S. Cohen
*Yale University School of Medicine and West Haven Veterans
Affairs, New Haven, Connecticut*

Michael D. Ezekowitz
*Yale University School of Medicine, West Haven Veterans Affairs,
and Cardiovascular Thrombosis Research Laboratory,
New Haven, Connecticut*

Kenneth L. Franco
Yale University School of Medicine, New Haven, Connecticut

I. INTRODUCTION

The diagnosis of thromboembolism originating either from a diseased valve or from the associated altered hemodynamics is often a presumptive one, based on the history of an acute event, the exclusion of other cardiac and noncardiac causes, and the demonstration, if possible, of an abnormality of a native or prosthetic valve. The incidence of embolism in patients with valvular heart disease is difficult to assess from published reports, because the length of patient follow-up often is not specified, and data relating to the degree of anticoagulation and the presence of other risk factors are seldom given; thus, comparisons of thromboembolic rates from different institutions must be made cautiously (1). The same considerations apply to prosthetic heart valves. For this reason, comparison of embolic rates, where possible, is made on the basis of reported first events per 100 patient-years (percentage of patients with a first thromboembolic event per year of exposure) (1). The valvular conditions listed in Table 1 predispose to systemic embolization. The approach to diagnosis and management of each condition will be considered separately.

II. NATIVE VALVES

A. Mitral Valve Disease

1. Mitral Stenosis/Regurgitation

Thromboembolism is most common in patients with isolated mitral stenosis and in those with mitral stenosis combined with mitral regurgitation (1), largely as a consequence of associated left atrial dilatation, stasis, and clot formation (see Chap. 14). The embolic rate for mitral stenosis is between one and four events per 100 patient-years (2,3), which is consistent with a lifetime embolic prevalence rate of 15–20% (2,4). Up to 16% of such events may be

Table 1 Conditions of Cardiac Valves Predisposing to Systemic Embolization

I. Mitral valve Mitral stenosis Mitral stenosis/regurgitation ?Pure mitral regurgitation Mitral prolapse	II. Aortic valve Sclerosis/stenosis III. Prosthetic valve IV. Precipitating factors Atrial fibrillation Endocarditis

fatal (5). Thromboembolism is usually reported to be much less common in patients with mitral regurgitation than in those with mitral stenosis, with an embolic rate between one and two events per 100 patient-years (2,3), affecting 3% of patients over their lifetime (5). This observation may be due to the turbulence produced in the left atrium by the regurgitant jet, resulting in a reduction in left atrial stasis. In the Mayo Clinic series, with a minimum 10-year follow-up, the rate of embolism among 65 patients with severe mitral regurgitation was 2.9 events per 100 patient-years (6). Higher rates are reported in patients with a combination of mitral regurgitation and mitral stenosis—up to four events per 100 patient-years (2) affecting 14–18% of patients over their lifetime (2,3). There are no rigorous clinical trials to support the use of pharmacological prophylaxis in patients with rheumatic mitral disease who are in sinus rhythm. However, for patients with mitral stenosis and sinus rhythm, an argument can be made in favor of low-dose warfarin anticoagulation in those with low risk for bleeding complications.

2. Mitral Prolapse

The association of nonejection clicks and late systolic murmurs with billowing mitral leaflets as identified by pathologic and angiographic correlation was made in the 1960s by Reid (7) and by Barlow and Bosman (8). An etiologic link between cerebral ischemic events and a prolapsing mitral valve was first proposed by Barnett et al. (9). Since then, isolated reports in the literature have also suggested such a connection, and an increased incidence of echocardiographically defined prolapse in patients under age 45 with both transient and fixed cerebrovascular events has been noted (10,11). The estimated prevalence of a mildly prolapsing mitral valve leaflet in the general population is between 5% and 10%, and it is probably as high as 20% if only a single clinical or echocardiographic criterion is required for the diagnosis. The incidence of embolism appears to be very low in this large population with mitral valve prolapse so defined. However, because the risk of embolization in the general population of patients with mitral valve prolapse is low (1 of 6000 adults with prolapse per year) and because there are no supporting trials to direct practice, it is not usual to anticoagulate these patients (12). Treatment with aspirin is a reasonable but untested compromise in patients with suspected embolic episodes. Warfarin therapy should be considered only for patients with recurrent symptoms, and it too is untested.

Prolapse as an etiology for cerebrovascular events remains a diagnosis requiring exclusion of other potential etiologies. Mitral valve prolapse has provided a major impetus to the popularization of diagnostic M-mode and two-dimensional echocardiographic techniques. It has also reinforced the need for rigorous clinicopathologic correlation. M-mode echocardiographic correlation of midsystolic M-mode mitral prolapse to the classic auscultatory findings remains a highly specific finding (13,14). Inclusion of less specific findings of pansystolic hammocking on M-mode echocardiography and the understandable but arbitrary "definition" of superior displacement of the anterior mitral leaflet in the apical two-dimensional echocardiographic view (15) made mitral valve prolapse an "epidemic" disease. The recognition by Levine et al. (16) that the saddle-shaped configuration of the mitral annulus can create an apparent superior displacement of the mitral leaflets in the apical view led to an attempt at establishing a more critical approach to this echocardiographic diagnosis. Cohen (17) showed that clinically significant symptoms were more common in those patients with severe degrees of prolapse as identified by two-dimensional echocardiography. The echocardiographic criteria for the diagnosis of prolapse are still controversial. An emerging consensus view is that evidence of prolapse in the parasternal view is the most specific echocardiographic finding and that correlation with both physical findings and Doppler interrogation is essential. What is clear is that displacement of the mitral leaflets above the mitral valve plane, restricted to the apical views, particularly if limited to the anterior leaflet, is a poor diagnostic criterion. Diagnostic criteria for prolapse by transesophageal echocardiography have not been defined, even though valve details are generally better seen in comparison with the transthoracic approach.

Several pathophysiologic aspects of the prolapse syndrome may explain its apparent association with cerebrovascular events. Platelet abnormalities including increased aggregation in the peripheral blood, increased aggregability in response to epinephrine stimulation, and decreased platelet survival times have been noted in patients with prolapse (18,19). Hyperadrenergic states have been noted in patients with symptomatic prolapse (20) and might theoretically increase platelet aggregation. Histologically, endothelial denudation has been observed in some individuals with prolapse and may be related to physical abrasion of adjacent tissues by the redundant valvular tissue (21). Fibrin and platelets are deposited on these abraded surfaces and may serve as potential embolic sources.

B. Aortic Valve Disease

Thromboembolism is much less common in patients with aortic as compared with mitral valve disease and is most frequently associated with superimposed infective endocarditis. The precise incidence is difficult to document. In a Mayo Clinic series of 68 medically treated patients, followed for at least 10 years, most emboli occurring in patients with aortic stenosis were calcareous, and many were clinically silent (22,23). The risk of embolism does not increase with the severity of the valvular lesion, and an embolus may be the first indication of calcific aortic stenosis. In addition, emboli dislodged during cardiac catheterization or at surgery may constitute a potential problem unless care is exercised. It is important to emphasize that the data with regard to embolic complications in patients with aortic valve disease are very limited. Specific treatment for prophylaxis is not usually advised.

III. PROSTHETIC VALVES

Prosthetic cardiac valve replacement remains one of the most important contributions in the field of cardiac surgery. It is estimated that approximately 40,000 prosthetic valves are implanted annually in the United States. The length and quality of life after valve replacement are related to the hemodynamic function of the prosthetic valve; the durability of the valve; various complications that may be associated with prosthetic valve dysfunction, including thrombosis, thromboemboli, and endocarditis; and preoperative left ventricular function. The operative mortality from cardiac valve replacement has continued to decrease (3–5% for aortic valve replacement and 5–10% for mitral valve replacement) because of better patient selection, earlier operation, improved techniques of myocardial protection, and concomitant coronary artery bypass procedures.

The characteristics of an ideal prosthetic valve include central flow, minimal transvalvular gradients, low thrombogenicity, resistance to infection, longevity, ease of implantability, wide availability, and a low noise level (24). Numerous prostheses have been introduced through the years, but none of the valves available today fulfills all of the criteria mentioned above. Patients with prosthetic valves require close follow-up so that potential problems can be recognized and appropriately treated. Successful management requires an understanding of the special design characteristics of the various prostheses as well as the complications common to all cardiac prostheses.

Prosthetic cardiac valves are divided into two major groups: mechanical and biopros-

Mechanical Valves

1. Starr Edwards Ball Valve

2. Bjork Shiley

3. St. Jude Medical

4. Omniscience

5. Medtronic - Hall

Bioprosthetic Valves

1. Carpentier - Edwards

2. Hancock

3. Ionescu - Shiley

4. Homograft

Figure 1 Prosthetic cardiac valves available for implantation over the last 10 years.

thetic. Mechanical valves are constructed of metal and synthetic materials, and bioprosthetic or tissue valves are constructed of biologic material treated chemically to reduce antigenicity and increase tissue strength, or of native tissue such as the aortic homograft (25) (Fig. 1). The most frequently used mechanical valves include the Starr-Edwards ball-and-cage valve, the Bjork-Shiley and Medtronic-Hall tilting-disc valves, and the St. Jude bileaflet valve. The most popular tissue valves include the Carpentier-Edwards and Hancock porcine valves, the Ionescu-Shiley bovine pericardial valve, and the aortic homograft.

A. Mechanical Cardiac Valves

The caged-ball valve was the first introduced in the late 1950s and has undergone several modifications. In its current configuration this mechanical valve consists of a Silastic ball in a non-cloth covered cage—the Starr-Edwards model 1260 aortic (Fig. 2) and 6120 mitral valves are currently the most frequently used caged-ball valves. These models have not undergone any modifications since 1966. Their major advantage lies in their proven long-term durability, which extends to over 25 years. The major disadvantage of the caged-ball valve and other mechanical valves is the need for lifelong anticoagulant therapy. A second disadvantage with this valve is the moderate transvalvular gradient. Its bulky ball-and-cage design is a distinct liability in patients with small left ventricles and/or small aortic roots (26). At one point in its development, in an effort to reduce the incidence of thromboembolic events, the struts of the Starr-Edwards valve were covered with cloth. This created additional problems with cloth wear, hemolysis, and embolization of the cloth material, as well as fibrin buildup on the struts (Fig. 3). This particular valve has been discontinued and is no longer available.

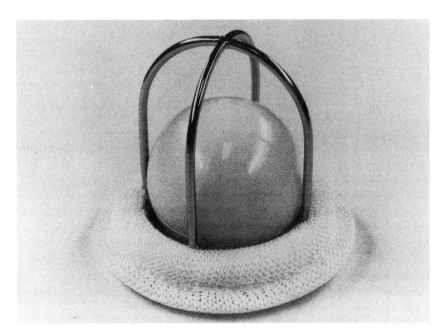

Figure 2   Starr-Edwards aortic prosthesis with silicone rubber ball and bare metal cage. (From McGoon DC et al., eds. Cardiac surgery 2. Philadelphia: F.A. Davis, 1987:108.)

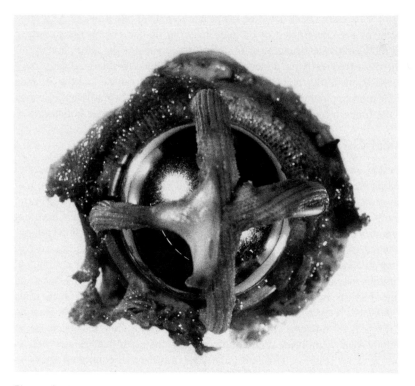

Figure 3 Starr-Edwards cloth-covered aortic prosthesis with metal ball. Fibrin buildup is seen in addition to an exposed strut from cloth wear.

The Bjork-Shiley and Medtronic-Hall were the most commonly employed tilting-disc valves (27). The primary advantage of the tilting-disc valve is to minimize transvalvular gradients and obtain a flow pattern that approaches central flow. The Bjork-Shiley valve was first introduced in 1969. It has undergone several modifications since that time. The valve has a low profile. The occluder is a tilting disc that opens to 60° and allows flow through major and minor orifices. In an effort to reduce the incidence of in situ thrombosis, the disc was modified in 1976 to form a slight convex-concave profile allowing the valve to open more widely by moving out of the orifice slightly (Fig. 4). The configuration diverts 40% more flow through the minor orifice, lessening stasis by eliminating contact between the open disc and the base of the valve (27). This change, unfortunately, was associated with a higher incidence of strut fractures in larger valves. As a result, the valve was withdrawn from the market in the mid-1980s. To completely eliminate the possibility of strut fracture, the Shiley corporation has developed a Monostrut valve with the entire valve housing constructed from a single piece of metal alloy, eliminating all welded struts. The convex-concave disc opens to 70° and provides nearly equal flow on both sides of the disc. This valve has been implanted in several thousand patients overseas but has not yet been approved by the Food and Drug Administration for use in the United States.

The St. Jude Medical valve was introduced in 1977. It is a bileaflet valve with two half-circle–shaped leaflets that open to an angle of 85° (Fig. 5). The hemodynamic characteristics of this prosthesis are excellent, with near-central laminar flow. It enjoys the lowest trans-

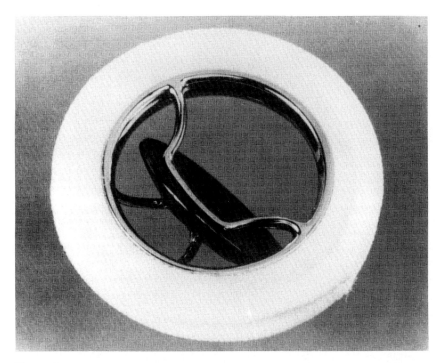

Figure 4 Bjork-Shiley prosthesis with convex-concave disc of pyrolite carbon. (From McGoon DC et al., eds. Cardiac Surgery 2. Philadelphia: F.A. Davis, 1987:110.)

valvular gradients, especially in smaller valves. This particular valve is well suited for replacement in patients with a small aortic root and/or left ventricle. A low-profile disc valve is often mildly regurgitant. Generally this is hemodynamically insignificant. It does decrease the problem of periprosthetic flow stagnation and might lead to a lower incidence of thrombosis (28). At the present time, the St. Jude valve is the most popular mechanical prosthesis used worldwide. A small buildup of thrombus or pannus ingrowth on the delicate mechanism may occasionally interfere with valve function by preventing opening or closing of the discs (29).

Two less commonly used tilting-disc valves also have the advantages of low-profile design and excellent durability. These are the Medtronic-Hall and Omniscience valves. Both have been available since the late 1970s.

B. Bioprosthetic Valves

Bioprosthetic valves (tissue valves) include homografts of cadaver aortic valves and glutaraldehyde-preserved porcine aortic and pericardial prostheses. The major advantage of bioprosthetic valves is low thrombogenicity in comparison with mechanical valves. These are ideal for patients who cannot be anticoagulated (30). Despite their natural configuration and central flow, they do have significant transvalvular gradients, especially in the smaller valves. The major disadvantage of these valves is their limited long-term durability. The glutaraldehyde-preserved porcine bioprostheses degenerate and calcify at 7 to 10 years after implantation (31). Clinically this is manifested by torn leaflets with resulting valvular

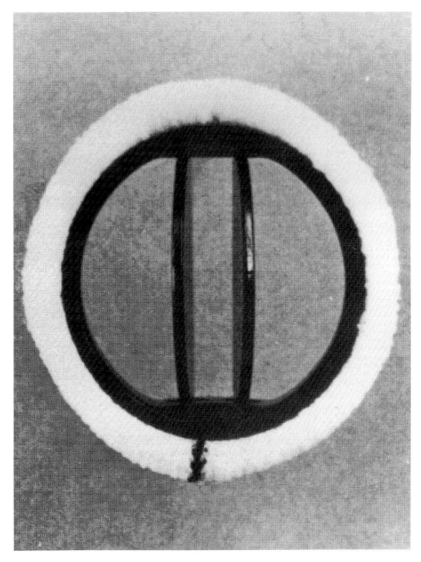

Figure 5   St. Jude aortic prosthesis. (From Frankl WS et al., eds. Valvular heart disease: comprehensive evaluation and management. Philadelphia: F.A. Davis, 1986:403.)

insufficiency, and by development of stenosis related to calcification of the cusps (31). The mitral bioprosthesis has a higher failure rate than the aortic tissue valves, probably because of the high shear forces that occur with left ventricular contraction and the pressure gradients between the left atrium and the left ventricle (31). The two commercially available porcine valves include the Hancock and the Carpentier-Edwards valves (Fig. 6). Both of these valves have been available since the mid-1970s.

The Ionescu-Shiley bovine pericardial valve was introduced in the early 1980s. It provided improved hemodynamic characteristics, especially in the smaller valves, but had a much larger stent, which impacted on the aortic and ventricular wall after either aortic or

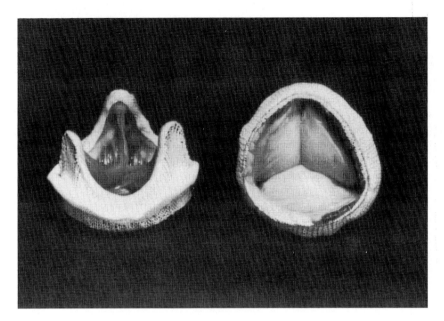

Figure 6 Carpentier-Edwards porcine aortic bioprosthesis. (From Frankl WS et al., eds. Valvular heart disease: comprehensive evaluation and management. Philadelphia: F.A. Davis, 1986:408.)

mitral valve replacement. The Ionescu-Shiley valve has been removed from the market because of early failure due to calcification and tissue degeneration (32). Early enthusiasm for the use of bioprostheses in children has waned because of early failure and rapid calcification.

The homograft aortic valve has been used in orthotopic aortic valve replacement since the early 1960s. Longevity of the homograft is related to cellular viability. Fresh homografts have excellent long-term viability, but for obvious reasons their availability is extremely limited. The current cryopreserved homograft aortic valve fulfills the criteria of central flow, minimal gradients, low thrombogenicity, and durability (Fig. 7). Implantation of this particular valve is technically demanding. Availability remains the main factor limiting its increased use in the United States. The cryopreserved valve is soaked in an antibiotic solution and cooled to $-196°C$ in a container of liquid nitrogen. The valves are harvested by procurement teams experienced in solid organ transplantation, packaged, and transported to Cryolife for preservation. Cryogenic preservation has demonstrated nearly 90% viability at the cellular level at the time of implantation of these particular valves (33). The homograft aortic valve is especially useful in children and adults with a small aortic root and in patients who cannot be anticoagulated (because of its low incidence of thromboemboli) and in patients with recurrent endocarditis (because of its low incidence of valve-related endocarditis) (34).

C. Assessment of Prosthetic Valve Function

Clinical evidence of prosthetic valve dysfunction varies, to some extent, with the different types of prostheses. The major complications of valve replacement are infection, thrombosis, thromboembolism, and mechanical failure of the valve itself. Incomplete relief of preoperative symptoms, the reappearance of preoperative symptoms, or the onset of new

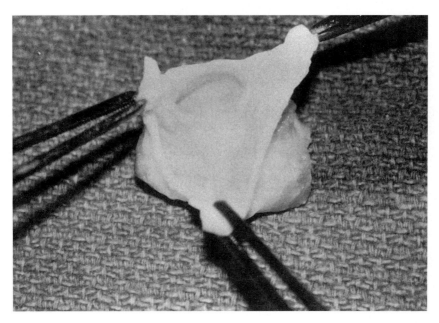

Figure 7   Aortic valve homograft. (Courtesy of Cryolife.)

symptoms may indicate prosthetic valve dysfunction or complication. Symptoms of congestive heart failure may result from valve obstruction or valvular regurgitation. New-onset
angina may result from prosthetic dysfunction or from coronary artery obstruction caused
by emboli to the coronary vessels or traumatic stenosis of the coronary ostia. Transient
ischemic attacks or stroke are usually due to emboli, but the presence of systemic emboli
should always raise the suspicion of prosthetic valve endocarditis. Unexplained fever or
"flulike symptoms" with or without new cardiac murmurs, splenomegaly, leukocytosis, and
positive blood cultures suggest the possibility of prosthetic valve endocarditis, particularly
in patients who have undergone recent dental manipulation or other instrumentation,
including cystoscopy and colonoscopy. Any alteration in the normal auscultatory characteristics of the specific prosthesis or the appearance of a new murmur (either systolic or
diastolic) may be an important sign of prosthetic valve malfunction. Hematuria, melena,
ecchymosis, and bleeding may result from excessive and poorly controlled anticoagulant
therapy. However, subclinical pathologic conditions occasionally are manifested in this
way, and appropriate workup is indicated.

Several imaging techniques may be usefully applied in the assessment of prosthetic valve
dysfunction. Cineradiographic techniques require that the prosthesis incorporate radiopaque
materials as part of its design to allow assessment of poppet motion and sewing ring stability
and mobility. The popular bileaflet St. Jude valve can be difficult to evaluate because its
ring is not radiopaque. Bioprosthetic struts and annular components of many prostheses
contain radiopaque materials, as do some metallic occluders. Restricted motion of the disc
or poppet of a mechanical prosthesis may cause thrombosis or infection. Exaggerated
mobility of the annulus may suggest a partially dehisced prosthesis (34). A change in the
degree of tilting motion between two examinations is more significant than the degree of
tilting on a single examination. The sewing ring of prosthetic heart valves has been imaged

by ^{111}In-labeled platelet scintigraphy in an animal model. Similar success has not been achieved in patients because of the large central blood pool and greater tissue attenuation.

Both transthoracic and transesophageal two-dimensional echocardiography are the predominant clinical tools currently used in assessment of prosthetic valve morphology and function. Both are useful in the assessment of ventricular function and detection of calcification of bioprosthetic valves, the presence of vegetations and ring abscesses, and of the rocking motion noted with ring dehiscence (35). Echocardiography has largely replaced phonocardiography for assessment of prosthetic valve dysfunction (36), although useful information can sometimes be obtained by combining both techniques (37). It should be recognized that prosthetic valves pose a special problem for the echographer because of the acoustic shadowing from the highly echo-reflective metallic surfaces. As a result, detailed imaging of the components of the prostheses by transthoracic echocardiography (TTE) is often limited (38). Thus, the presence of thrombi on prosthetic heart valves may have to be inferred on the basis of a clinical suspicion of dysfunction (e.g., increasing dyspnea, chest pain, embolic episodes, worsening heart failure, or changes in prosthetic sounds), in combination with evidence of abnormal motion of the valve detected by echocardiography, fluoroscopy, and/or heart catheterization, and/or Doppler echocardiographic evidence of a change in valvular dynamics (38).

However, the cause and mechanism of prosthetic valve dysfunction is generally better assessed by transesophageal echocardiography (TEE) than by TTE (Fig. 8). The esophageal window eliminates the acoustic shadow encountered in the transthoracic approach by imaging from behind the prosthesis. The combination of close proximity to the prosthesis and use of the higher-frequency TEE transducer permits visualization of a remarkable

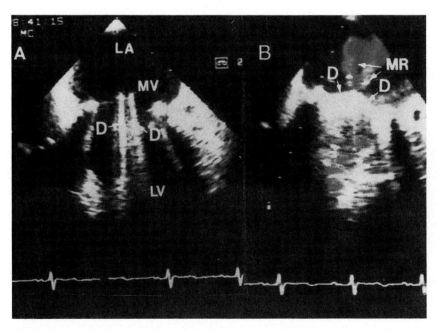

Figure 8   Transesophageal four-chamber view from a patient with a St. Jude mitral valve. (A) Disks are open and parallel to each other in diastole. (B) Disks are closed in systole with trace mitral regurgitation. (From Ref. 35.)

amount of detail of prosthetic valve structure. It also more accurately detects regurgitant flow, which can be masked by acoustic shadowing to such a degree that even severe mitral insufficiency may not be detectable by TTE (Fig. 8). It is important to note that a Carpentier ring, increasingly used in atrioventricular valvuloplasty, can also cause significant acoustic shadowing and a comparable degree of underestimation of the severity of mitral regurgitation as determined by TTE. Transesophageal echocardiography is also useful in the detection of thrombus and vegetations and in the evaluation of certain complications of endocarditis such as ring dehiscence or ring abscess. The anatomic assessment of mitral and tricuspid prostheses is best achieved by TEE imaging, and echocardiographic evaluation of these is incomplete without it, particularly when assessing potential insufficiency.

The initial TEE assessment of both mitral and tricuspid prostheses is performed from the standard four-chamber TEE view. The mitral prosthesis can often be visualized in its short axis by slow withdrawal from a left ventricular transgastric short-axis transverse- and vertical-plane view with a biplane transducer. Low esophageal and higher horizontal and vertical biplane views are particularly useful for the tricuspid valve and annulus. Aortic prostheses are seen in both a TEE long-axis view and by antegrade flexion from this position with or without advancement or withdrawal of the probe. The slight increase in distance from the probe is often sufficient to reduce the amount of detail that can be seen in aortic prostheses, although, in general, more detail is seen than with transthoracic imaging. Ring abscess visualization is clearly superior by TEE.

We recently reported a case (39) of thrombotic obstruction of a mitral bioprosthetic valve diagnosed by TEE in which a change was noted in TTE prosthetic appearance (Fig. 9). The diagnosis of a thrombosed prosthesis calls for thrombolytic therapy (40,41) or urgent surgery (42,43). When there is a question of mitral prosthetic malfunction, TEE should routinely be planned (44).

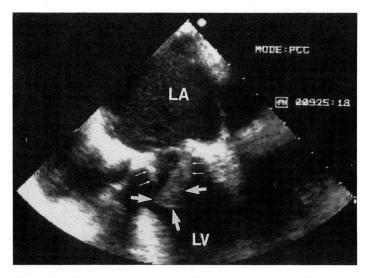

Figure 9   TEE of thrombosed mitral bioprosthesis (four chamber view). A large thrombus (large arrows) partially obstructs the prosthetic orifice. The LA is dilated and shows spontaneous echo contrast. The small arrows identify the prosthetic struts. LV = left ventricle.

Doppler echocardiographic techniques are now used as the method of choice for assessing the hemodynamic function of prosthetic valves, although there are caveats to be observed in its use and clinical correlation is essential. The placement of a prosthetic valve ring inherently reduces the cross-sectional area of the native valve annulus to some degree, and its presence establishes an irreducible resting gradient that varies by prosthesis and size. Application of basic Doppler echocardiographic principles allows measurement of these gradients and estimation of the effective area of the prosthesis, and has permitted the establishment of normal values for most valves and valve sizes (45).

Continuous-wave Doppler echocardiography provides the most useful assessment of prosthetic valves (46). Color Doppler is useful for screening for regurgitant lesions (if these are not acoustically shadowed by the prosthesis) and for the anatomic localization of leaks as valvular or paravalvular. Both pulsed-wave and continuous- wave Doppler are useful for detecting regurgitation and for measurement of velocity across prostheses. The use of pulsed-wave Doppler is largely limited to atrioventricular valves, where maximal gradients are inherently low. Aortic gradients must be assessed by continuous-wave Doppler, because the higher velocities cannot be resolved by pulsed wave Doppler.

Accurate determination of the gradient across a prosthesis is determined using a modified Bernoulli equation (instantaneous gradient $= 4$ [peak velocity]^2). Both peak instantaneous and mean gradients across the prosthesis can be reassessed. Pressure half-time methods are used for determination of the valve area across atrioventricular prostheses (47). Normal valves of Doppler-derived gradients have a wide variation, mainly because of their marked flow-dependence. At high flow rates Doppler gradients may approach the range ordinarily considered to represent stenotic values. Thus, accurate evaluation of prosthetic valve function demands information on flow rate at the time that the gradient is measured, especially when valves with small orifices are being evaluated. In general, prosthetic valve design, valve size, and flow conditions must all be considered when interpreting Doppler data from prosthetic valves.

There are several general sources of error which may be present when the Doppler principle is used to calculate pressure gradient (Table 2). Overestimation of the gradient by Doppler may be caused by nonuniform flow patterns across a normally functioning prosthesis or by regional variation in flow, which may lead to overestimation of the peak valve gradient (44). The Doppler measurement is in fact accurate but detects regional flow anomalies that are not representative of the true net flow across the prosthesis. An important cause of overestimation occurs when there is increased flow velocity proximal to the valve. This measurement is usually correctly ignored with velocities less than 1.5 m/s (48). In the St. Jude bileaflet valve and the Starr-Edwards valve, Doppler gradient systematically exceeds catheter gradients (49,50). Studies have shown that the two leaflets of the St.

Table 2 Sources of Error in Measuring
Doppler Gradients Across Prosthetic Valves

Overestimation
  Nonuniform flow patterns
  Increased flow velocities proximal to the valve
  Small valves
Underestimation
  Malalignment of the Doppler beam

Jude valve create a tunnel-like geometry that results in high velocities and therefore high gradients between the two leaflets (44), but actual flow through the effective orifice is lower in velocity and nonobstructive. The continuous-wave Doppler flow profile may provide adjunctive information. A high peak velocity with a rapid falloff in velocity during systole is more suggestive of prosthetic design–related flow anomalies than of hemodynamically significant flow obstruction and represents a lower mean than peak gradient. In general, the differences between Doppler gradient and catheter gradient are not significant in large valves, but significant differences can be seen with smaller valves. In addition, Doppler gradients across bioprosthetic valves seem, in general, to be more accurate than those across mechanical prostheses (51). Misinterpretation of a mitral regurgitant jet as an aortic flow jet is an important source of error. It should be carefully noted that the onset of mitral flow occurs during isovolumic contraction, while aortic flow starts later.

The main reason for underestimating pressure gradient by Doppler is misalignment of the Doppler beam with blood flow direction. The angle between the ultrasound beam and blood flow in the Doppler equation is usually assumed to be $0°$. If the angle is more than about $30°$, the true blood flow velocity will be underestimated as a function of the cosine of the angle of incidence. Pressure half-time determinations of mitral valve area are also subject to error and are affected by many variables (52). Left ventricular hypertrophy and/or aortic insufficiency can shorten pressure half-time and cause underestimation of the severity of mitral stenosis. Application of the continuity equation usually provides accurate estimates of mitral prosthetic valve area (53).

Echocardiography provides the unique benefit of allowing patients to serve as their own controls. Regardless of the absolute validity of the determined values, a definite change suggests an alteration in valve function. Although the diagnosis of prosthetic valve dysfunction may be made quite accurately by the history and physical examination and noninvasive studies, cardiac catheterization is often indicated to confirm the clinical findings and to provide complete assessment of the cardiac status, including that of the coronary arteries. Moreover, when symptoms suggest the possibility of valve dysfunction, but there is an absence of supporting physical and noninvasive findings, valve dysfunction should not be excluded without a cardiac catheterization.

D. Thromboembolism

Thomboembolism is suggested clinically by any new, permanent or transient, focal or global neurologic deficit, exclusive of hemorrhage, and by any peripheral arterial embolus, unless these are proved to have resulted from another cause (54). It remains the leading cause of morbidity and mortality following valve replacement. It is quite likely that the incidence of thromboembolism is underreported because the presentation is not specific. Local thrombosis, which may embolize, is caused by a combination of stasis at hinge points and the sewing ring and the failure of endothelialization of the device (54). Many observers have noted that the highest risk of thromboembolism occurs in the first 12 months following valve replacement and that the incidence appears to decrease at a fairly steady rate thereafter.

Thromboembolic phenomena are more common with mechanical valves than with bioprosthetic valves. However, embolic complications are not rare with bioprosthetic valves, particularly in the mitral portion (54). All mechanical valves have approximately the same risk for thromboembolic events when anticoagulation with warfarin is used indefinitely (55) (Fig. 10). The risk is greater for mitral valve replacement than for aortic valve replacement. Without warfarin, the incidence of thromboembolism increases four- to eightfold in patients

Type	Model	Reports	Pt-yrs	TE rate
Mechanical	Starr-Edwards	7	21,760	2.3
	Bjork-Shiley	9	7,753	1.9
	St. Jude	11	5,418	1.4
	Medtronic Hall	6	6,570	1.8
	Omniscience	4	753	2.7
Tissue	Carpentier	3	3,513	1.4
	Hancock	5	1,890	1.0
	Ionescu	10	9,296	0.8

Figure 10 Thromboembolic rates for prosthetic aortic valves. (From Ref. 56.)

with mechanical aortic valves and is probably even higher in those with mechanical mitral valves (56) (Fig. 11). Platelet inhibitors without warfarin are ineffective. All patients with mechanical valves should be treated for life with warfarin at a prothrombin time of about 1.5 times the control value (57–59). Inadequate anticoagulant therapy, atrial fibrillation, low cardiac output, history of previous embolization, multiple valve replacements, sepsis, or endocarditis may increase the incidence of thromboembolic events. Patients with a mechanical valve with a need for surgery require interruption of anticoagulant therapy with warfarin for as short a time as possible. Heparin should be used for initiation of anticoagulation until warfarin can be introduced and readjusted into the therapeutic range.

Thromboembolic events are less common in patients with bioprosthetic valves than in those with mechanical valves. This complication, for all type of valves, is more common

Type	Model	Reports	Pt-yrs	TE rate
Mechanical	Starr-Edwards	9	19,949	4.4
	Bjork-Shiley	9	6,188	3.3
	St. Jude	11	4,104	1.6
	Medtronic Hall	7	4,053	2.6
	Omniscience	5	1,017	2.8
Tissue	Carpentier	3	3,363	2.0
	Hancock	6	4,831	2.4
	Ionescu	8	3,702	1.8

Figure 11 Thromboembolic rates for prosthetic mitral valves. (From Ref. 56.)

with mitral valve replacement (56) (Figs. 10 and 11). For bioprosthetic valves anticoagulant therapy is recommended initially for both aortic and mitral valve replacement. It may safely be discontinued after 3 months, at which time the sewing ring is usually endothelialized. Anticoagulant therapy should be continued indefinitely, if possible, when any of the following conditions exists: chronic atrial fibrillation, a large left atrium, presence of a clot in the left atrium at surgery, history of a thromboembolic event within 6 months of mitral valve replacement, low cardiac output states, poor left ventricular function, and the use of a small prosthesis (Fig. 12). In these patients it may be better to use a mechanical valve with known durability rather than a bioprosthesis. An advantage of the aortic valve homograft is that it enjoys freedom from thromboembolic events, i.e., freedom from thromboembolism has been reported as 97% at 10 years without the use of anticoagulant therapy (33) (Fig. 13).

In most studies anticoagulant-related hemorrhage is defined as any episode of internal or external bleeding that causes death, stroke, operation, or hospitalization or requires transfusion (56). The incidence of bleeding complications among patients receiving anticoagulant therapy is between 1% and 4% per patient per year. The variability of criteria for reporting bleeding complications makes comparison of reports difficult. The incidence of fatal bleeding episodes approaches 1% per patient per year. Bleeding complications most frequently involve the central nervous system, the retroperitoneal area, and the gastrointestinal tract. Factors that may increase the incidence of bleeding complications include age over 70 (58,59), history of gait disturbance, history of previous stroke or episode of gastrointestinal bleeding (including peptic ulcer disease or diverticulitis), the use of a mechanical valve, low cardiac output or poor ventricular function, liver dysfunction, poor compliance, and the use of combinations of drugs including warfarin, aspirin, and dipyridamole. Recent data (unpublished) suggest that low doses of warfarin INR 2.0–3.0 with low-dose aspirin carries a low risk of hemorrhage.

The current recommendations for patients with mechanical heart valves include administration of warfarin alone or with aspirin or dipyridamole (57,60).

1.   Chronic A-fib

2.   Large LA

3.   Clot in LA

4.   Hx of TE event within 6 months MVR

5.   LCO or poor LV function

6.   Small- sized prosthesis

Figure 12 Indications for anticoagulation in patients with mitral bioprostheses. A-fib = atrial fibrillation; LA = left atrium; TE = thromboembolic; MVR = mitral valve replacement; LCO = low cardiac output; LV = left ventricular.

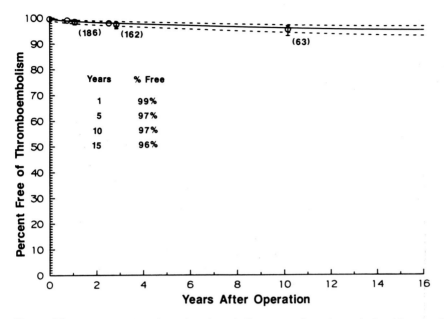

Figure 13 Percent freedom from thromboembolic events after primary isolated homograft aortic valve replacement. (From Ref. 33.)

E. Thrombosis

Thrombosis of mechanical prosthetic valves, especially the tilting-disc valve, is one of the most serious complications of valve replacement, with an incidence ranging from 0.5% to 4% per patient per year (61) (Figs. 14 and 15). The clinical presentation may vary from an insidious onset of mild symptoms to acute circulatory decompensation often resulting in death. The acute onset of valve dysfunction should suggest the possibility of valve thrombosis, especially in a patient who has received inadequate anticoagulant therapy. Immediate diagnosis and prompt intervention decreases the mortality associated with this complication. The risk of valve thrombosis is dependent largely on valve site. Mechanical prostheses in the tricuspid position have the highest incidence of thrombosis, whereas this complication is least common in the aortic position (62).

The treatment for a partially thrombosed aortic valve is replacement of the valve, thrombectomy, or the use of thrombolytic therapy (61) (Fig. 16). The greatest value of thrombolytic therapy is in the stabilization of a patient before surgery, allowing an elective, safer operation. Surprisingly, systemic embolization and permanent severe neurologic defect have been uncommon, but this remains the major risk for patients undergoing prosthetic valve thrombolysis (63,64).

Thrombosis of a mechanical mitral valve can occur in the early postoperative period in a patient who has low cardiac output and has been inadequately anticoagulated (Fig. 17). Thrombosis of a mechanical mitral valve is manifested by low cardiac output refractory to all pharmacologic support and must be differentiated from other possible causes such as cardiac tamponade. A thrombosed mechanical prosthesis requires immediate operation. Thrombolytic therapy is another option (64), but may increase the risk of reoperation if it fails. At operation a decision has to be made whether to replace the valve or to perform a

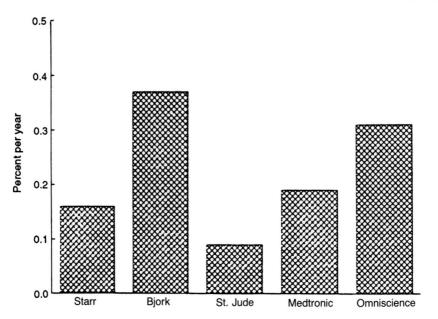

Figure 14 Pooled thrombosis rates for mechanical aortic valves, 1983–1987. (From Ref. 56.)

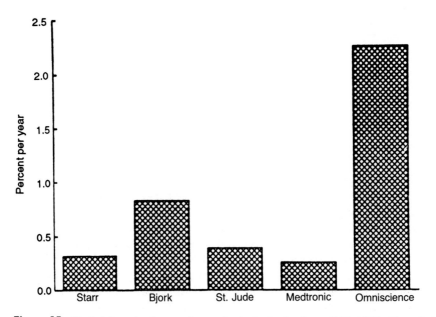

Figure 15 Pooled thrombosis rates for mechanical mitral valves, 1983–1987. (From Ref. 56.)

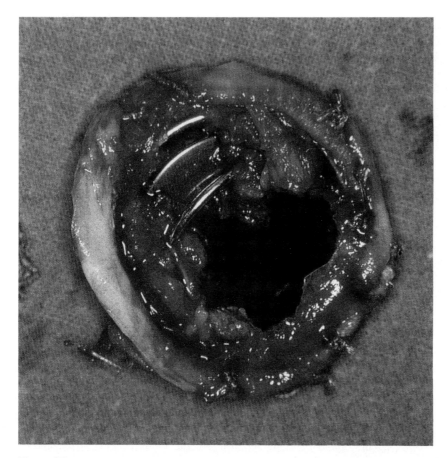

Figure 16   Thrombosed Bjork-Shiley aortic valve. (Removed at operation.)

thrombectomy. Thrombectomy may be sufficient therapy if the clot is of recent origin and can be removed safely without residual thrombus, and the valve appears to be functioning normally. Prevention of valve thrombosis requires adequate anticoagulation, which should be instituted early in the perioperative period, with the addition of heparin until the prothrombin time comes into therapeutic range.

F.   Endocarditis

Patients with prosthetic valves are at a higher risk of developing valve-related endocarditis than patients with congenital or acquired valvular heart disease (65). Antibiotic prophylaxis at the time of procedures or illnesses that may cause bacteremia is imperative in patients with prosthetic valves. The incidence of prosthetic valve endocarditis is similar for all types of prosthetic valves (1% to 4% per patient per year). Prosthetic valve endocarditis can occur early (<60 days after replacement) or late (>60 days after replacement) (66). Early prosthetic valve endocarditis is believed to result from intraoperative contamination or postoperative wound or urinary tract infections. Common etiologic organisms include *Staphylococcus aureus*, *Staphylococcus epidermidis*, gram-negative enterobacteria, and

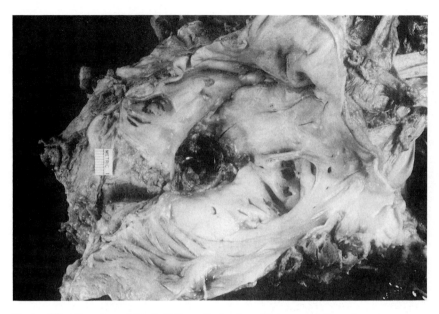

Figure 17 Thrombosed Bjork-Shiley mitral valve. (Autopsy specimen.)

fungi, especially *Candida* and *Aspergillus*. Most patients with early prosthetic valve endocarditis will require valve replacement. The mortality associated with early prosthetic valve endocarditis is high, and most deaths are due to septic shock. Late prosthetic valve endocarditis resembles native valve endocarditis, with trauma and dental and genitourinary manipulations being responsible for most cases. Organisms commonly involved include *Streptococcus viridans*, *Staphylococcus epidermidis*, and gram-negative *Hemophilus* or *Actinobacillus*. Approximately 50% of cases will require valve replacement. Prosthetic valves in the aortic position are more commonly involved than other valves, and in patients with multiple prosthetic valves, infection is usually confined to the most downstream valve. The clinical picture of late prosthetic valve endocarditis may be subtle, with vague flulike symptoms, or it may be dominated by fever, malaise, fatigue, anorexia, sweating, and chills. The development of a new regurgitant murmur, splenomegaly, leukocytosis, and petechiae are common. Episodes of systemic embolization should always suggest the diagnosis (Fig. 18). After appropriate blood cultures have been taken, antibiotic therapy is initiated. Surgery should be considered early in the course of prosthetic valve endocarditis if any of the following are present: uncontrolled infection resistant to medical therapy, persistent or recurrent fever, moderately severe congestive heart failure, evidence of systemic emboliza- tion, large vegetations seen on two-dimensional echocardiography, atrioventricular conduc- tion disturbances, nonstreptococcal or fungal etiology, and evidence of prosthetic valve dysfunction (for example, clinical findings suggesting valve thrombosis or valve insuffi- ciency secondary to valve dehiscence) (Fig. 19). It has been recommended that anti- coagulants be continued during treatment of the infection unless major cerebral emboliza- tion occurs, in which case the possibility of hemorrhage exists (65,66).

  Mechanical valve endocarditis usually involves the suture line and the subvalvular cardiac tissue, with the development of ring abscesses in about 65% of cases (65). With aortic prostheses, complications lead to conduction disturbances, dehiscence with or with- out regurgitation. Vegetations on a mitral prosthesis usually lead to obstruction.

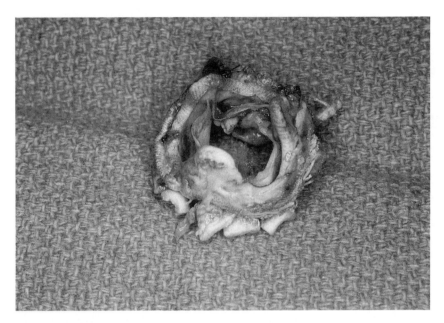

Figure 18 Carpentier-Edwards bioprosthetic aortic valve removed at operation from a patient with *Pseudomonas* endocarditis and systemic emboli.

1. Uncontrolled infection resistant to medical therapy

2. Persistent or recurrent fever

3. Moderate severe CHF

4. Systemic emboli

5. Large mobile vegetations on 2D-ECHO

6. Atrioventricular conduction disturbance

7. Nonstreptococcal or fungal etiology

8. Prosthetic valve dysfunction

Figure 19 Indications for open heart surgery in patients with prosthetic valve endocarditis. CHF = congestive heart failure.

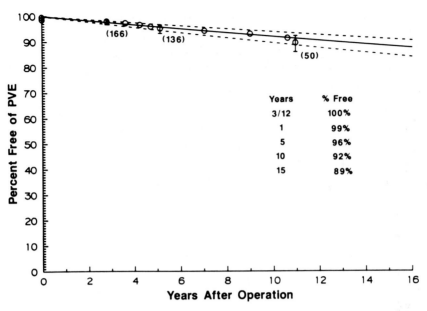

Figure 20 Percent freedom from allograft valve endocarditis in a group of patients undergoing primary isolated homograft aortic valve replacement. (From Ref. 33.)

Bioprosthetic valve endocarditis frequently involves the valve cusp initially and may result in localized perforation and regurgitation, especially in the aortic position (66). The infection may also spread to involve the sewing ring, with the development of ring abscess. However, ring abscesses appear to occur less frequently with tissue valves, perhaps because valve dysfunction secondary to cusp perforation occurs earlier. Tissue valves in the mitral position tend to become stenotic due to the development of obstructive vegetations or may tear or perforate, becoming regurgitant. Surgical treatment of prosthetic valve endocarditis involves early aggressive intervention, with removal of all infected tissue including the prosthesis, extensive debridement of necrotic material, restoration of valve function, and the correction of abnormal communications between chambers. Ring abscesses should be debrided but left in communication with the blood stream. Suturing of a prosthetic valve in an infected area may require alteration of the usual technique employed with valve insertion, and in some instances it has been necessary to suture the prosthesis in the ascending aorta when placement in a severely necrotic annulus was not possible. Placement of the valve in the ascending aorta requires concomitant coronary artery bypass grafting. Aortic valve homograft has been used in patients with aortoventricular discontinuity to reestablish the left ventricular outflow tract. The homograft valve has been shown to have a very low incidence of valve-related endocarditis at ten years (33) (Fig. 20).

IV. FACTORS PRECIPITATING EMBOLISM IN PATIENTS WITH VALVULAR DISEASE

A. Atrial Fibrillation

Atrial fibrillation is the single most important factor predisposing to thromboembolism in patients with valvular heart disease (1,4,67,68), and it is discussed in detail in the Chapter

14. Embolic episodes often occur shortly after fibrillation first develops. Szekely (3) reported that 33% of emboli occurred within 1 month and 66% within 12 months after its onset. Enlargement of the left atrium is found mainly with mitral valve disease. However, the degree of left atrial enlargement as assessed by M-mode echocardiography was not found to be an additional risk factor for emboli in patients with mitral valve disease and atrial fibrillation (66). In the presence of atrial fibrillation, the embolic rate was not higher among patients with very large atria (>55 mm) than among those with less large atria (45–55 mm). Enlargement of the left atrium in patients with sinus rhythm may indirectly lead to thromboembolism by predisposing to atrial fibrillation. Therefore, these patients are liable to atrial fibrillation, and a case could be made for prophylactic anticoagulation. Contrary to earlier reports (69), it now appears that atrial appendectomy during mitral valvotomy does not influence subsequent risk of embolism.

A history of previous embolism is a risk factor for recurrent emboli, which can occur in up to 20% (3) of patients with mitral stenosis. The mortality associated with a second embolus is as high as 42% (2,3). The likelihood of embolism correlates only slightly with the severity of the patient's symptoms (2,4), and the relief of symptoms by successful mitral valvotomy does not eliminate the risk of recurrence. Thus, even asymptomatic patients require prophylactic anticoagulation. Low cardiac output may be an important risk factor (3). Age may be an independent risk factor (2,3); the first embolus most commonly occurs in the fourth decade of life, and the incidence of emboli increases to 38% among patients in the seventh decade (70).

B. Endocarditis as an Embolic Source

Details regarding prosthetic valve endocarditis are found earlier in this chapter. An embolic episode occurring in the context of a fever in a patient with or without a heart murmur should alert the clinician to the possible diagnosis of endocarditis. In a review of 10 echocardiographic studies, Hagen and DeMaria noted a 32% incidence of embolus among 249 patients with vegetations on echocardiography, as opposed to a 14% incidence among 220 patients with endocarditis but without a vegetation (71). Most of these studies were performed in tertiary centers and consequently drew from a skewed study cohort. Of interest, however, is the observation that embolic events were found to be more common in patients with echocardiographically detected vegetations in 8 out of 10 studies (69). It is likely that the presence of vegetations on an echocardiogram identifies a group at increased risk of embolization. The prognostic significance of echocardiographically determined vegetation size remains uncertain. Although the older literature is variable in its conclusions, several more recent studies suggest that the presence of a vegetation of 1 cm or more in diameter on a native mitral valve may predict increased embolic risk (72,73). However, the number of patients studied is small, and validation in a larger cohort is necessary before a more aggressive approach toward early surgical intervention can be considered.

The risk of prosthetic endocarditis is similar for both aortic and mitral prostheses (see above). Mechanical valves tend to present a greater risk in the first 3 months after surgery, while the risk for porcine valves is higher after 12 months. By 5 years cumulative risk is the same for both types of prosthesis (74). Vegetations on prosthetic valves tend to be smaller than on native valves and are generally obscured by acoustic shadowing (71). For native valve infections, TEE is reported to enhance the ability to distinguish between "possible" and "definite" vegetations (71) and increases the detection rate in comparison with TTE (75). Its superiority in the detection of abscesses associated with endocarditis is well established (76). Transesophageal echocardiography provides additional information with regard to the degree of valvular damage and disruption of valvular supporting structures not evident on simultaneous TTE study. Thus, the major advantage of TEE is in the higher detection rate of vegetations or of associated complications in patients with diagnosed endocarditis who are not doing well. Recognition of processes such as abscesses and of major changes in the competency of the valve may mandate a more aggressive approach.

C. Associated Thrombi

In patients with mitral valve disease or prosthetic mitral valves, thrombi most often form in the left atrium or, in the case of a prosthetic heart valve, within the valve mechanism. Thrombi may also form in the left ventricle if there is severe left ventricular function/ dysfunction (discussion related to the left ventricle is found in Chap. 11). Four methods have been used for the detection of left atrial thrombi: two-dimensional echocardiography, computed tomography, magnetic resonance imaging, and ^{111}In-scintigraphy. Of these, echocardiography has been the most widely evaluated. An important advance has been the development of TEE.

The yield for the detection of atrial thrombus by TTE is low because of difficulty in visualizing the left atrial appendage. The highest reported detection rate for left atrial thrombi by TTE in rheumatic mitral disease is from the Philippines, where 30 clots were detected and confirmed at surgery and/or autopsy in a series of 293 patients. However, 21 thrombi (41.0% of the total) were missed, including all 11 located in the left atrial appendage, and in three patients diagnosed as "positive" for thrombus the diagnosis was not confirmed at surgery. In the third world, patients tend to be thin and image quality is usually excellent. Western experience for atrial clot detection by TTE has been much less rewarding.

The observation of a sixfold increased risk of cerebrovascular events in patients with chronic atrial fibrillation, regardless of associated clinical conditions, has increased interest in the atrium as a potential embolic source in these patients. The emergence of TEE represents a major improvement in the accessibility of the left atrium and other basal cardiac structures and of the aorta to high-resolution imaging and is modifying both the approach to the noninvasive investigation of cerebral and peripheral embolic disease and the range of diagnostic entities reportedly associated with them.

While TEE has obvious advantages in identifying thrombus in the left atrium and its frequently associated spontaneous echo contrast, its clinical value in stratifying risk and guiding anticoagulant therapy needs additional assessment.

D. Recommendations for Preventing Thrombotic and Embolic Complications in Patients with Artificial Heart Valves

These recommendations are adapted from the Third American College of Chest Physicians Consensus Conference on Antithrombotic Therapy, published as a supplement to Chest in 1992 (77).

It is strongly recommended that all patients with mechanical prosthetic heart valves receive warfarin therapy (international normalized ratio [INR] 2.5–3.5) (59,78–81). These levels are satisfactory for tilting disc valves (76–79). The experience with ball valves is limited for INRs below 4.5. Levels of warfarin with an INR between 2.2 and 3.3 are probably adequate for ball valves. Aspirin 160 mg/day in addition to warfarin (INR 3.0–4.5) may offer additional protection without an increased risk of bleeding (82). Aspirin at a dosage of 500 mg/day in addition to warfarin increased the bleeding risk without a corresponding increase in efficacy.

Dipyridamole (400 mg/day) added to warfarin produced a variable level of added protection (83–86).

Patients who have suffered a systemic embolization in spite of adequate therapy, and who also have a mechanical prosthetic heart valve, may benefit from aspirin 160 mg/day in addition to warfarin (80). Dipyridamole 400 mg/day is an alternative option (13,34). In patients for whom warfarin is contraindicated, dipyridamole 150 mg/day and aspirin 600 mg/day may be used (87).

It is recommended that all patients with bioprosthetic valves in the mitral position who are also in sinus rhythm be treated for the first 3 months after valve insertion with warfarin at an INR of 2.0–3.0 (87). Those with bioprosthetic valves in the aortic position who are also in sinus rhythm do not require anticoagulation. Patients with bioprosthetic valves who are in atrial fibrillation require anticoagulation with warfarin at an INR of 2.0–3.0. This recommendation is extrapolated from the five atrial fibrillation studies that have recently been completed and which are discussed in detail in Chapter 14.

REFERENCES

1. Cheseboro JH, Ezekowitz MD, Badimon L, Fuster V. Intracardiac thrombi and systemic thromboembolism: detection, incidence, and treatment. Annu Rev Med 1985; 36:579–605.
2. Coulshed N, Epstein EJ, McKendrick CS, Galloway RW, Walker E. Systemic embolism in mitral valve disease. Br Heart J 1970; 32:26–34.
3. Szekely P. Systemic embolization and anticoagulant prophylaxis in rheumatic heart disease. Br Med J 1964; 1:1209–12.
4. Neilsen GH, Galea EG, Hossack KF. Thromboembolic complications of mitral valve disease. Aust NZ J Med 1978; 8:372.
5. Askey JM, Berstein S. The management of rheumatic heart disease in relation to systemic arterial embolism. Prog Cardiovasc Dis 1960; 3:220.
6. Fuster V, Pumphrey CW, McGoon MD, Chesebro JH, Pluth JR, McGoon DC. Systemic thromboembolism in mitral and aortic Starr-Edwards prostheses: A 10–19 year follow-up. Circulation 66 (Suppl I), 1982; I157–I161.
7. Reid JV. Midsystolic clicks. S Afr Med J 1961; 35:353–55.
8. Barlow JB, Bosman CK. Aneurysmal protrusion of the posterior leaflet of the mitral valve. Am Heart J 1966; 71:166–78.
9. Barnett HJM, Jones MW, Boughner DR, Kostuk WJ. Cerebral ischemic events associated with prolapsing mitral valve. Arch Neurol 1976; 33:771–82.
10. Barnett HJ, Boughner DR, Taylor DW, Cooper PE, Kostuk WJ, Nichol PM. Further evidence relating mitral-valve prolapse to cerebral ischemic events. N Engl J Med 1980; 302:139–44.
11. Sandok BA, Guiliani ER. Cerebral ischemic events in patients with mitral valve prolapse. Stroke 1982; 13:448–50.
12. Hart RG, Easton JD. Mitral valve prolapse and cerebral infarction. Stroke 1982; 13:429–30.
13. Dillon JC, Hain CL, Chang S, Feigenbaum H. Use of echocardiography in patients with prolapsed mitral valve. Circulation 1971; 43–4:503–8.
14. Kerber RE, Isaeff DM, Hancock EW. Echocardiographic patterns in patients with the syndrome of systolic click and late systolic murmur. N Engl J Med 1971; 284:691–3.
15. Gilbert BW, Schatz RA, Von Ramm OT, Behar VS, Kisslo JA. Mitral valve prolapse: two-dimensional echocardiographic and angiographic correlation. Circulation 1976; 54:716–723.
16. Levine RA, Triulzi MO, Harrigan P, Weyman AE. The relationship of mitral anular shape to the diagnosis of mitral valve prolapse. Circulation 1987; 75:756–67.

17. Cohen IS. Two-dimensional echocardiographic mitral valve prolapse: evidence for a relationship of echocardiographic morphology to clinical findings and to mitral anular size. Am Heart J 1987; 113:859–68.

18. Walsh PN, Kansu TA, Corbett JJ, Savino PJ, Goldburgh WP, Schatz NJ. Platelets, thromboembolism and mitral valve prolapse. Circulation 1981; 63:552–559.

19. Steele P, Weily H, Raqinwater J, Vogel R. Platelets survival time and thromboembolism in patients with mitral valve prolapse. Circulation 1979; 60:43–5.

20. Pasternac A, Tubau JF, Puddu PE, Krol RB, DeChamplain J. Increased plasma catecholamine levels in patients with symptomatic mitral valve prolapse. Am J Med 1982; 73:783–90.

21. Chesler E, King RA, Edwards JE. The myxomatous mitral valve and sudden death. Circulation 1983; 67:632–9.

22. Brockmeier LB, Adolph RJ, Gustin BW, Holmes JC, Sacks JG. Calcium emboli to the retinal artery in calcific aortic stenosis. Am Heart J 1981; 101:32–37.

23. Holley KE, Bahn RC, McGoon DC, Mankin HT. Spontaneous calcific embolization associated with calcific aortic stenosis. Circulation 1963; 27:197–202.

24. McClung JA, Stein JH, Ambrose JA, Herman MV, Reed GE. Prosthetic heart valves: a review. Progr Cardiovasc Dis 1983; 26:237–70.

25. Grunkemeier GL, Rahmtoola SH, et al. Artificial heart valves. Annu Rev Med 1990; 41:251.

26. Bonchek BI. Basis for selecting a valve prosthesis. In Cardiac surgery 2. Philadelphia: F.A. Davis, 1986:109.

27. Bjork VO: Development of an artificial heart valve. Ann Thorac Surg 1990; 50:151–54.

28. Whittlesey D, Geha AS. Selection and complications of cardiac valvular Prostheses. Thoracic and cardiovascular surgery (WWL Glenn, Ed.). Norwalk, Connecticut: Appleton & Lange, 1991:1719.

29. Nair CK, Mohiuddin SM, Hilleman DE, Schultz R, Bailey RT, Cook CT, Sketch MH. Ten year results with the St. Jude Medical prosthesis. Am J Cardiol 1990; 65:217–25.

30. Jamieson WR, Allen P, Miyagishima RT, Gerein AN, Munro AI, Burr LH, Tyers GFO. The Carpentier-Edwards standard porcine bioprosthesis. Thorac Cardiovasc Surg 1990; 99:543–61.

31. Gallo I, Nistal F, Blasquez R, Arbe E, Artiñano E. Incidence of primary tissue valve failure in porcine bioprosthetic heart valves. Ann Thorac Surg 1988; 45:66–70.

32. Reul GJ, Cooley DA, Duncan J, et al. Valve failure with the Ionescu-Shiley bovine pericardial bioprosthesis. J Vasc Surg 1985; 2:191.

33. O'Brien MF, Stafford EG, Gardner MAH, Pohlner PG, McGriffin DC, Kirklin JW. A comparison of aortic valve replacement with viable cryopreserved and fresh allograft valves, with a note on chromosomal studies. J Thorac Cardiovasc Surg 1987; 94:812–23.

34. Morris DC. Management of patients with prosthetic heart valves. Curr Prob Cardiol 1982; 7:15.

35. Bansal RC, Shah PM, et al. Transesophageal echocardiography. Curr Prob Cardiol 1990; 15:698.

36. Kotler MN, Minitz GS, Panidis I, Morganroth J, Segal BL, Ross J. Non-invasive evaluation of normal and abnormal prosthetic valve function. J Am Coll Cardiol 1983; 2:151–73.

37. Cunha CLP, Giuliani ER, Callahan JA, et al. Echophonocardiographic findings in patients with prosthetic heart valve malfunction. Mayo Clin Proc 1980; 55:231–42.

38. Come PC. Pitfalls in the diagnosis of periprosthetic valvular regurgitation by pulsed Doppler echocardiography. J Am Coll Cardiol 1987; 9:1176–9.

39. Lanzieri M, Michaelson S, Cohen IS. Transesophageal echocardiography in the diagnosis of mitral bioprosthetic obstruction. Crit Care Med 1991; 19:979–81.

40. Ledain LD, Ohayon JP, Colle JP, Lorient-Roudant FM, Roudant RP, Besse PM. Acute thrombotic obstruction with disc valve prostheses: diagnostic considerations and fibrinolytic treatment. J Am Coll Cardiol 1986; 7:743–51.

41. Graver LM, Gelber PM, Tyras DH. The risks and benefits of thrombolytic therapy in acute

aortic and mitral prosthetic valve dysfunction: report of a case and review of the literature. Ann Thorac Surg 1988; 46:85–88.

42. Copans H, Lakier JB, Kinsley RH, Colsen PR, Fritz VU, Barlow JB. Thrombosed Bjork-Shiley prostheses. Circulation 1980; 61:169–174.

43. Alvarez-Ayuso L, Juffe A, Rufilanchas JJ, Babin F, Burgos R, Figuera D. Thrombectomy: surgical treatment of the thrombosed Björk-Shiley prosthesis: Report of seven cases and review of the literature. Thorac Cardiovasc Surg 1982; 84:906–10.

44. Currie PH, Calafiore P, Stewart WJ, et al. Transesophageal echo in mitral prosthetic dysfunction. J Am Coll Cardiol 1989; 13:69.

45. Reisner SA, Meltzer RS. Normal values of prosthetic valve Doppler echocardiographic parameters: a review. J Am Soc Echocardiogr 1988; 3:201–10.

46. Ramirez ML, Wong M, Sadler N, Shah PM. Doppler evaluation of bioprosthetic and mechanical aortic valves: data from four models in 107 stable, ambulatory patients. Am Heart J 1988; 115:418–425.

47. Hatle L, Bjorn B, eds. Doppler ultrasound in cardiology: physical principles and clinical applications. Philadelphia: Lea and Febiger, 1985:pp. 110–143.

48. Hegreneas L, Hatle L. Aortic stenosis in adults—noninvasive estimation of pressure differences by continuous wave Doppler echocardiography. Br Heart J 1985; 54:396–404.

49. Baumgartner H, Khan S, DeRobertis M, Czer L, Maurer G. Effect of prosthetic valve design on the Doppler-catheter gradient correlation: an in vitro study of normal St. Jude, Medtronic-Hall, Starr-Edwards, and Hancock valves. J Am Coll Cardio 1992; 19:324–32.

50. Baumgartner H, Khan S, DeRobertis M, Czer L, Maurer G. Discrepancies between Doppler and catheter gradients in aortic prosthetic valves in vitro: A manifestation of localized gradients and pressure recovery. Circulation 1990; 82:1467–75.

51. Baumgartber H, Czer L, DeRobertis M, et al. Doppler gradients across prosthetic heart valves: limitations and pitfalls. American College of Cardiology Learning Center Highlights 1992; 7: 1–7.

52. Thomas JD, Weyman AE. Doppler mitral pressure half time: a clinical tool in search of theoretical justification. J Am Coll Cardiol 1987; 10:923–9.

53. Dumesnil JG, Honos GN, Lemiuex M, Beauchemin J. Validation and applications of mitral prosthetic valvular areas calculated by Doppler echocardiography. Am J Cardiol 1990; 65: 1443–8.

54. Schoen FJ. Surgical pathology of removed natural and prosthetic heart valves. Hum Pathol 1987; 18:558–67.

55. Edmunds LH, Clark RE, Cohn LH, Miller DC, Weisel RD. Guidelines for reporting morbidity and mortality after cardiac valvular operations. J Thorac Cardiovasc Surg 1988; 96:351–53.

56. Starr A, et al. Tissue and mechanical valves. J Cardiac Surg 1988; 3:442.

57. Edmunds LH. Thrombotic and bleeding complications of prosthetic heart valves. Ann Thorac Surg 1987; 44:430–45.

58. Penny WJ, Chesebro JH, Fuster V, et al. Antithrombotic therapy for patients with cardiac disease. Curr Prob Cardiol 1988; 13:439.

59. Stein PD, Kantrowitz A, et al. Antithrombotic therapy in mechanical and biological prosthetic heart valves and saphenous vein bypass grafts. Chest 1989; 95:107.

60. Saour JN, Sieck JO, Mamo LA, Gallus AS. Trial of different intensities of anticoagulation in patients with prosthetic heart valves. N Engl J Med 1990; 322:428–32.

61. Deviri E, Sareli P, Wisenbaugh T, Cronje SL. Obstruction of mechanical heart valve prostheses: clinical aspects and surgical management. J Am Coll Cardiol 1991; 17:646–50.

62. Kontos GJ, Schaff HV. Thrombotic occlusion of a prosthetic heart valve: diagnosis and management. Mayo Clin Proc 1985; 60:118–122.

63. Graver LM, Gelber PM, Tyras DH. The risks and benefits of thrombolytic therapy in acute aortic and mitral prosthetic dysfunction. Ann Thorac Surg 1988; 46:85–88.

64. Silber H, Khan SS, Matloff JM, Chaux A, DeRobertis M, Gray R. The St. Jude valve: thrombolysis as the first line of therapy for cardiac valve thrombosis. Circulation 1993; 87: 30–7.

65. Wilson WR, Danielson GK, Giuliani ER, Geraci JE. Prosthetic valve endocarditis. Mayo Clin Proc 1982; 57:155–161.

66. Watanakunakorn C. Prosthetic valve infective endocarditis. Prog Cardiovasc Dis 1979; 22: 181–192.

67. Rogers PH, Sherry S. Current status of antithrombotic therapy in cardiovascular disease. Prog Cardiovasc Dis 1976; 19:235–53.

68. Sherrid MR, Clark RD, Cohn K. Echocardiographic analysis of left atrial size before and after operation in mitral valve disease. Am J Cardiol 1979; 43:171–8.

69. Sommerville W, Chambers RJ. Systemic embolism in mitral stenosis: relation to the size of the left atrial appendix. Br Med J 1964; 2:116.

70. Casella L, Abelmann WH, Ellis LB. Patients with mitral stenosis and systemic emboli. Arch Intern Med 1964; 114:773–81.

71. Infective endocarditis. In: Hagan AD, DeMaria AN, eds. Clinical applications of two-dimensional echocardiography and cardiac Doppler. 2d ed. Boston: Little, Brown, 1989: 161–78.

72. Jaffee WM, Morgan DE, Pearlman AS, Otto CM. Infective endocarditis, 1983–1988: Echocardiographic findings and factors influencing morbidity and mortality. J Am Coll Cardiol 1990; 15:1227–33.

73. Mügge A, Daniel WG, Frank G, Lichtlen PR. Echocardiography in infective endocarditis: reassessment of prognostic implications of vegetation size determined by the transthoracic and transesophageal approach. J Am Coll Cardiol 1989; 14:631–8.

74. Calderwood SB, Swinski LA, Waternaux CM, Karchmer AW, Buckley MJ. Risk factors for the development of prosthetic valve endocarditis. Circulation 1985; 72:31–7.

75. Shively BK, Gurule FT, Roldan CA, et al. Diagnostic value of transesophageal compared with transthoracic echocardiography in infective endocarditis. J Am Coll Cardiol 1991; 18:391–7.

76. Daniel WG, Mügge A, Martin RP, Lindert O, Hausmann D, Nonnast-Daniel B, Laas J, Lichtlen PR. Improvement in the diagnosis of abscesses associated with endocarditis by transesophageal echocardiography. N Engl J Med 1991; 324:795–800.

77. Stein PD, Alpert JS, Copeland J, Dalen JE, Goldman S, Turpie AGG: Antithrombotic therapy in patients with mechanical and biological prosthetic heart valves. Chest 1992; 102 (Suppl 4): 445–55.

78. Sethia B, Turner MA, Lewis S, Rodger RA, Bain WH, Kouchoukos NT. Fourteen years' experience with the Bjork-Shiley tilting disc prosthesis. J Thorac Cardiovasc Surg 1986; 91: 350–61.

79. Vogt S, Hoffman A, Roth J, et al. Heart valve replacement with the Bjork-Shiley and St. Jude Medical prostheses: a randomized comparison in 178 patients. Eur Heart J 1990; 11:583–91.

80. DiSosa VJ, Collins JJ Jr, Cohn LH. Hematological complications with the St. Jude valve and reduced dose coumadin. Ann Thorac Surg 1989; 48:280–3.

81. Kopf GS, Hammond GL, Geha AS, Elefteriades J, Hashim SW. Long-term performance of the St. Jude Medical valve: low incidence of thromboembolism and hemorrhagic complications with modest doses of warfarin. Circulation 1987; 76(suppl 3):132–136.

82. Turpie AGG, Gent M, Laupacis A, Latoury, Gunstensen J, Basile F, Klimek M, Hirsh J. Reduction in mortality by adding aspirin (100mg) to oral anticoagulants in patients with heart valve replacement (abstr). J Am Coll Cardiol 1992; 19(suppl A):103A.

83. Sullivan JM, Harken DE, Gorlin R. Effect of dipyridamole on the incidence of arterial emboli after cardiac valve replacement. Circulation 1969; 39–40(suppl 1):I149–53.

84. Rajah SM, Sreeharon N, Joseph A, et al. Prospective trial of dipyridamole and warfarin in heart valve patients (abstr). Acta Ther (Brussels) 1980; 6:54.

85. Groupe de Recherche P.A.C.T.E. Prévention des accidents thromboemboliques systémiques chez les porteurs de prothèses valvulaires artificielles. Coeur 1978; 9:915–69.

86. Altman R, Rouvier J, Gurfinkel E, D'Ortencio O, Manzanel R, deLaFuente L, Favaloro R. Comparison of two levels of anticoagulant therapy in patients with substitute heart valves. J Thorac Cardiovasc Surg 1991; 101:427–31.

87. Turpie AGG, Gunstensen J, Hirsh J, Nelson H, Gent M. Randomized comparison of two intensities of oral anticoagulant therapy after tissue heart valve replacement. Lancet 1988; 1:1242–5.

14

The Left Atrium

Michael D. Ezekowitz
*Yale University School of Medicine, West Haven Veterans Affairs,
and Cardiovascular Thrombosis Research Laboratory,
New Haven, Connecticut*

Ira S. Cohen
*Yale University School of Medicine and West Haven Veterans
Affairs, New Haven, Connecticut*

Charles C. Gornick
*Veterans Affairs Medical Center and University of Minnesota,
Minneapolis, Minnesota*

I. INTRODUCTION

As in any other part of the body, the formation of thrombus in the left atrium is related to blood stasis. Factors contributing to left atrial stasis are left atrial enlargement and reduced atrial flow velocities due to atrial fibrillation, mitral stenosis, or a low cardiac output state (1–5). The peripheral position of the left atrial appendage makes it particularly prone to low blood flow velocities (1,6). Recently, a new echocardiographic finding—spontaneous echocardiographic contrast (SEC) or "smoke"—has been associated with left atrial thrombus and/or embolus (1–5,7,8). It appears to be a marker of low-velocity blood flow as well as of red cell rouleaux formation (clumping) and requires the presence of fibrinogen (9,10).

Mitral stenosis and valvular disease are considered in detail in Chapter 12. This chapter will evaluate the left atrium as a potential embolic source and address ancillary factors contributing to atrial thrombogenesis. The problem of nonrheumatic atrial fibrillation and its management will be emphasized. The assumption will be made that the left atrium is the source of *embolization* in patients with atrial fibrillation. It is recognized, however, that nonrheumatic atrial fibrillation is a marker of associated heart and vascular disease, such as atherosclerosis, that may independently predispose the patient to embolization (11). In addition, it is possible that in situ intracerebral thrombosis precipitated by a local event such as plaque rupture and/or a reduction in cardiac output may constitute a third mechanism for stroke in patients with atrial fibrillation.

Before the early 1900s, atrial fibrillation, as a clinical disorder, was poorly understood. In 1906, Einthoven (12) made the first electrocardiographic demonstration of atrial fibrillation. There was controversy concerning the origin of the arrhythmia. Simultaneous reports by Lewis (13,14) and by Rothberger and Winterberg (15,16) confirmed the relationship between electrocardiographically documented atrial fibrillation and the clinical disorder of a chronic irregularly irregular pulse.

II. ECHOCARDIOGRAPHIC APPROACHES TO THE DIAGNOSIS OF LEFT ATRIAL THROMBUS

A. Spontaneous Echocardiographic Contrast

Prominent intracavitary echoes—so-called echo contrast—can be visualized in the right heart chambers after the intravenous injection of a variety of physiologic solutions that have been agitated to produce microcavitations (17). Right-sided bubbles are often seen in patients with intravenous and/or central lines when the infusate reaches the heart (18). These are thought to be small air bubbles in suspension that are imaged as mobile spherical echoes, 0.5–2.0 mm in diameter, that clear from the normal heart over several cardiac cycles. "Bubble" or "echo contrast" studies that are useful diagnostically are produced by the intravenous injection of agitated saline and can be used to opacify the right heart as a means of detecting intracardiac shunts, delineating right-sided endocardial borders, enhancing Doppler signals, and assessing the severity of tricuspid regurgitation. Spontaneous echoes of this size have also been identified in patients with right- and left-sided prosthetic heart valves (19), in the false lumen of the descending aorta in type III dissection (20), and in the inferior vena cava in pericardial constriction (21).

In contrast, the echoes characterized as SEC are of a significantly finer order of magnitude than contrast echoes and, as a result, are barely visible as discrete elements (Fig. 1). Their small size accounts for the observation that SEC is commonly visualized in the left atrium using a 5-MHz transesophageal echocardiographic (TEE) probe but is only rarely visualized using a longer-wave-length 2.5-MHz transthoracic echocardiographic (TTE) probe (1,3–5).

Spontaneous echocardiographic contrast was first noted within ventricular aneurysms (22) and in myopathic ventricles and was related both to low blood flow velocities and to an increased risk of left ventricular thrombus formation (23). Patients with apical thrombus have lower ventricular inflow and outflow velocities (as measured by Doppler) than similar patients without thrombus. Mitral regurgitation seems to confer a protective effect— perhaps because of its association with higher ventricular and, consequently, apical inflow velocities (23). Spontaneous echocardiographic contrast may clear with clinical improvement of ventricular function and after aneurysmectomy (24). Spontaneous echocardiographic contrast as an incidental finding has also been identified in the true lumen of the descending thoracic aorta (25).

In vitro studies suggest that SEC is due to stasis (reduced shear rates) (1), and that its particulate elements are red blood cells that have undergone rouleaux formation (1,9,22) and/or agglutinated platelets (26). Its presence is also related to serum fibrinogen or fibrin concentration. Spontaneous echocardiographic contrast has been reported in patients with multiple myeloma, a condition associated with red blood cell rouleaux formation (24). Anticoagulants do not have an effect (3). Therapeutic interventions that significantly change atrial flow dynamics (e.g., mitral valve surgery) may cause resolution of SEC (1). Its response to the administration of platelet deaggregating agents is controversial (27). The gain setting of the instrument is an important factor when attempts are made to quantify the intensity of the contrast. Increasing the gain alone may generate a cloudy image. This effect, however, traverses anatomical borders. More important, the characteristic swirling nature of SEC motion, aptly described as "echo smoke," cannot be reproduced solely by increasing gain settings. The use of a biplanar probe, having fewer elements for each plane than a dedicated single-plane probe, may theoretically decrease sensitivity for visualization of SEC. When evaluating the atrium for SEC it is essential to systematically explore the

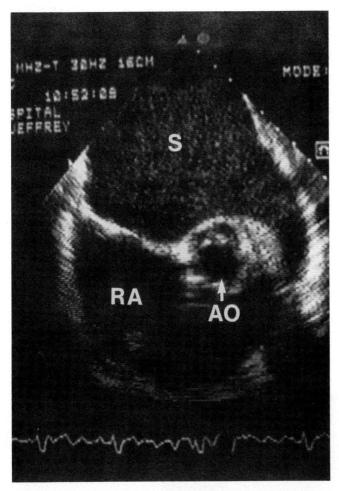

Figure 1   Spontaneous echo contrast (SEC). In this transesophageal echocardiogram SEC is seen as fine particulate echoes (S) in the left atrium. The left atrial appendage is the comma-shaped outpouching of the atrium at 3 o'clock. RA = right atrium separated from the left atrium by the transversely oriented interatrial septum at 9 o'clock, AO = the aortic valve in cross section.

chamber in multiple planes, starting with high initial gain settings. Spontaneous echocardiographic contrast may be visualized in certain imaging planes and not in others. The left atrial appendage is the most common site for SEC (2). Observations at our institution suggest that its presence requires an enlarged left atrial chamber ($\geq$4.5 cm in diameter) and low mitral flow velocities at the level of the mitral annulus.

The presence of SEC in the left atrium is associated with intracavitary left atrial thrombi (1–4) and embolic episodes in patients with underlying mitral valve disease, mitral prostheses, and nonrheumatic atrial fibrillation (3–5,7,8). Two studies suggest that SEC can occur in patients in sinus rhythm who also have low cardiac flow velocities, even in the absence of mitral valve disease, and that its presence is an independent marker of increased risk for thromboembolism (7,8). Spontaneous echocardiographic contrast has been seen in the body of the atrium during paroxysmal atrial fibrillation with subsequent confinement to the atrial appendage after resumption of sinus rhythm in a patient with a stroke and a normal mitral valve (6). We have seen SEC associated with biatrial thrombi in a patient in normal sinus rhythm with end-stage dilated cardiomyopathy; SEC has been noted to traverse a mitral valve prosthesis despite a flow velocity that was sufficiently high to cause color flow aliasing across the prosthesis. This finding suggests a particulate nature of SEC that is independent of flow. Our experience confirms that of others (3,4,7,8), that echocardiographically detectable left atrial thrombus is uncommon in the absence of SEC (28).

B. Left Atrial Thrombi—Transesophageal Echocardiographic Approach and Characteristics

Transthoracic echocardiographic evaluation for left atrial thrombus is usually unrewarding. At the very least, it requires the addition of supplemental views to image the left atrial appendage. From the parasternal short-axis view at the level of the aortic valve the transducer is aimed inferolaterally to image the pulmonary artery at its bifurcation. The left atrial appendage lies immediately inferior to the bifurcation, and slight inferior and lateral angulation of the probe will occasionally bring it into view (Fig. 2). However, even with adequate imaging of the appendage by TTE, thrombi in the left atrial appendage are only very infrequently visualized. Details of atrial wall anatomy and motion are virtually never seen by TTE but are commonly seen on TEE. We have seen on TEE a large thrombus filling

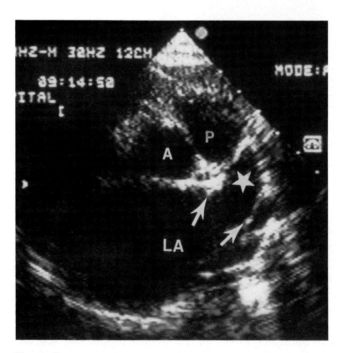

Figure 2 Transthoracic echo of the left atrial appendage. The asterisk indicates the appendage cavity. The arrows show its origin from the body of the left atrium (LA), which is dilated. A = aorta in cross section, P = main pulmonary artery.

the appendage and extending into the left atrial cavity that could not be visualized from the chest wall by TTE even in retrospect (Fig. 3).

The transesophageal approach is superior to transthoracic evaluation of the left atrium because it provides direct access to the posterior portion of the heart. To image the left atrial appendage, the TEE probe is advanced to a depth of 25 to 30 cm from the incisors. Occasionally the appendage is immediately apparent from this position. Usually, a four-chamber TEE imaging plane is obtained. The probe is then withdrawn slightly until the mitral valve is lost from the imaging plane. The inferior atrial border assumes an oval, truncated appearance. From this position the entire probe is rotated counterclockwise and anteflexed to bring the appendage into view. Occasionally, the anatomical relationship of the patient's esophagus to the atrium requires repositioning of the patient. The wall of the appendage is often muscular, with small protuberances caused by the musculi pectinati. These are either hemispherical, approximately 2–3 mm in width and height, or linear and of similar or greater length. They are often prominent at or near the apex of the appendage and should not be misinterpreted as thrombus (Fig. 4a and 4b). A prominent ridge may be present at the junction of the atrial wall with the left superior pulmonary veins. On occasion this ridge may produce a reverberation artifact that superficially resembles an intracavitary thrombus. However, this apparent "clot" is always in direct line with the ridge and at a depth twice that of the ridge from the top of the two-dimensional echo sector in any view in which

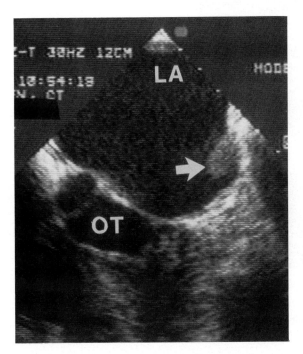

Figure 3 Transesophageal echo of the left atrium (LA) just above the mitral valve plane. The tip of a thrombus (white arrow) protrudes from the left atrial appendage into the left atrial cavity, which is filled with spontaneous echo contrast. After this study repeat attempts at visualizing this thrombus, which fills the appendage, by transthoracic echocardiography were unsuccessful. OT = left ventricular outflow tract.

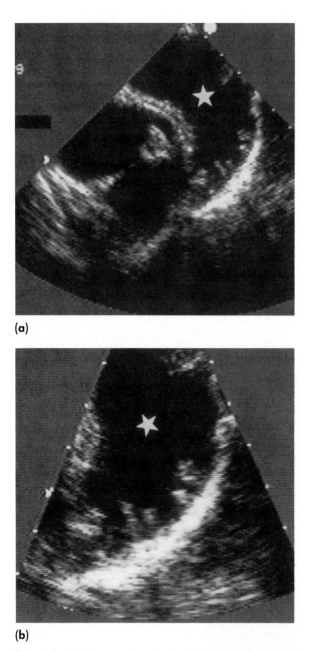

(a)

(b)

Figure 4   (a) Transesophageal echo of a normal atrial appendage. The asterisk lies in the cavity of the appendage, which has prominent pectinate muscles. (b) Detail of (a). The pectinate muscles are seen as discrete fingerlike ridges protruding into the appendage cavity from its inferolateral border.

it is imaged. Minor manipulations and rotation of the probe should be made to explore the appendage more fully, as the initial sector may not visualize the plane of a thrombus. There is substantial anatomical variability in the size and shape of the appendage. Infrequently, a single-plane probe may fail to allow visualization of the appendage. The use of a biplanar or multiplanar probe provides a more comprehensive examination, particularly in such cases. In most series 80–90% of patients with a thrombus in the left atrium have associated SEC (1,3,4,28). Its presence should intensify efforts to fully explore both the appendage and the superior portion of the atrium, between the inflow regions of the right and left pulmonary veins and along the interatrial septum below the right pulmonary vein entrance, for the presence of clots.

Left atrial thrombi may be intracavitary or mural and lie either within the body or within the left atrial appendage. In general, intracavitary atrial thrombi are imaged in subjects with severely reduced cardiac output (usually due to end-stage cardiomyopathy), in patients with extreme atrial enlargement due to rheumatic mitral stenosis in whom the flow, even with fairly normal cardiac outputs, is low per unit area of atrial chamber, or in patients with atrial fibrillation (1,2). Intracavitary thrombi show some predilection for the superior atrial wall between the entrance points of the pulmonary veins (Fig. 5), although we have seen clots on the interatrial septum (Fig. 6), and apparently free within the atrial cavity, as well as adjacent to the free wall of the atrium. Thrombi, if fresh, tend to have a homogeneous echo

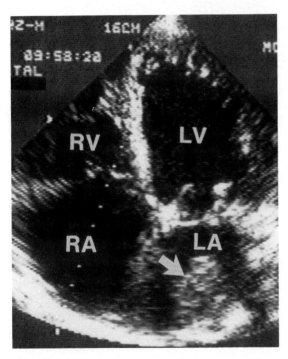

Figure 5   Transthoracic apical four-chamber echocardiogram. A large thrombus (white arrow) is present attached to the left atrial wall between the entrance points of the pulmonary veins. A mitral bioprosthetic valve lies between the left atrium (LA) and left ventricle (LV). RA = right atrium; RV = right ventricle.

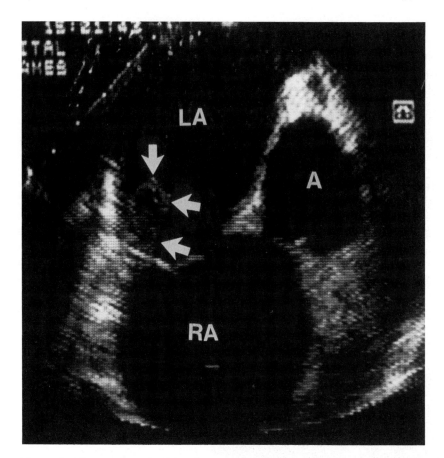

Figure 6 Transesophageal echocardiogram of a clot (arrow) on the atrial septum just below the entrance of the right pulmonary veins. There is faint spontaneous echo contrast in the left atrium, and both atria are dilated. This patient was in normal sinus rhythm with dilated cardiomyopathy. The apparent defect in the interatrial septum (horizontal structure between right atrium [RA] and left atrium [LA]) is an artifact. However, a patent foramen ovale was present (not shown). A = aorta in cross section.

reflectance, finely granular in character and similar in appearance to hepatic tissue as visualized in a subcostal TTE view. In general, atrial thrombus tends to be less echodense than ventricular thrombus. Chronicity can cause organization with increase in echo reflectance. Localization to the appendage appears to be related to several factors, the most important of which relates to its position at the periphery of flow (1). Doppler interrogation shows a reduced flow velocity in the appendage of persons with SEC (1). Other investigators have reported a reduction in appendage ejection fraction in patients with left atrial thrombus (29). Within the appendage, thrombi may be mural or intracavitary. Mural thrombi in the appendage tend to be elongated flat structures aligned along the wall and wider than the musculi pectinati (Fig. 7). Intracavitary appendicular thrombi are often rounded but may fill the appendage (Fig. 8). In our experience, intracavitary left atrial thrombus visible by TTE

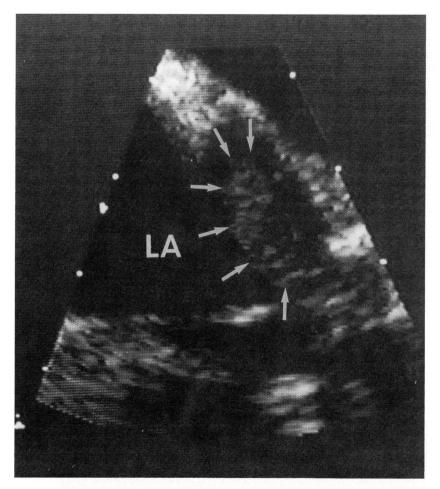

Figure 7 Transesophageal echocardiogram of a mural left atrial thrombus (small white arrows) tucked against the wall of the left atrial appendage just below the ridge separating the appendage from the entrance of left superior vein. LA = left atrium.

within the body of the chamber is rarely seen and then only in the presence of disease states associated with extremely low cardiac output states (e.g., end-stage cardiomyopathies).

C. Left Atrial Myxoma

The most important condition to differentiate from a left atrial clot is a left atrial myxoma (Fig. 9). Effert and Domanig reported the first case of left atrial myxoma diagnosed by ultrasound in 1959 (30). Echocardiography is the technique of choice for the diagnosis of myxoma—an entity that, like left atrial clot, is associated with peripheral embolic events. Myxomas typically arise from the interatrial septum and are attached to it by a stalk. Clots only rarely have stalks, tend to arise from the appendage or body of the chamber, and less

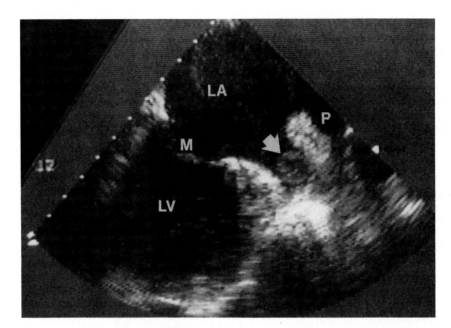

Figure 8 Transesophageal echocardiogram in the vertical plane showing an intracavitary thrombus in the cavity of the left atrial appendage (white arrow). The left atrium (LA) is filled with swirling spontaneous echo contrast. P = entrance of the left superior pulmonary vein; M = mitral valve plane with the valve leaflets immediately below; LV = left ventricle.

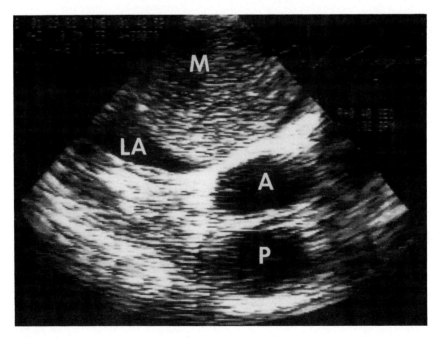

Figure 9 Transesophageal echocardiogram of a large left atrial myxoma (M). LA = residual left atrial cavity; A = aortic outflow tract; P = pulmonary outflow tract.

commonly are close to the interatrial septum (Fig. 6). On rare occasions, myxomas cannot be imaged by TTE techniques either because the mass is located in an inaccessible part of the heart or because of a small difference in the acoustic impedance between the tumor and blood (31,32). Color Doppler may be helpful in the detection of the tumor by defining the blood pool. The relative efficacy of TTE versus TEE in the detection of myxomas has recently been reported. Although the detection of structural details and stalk attachment to the atrial septum may be better with TEE, diagnostic accuracy is similar for both techniques (33). Occasionally, identification of structural detail by TEE is helpful in distinguishing tumor, clot, vegetations, and normal structural variants (34). Rarely, other tumors can invade the left atrium and mimic myxomas (35,36). The absence of SEC is more helpful than its presence. A large myxoma may reduce flow rates, causing SEC. Given the association of clot with SEC, its absence would suggest a nonthrombotic etiology for an unidentified mass lesion.

The clinical presentation of myxomas is quite characteristic. These tumors are associated with constitutional symptoms and may present in asymptomatic patients without structural heart disease and in patients who have unexplained syncope, episodic dyspnea, or a murmur, which may be intermittent.

III. ANEURYSM OF THE INTERATRIAL SEPTUM

Several investigators (36–38) have reported an increased incidence of atrial septal aneurysm (ASA)—a redundant, mobile outpouching of the fossa ovalis (septum primum)—and embolic events. There is an increased incidence of aneurysms of the atrial septum in patients referred for echocardiographic evaluation of a potential source for otherwise unexplained cerebrovascular events.

An arbitrary echocardiographic definition of ASA has been proposed, identifying it as an outpouching or redundancy of the atrial septum with an orifice of 1.5 cm or greater and a total to-and-fro excursion between the atria of at least 1.5 cm (38); other investigators have suggested smaller dimensions and/or excursions (39,40). Transesophageal echocardiography is superior to TTE in its detection (37,40).

Atrial septal aneurysm occurs as either a primary developmental anomaly (no pressure differential between the atria) or as a secondary phenomenon developing as a consequence of complex congenital heart lesions associated with pressure overload on the right atrium or, less commonly, the left atrium (41). Involvement of the entire septum is common in the secondary form. The incidence varies from 0.2% to 1% (42) of the population, and the reported association with embolic episodes is as high as 20–28% (38,39) in selected populations.

The pathophysiologic mechanism for the apparent association with embolic episodes may be multifactorial. Structurally, ASAs are commonly fenestrated (41,43) and associated with either a patent foramen ovale or an atrial septal defect that provides a potential path for paradoxical embolization. Atrial septal aneurysm may have deposits of fibrin and thrombin on its surface or interstices (41), and others have noted gross thrombus formation (44). In some subjects a remarkable degree of mobility of the aneurysm is evident on two-dimensional echocardiography, suggesting an obvious catapulting mechanism by which such deposits could embolize into the circulation. There is increased incidence of mitral valve prolapse in subjects with ASA (see Chap. 12). Mitral valve prolapse is reported to be associated with an increased incidence of cerebral infarction in young patients under age 45 (45,46). Treatment strategies for ASA have not been defined. In a preliminary report,

Sharma et al. (47) found a reduced embolic rate in patients receiving low-dose warfarin therapy; however, treatment with warfarin is as yet unproven therapy for this condition.

IV. NONRHEUMATIC ATRIAL FIBRILLATION

A. Prevalence and Significance as a Risk Factor for Embolic Disease

In western societies, nonrheumatic atrial fibrillation is a common condition in the elderly (Fig. 10). It is estimated that under the age of 50 it is unusual, occurring in a fraction of 1% of the total population (48). In this setting atrial fibrillation usually occurs as an isolated phenomenon, without evidence of structural heart disease, hypertension, or diabetes. These patients are termed lone atrial fibrillators and are at low risk for embolization as compared with other patients in atrial fibrillation (49). In the group aged 60 to 69 years the prevalence of atrial fibrillation is about 3.8% for men but somewhat less for women (50). Above the age of 70 the prevalence is estimated to be as high as 9% (51). In a community-based study in Minnesota, 16.1% of men and 12.2% of women older than 75 had atrial fibrillation (52). Atrial fibrillation is a marker both of a higher incidence of stroke (five times that of comparable patients in sinus rhythm) and of increased mortality (50,53). The high mortality may be related to an increased predisposition to serious ventricular arrhythmias, which may occur either spontaneously because of related structural heart disease or as a result of the proarrhythmic effect of drugs used to maintain sinus rhythm, e.g. quinidine (54), flecainide, and encainide (type 1A and 1C agents) (55). In Western societies it is anticipated that as the population ages the prevalence of atrial fibrillation will increase dramatically. Thus, the role of atrial fibrillation as a source for systemic embolization and resultant stroke will

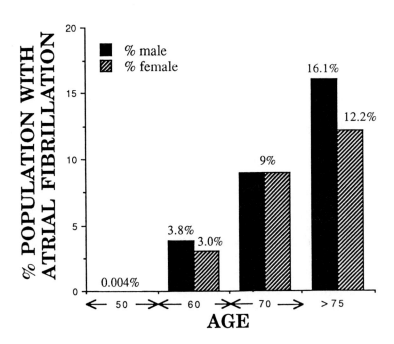

Figure 10   Prevalence of atrial fibrillation.

increase unless appropriate therapy is instituted. Conceivably, with better recognition and treatment of hypertension, nonrheumatic atrial fibrillation may eventually become the most important factor causing stroke in an aging population.

B. Etiology of Atrial Fibrillation

1. Electrophysiological Considerations (Fig. 11)

In most instances, reentry is the probable mechanism of atrial fibrillation. Other possible mechanisms include a rapid and continuously discharging automatic focus or foci (56). Reentry, consisting of multiple wavelets (57), is affected by tissue mass, refractory periods, and conduction velocity. Other factors such as stretch (58), autonomic stimulation (59), and a host of other modulating influences can affect the electrophysiologic properties of the atrium.

Atrial mapping studies have demonstrated that multiple intra-atrial reentry circuits form the basis of the arrhythmia. The reentry is random, with individual wavelets lasting only a few hundred milliseconds (60).

The onset of atrial fibrillation requires an initiating event in most instances, and this event is believed to be a premature atrial beat, supporting the concept that reentry is the underlying mechanism. Less commonly, a premature ventricular beat conducted retrograde into the atrium initiates fibrillation. Slowing of the rate of impulse generation within the sinus mode may precipitate the arrhythmia.

2. Clinical Considerations

Most cases of atrial fibrillation are idiopathic. An important minority of patients have an etiology that is directly treatable. These etiologies include thyrotoxicosis, acute coronary ischemic syndromes, pulmonary embolism, and acute hypoxia related to exacerbations of chronic pulmonary disease or the use of drugs such as bronchodilators (Table 1). Patients with mitral valve disease revert to sinus rhythm after valve replacement or repair as the left atrial size decreases with hemodynamic improvement. There are also irreversible causes of atrial fibrillation that require treatment of the arrhythmia rather than the cause (Table 1).

Although atrial fibrillation may occur as a transient and recurring paroxysmal arrhythmia, it is more commonly a chronic incessant arrhythmia associated with underlying heart disease. In some patients, paroxysmal atrial fibrillation is associated with the tachycardia-bradycardia syndrome (61). The transition from paroxysmal to chronic atrial fibrillation varies considerably and probably depends on the underlying etiology. Takahashi et al. (62) followed 94 patients with paroxysmal atrial fibrillation, 54.3% of whom had underlying hypertension and/or coronary artery disease. Over a period of 1 year 25% developed chronic atrial fibrillation.

Hyperthyroidism should always be considered in patients in whom atrial fibrillation occurs without apparent underlying cardiac cause, especially if the ventricular response during the arrhythmia is rapid (63). On occasion, atrial fibrillation occurs in the absence of any apparent cardiac or systemic disease ("lone atrial fibrillation"). Younger patients without concomitant diseases such as hypertension or diabetes who have lone atrial fibrillation are reported to have an excellent prognosis (64). Care must be taken, however, not to overlook the presence of associated early or subclinical cardiomyopathy.

C. Diagnosis of Atrial Fibrillation

The atria in patients with atrial fibrillation appear to be activated simultaneously in multiple areas with impulses following a variety of routes. Consequently, the surface electrocardio-

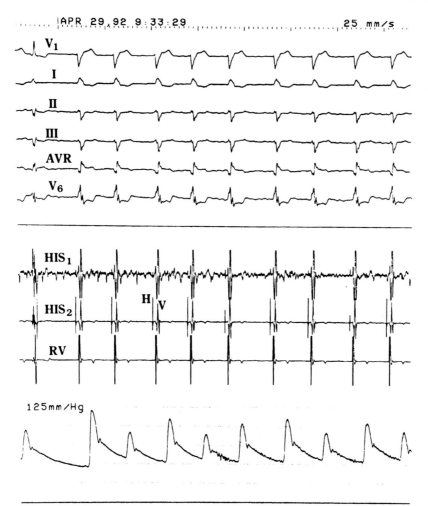

Figure 11 Electrocardiographic (ECG) and intracardiac recordings demonstrating typical findings in atrial fibrillation. Intracardiac tracing labeled His$_1$ demonstrates a baseline characterized by fractionated and irregular atrial electrograms. In the His$_2$ intracardiac tracing, the His bundle deflection (H) is followed by the ventricular electrogram (V). Tracings from top to bottom include standard ECG leads V$_1$, I, II, III, AVR, and V$_6$; intracardiac electrograms from the area of the His bundle (His$_1$, His$_2$); right ventricle; and aortic blood pressure (mm Hg).

gram demonstrates a markedly irregular and low-amplitude baseline (Figs. 11 and 12). Since the arrival of atrial electrical impulses at the AV node is erratic, an irregularly irregular ventricular response results. It is fortunate that the physiologic gating mechanism of the AV node blocks the majority of the atrial impulses and thereby prevents the development of rapid ventricular rates.

In patients with preexcitation (e.g., Wolff-Parkinson-White syndrome), an alternative pathway(s) to the ventricles besides the AV node is present. In such instances, extremely rapid ventricular rates can occur. On the surface electrocardiogram, QRS complexes can

Table 1 Conditions Associated with Atrial Fibrillation

Cardiac	Systemic
Cardiac surgery	Age
Cardiomyopathy	Alcohol
Congenital heart disease	Cerebrovascular accident
Hypertension	Chronic pulmonary disease
Ischemic heart disease (acute or chronic)	Electrocution
Lipomatous hypertrophy	Electrolyte abnormalities
Pericarditis	Fever
Preexcitation syndromes	Hypothermia
Tachycardia-bradycardia syndrome	Hypovolemia
Tumors	Pregnancy
Valvular heart disease	Sudden emotional change
Ventricular hypertrophy	Swallowing
Ventricular pacing	Thyrotoxicosis
	Trauma

appear wide and bizarre as a result of fusion of ventricular activation by antegrade conduction over an accessory connection(s) and the AV node (Figs. 13 and 14).

During atrial fibrillation, intracardiac electrograms are characterized by marked beat-to-beat variations in rate and morphology. In some instances, electrogram recordings can be discrete, with isoelectric baselines between each deflection. In others (including recordings from the same person at a different time), the intervening baseline can be chaotic, suggesting more rapid and disordered electrical activity. Although differences in intracardiac recordings during atrial fibrillation may not be of clinical significance, they may be indicators of different factors affecting the substrate of the arrhythmia.

D. Cardioversion

1. Predictors of Successful Cardioversion

Echocardiographically determined left atrial size has been proposed as a predictor of successful long-term maintenance of sinus rhythm after cardioversion of atrial fibrillation (65–67). The posterior wall of the left atrium lies in an area of the heart commonly obscured by side lobe artifacts from the posterior pericardium. Additionally, the angle of incidence of the interrogating echo beam may be tangential to the true anteroposterior atrial dimension. Both these factors create difficulties with respect to accurate and reproducible measurement of left atrial size. Two-dimensional guidance of the M-mode measurement lessens these potential sources of error and should be routinely used. In the era before two-dimensionally guided M-mode echocardiography, Henry et al. (65), using single-plane M-mode measurements of the left atrium in patients with mitral, aortic, or hypertrophic disease, concluded that if left atrial size was greater than 4.5 cm maintenance of sinus rhythm was unlikely at 6 months after cardioversion, with 75% of successfully cardioverted patients again in atrial fibrillation at that time. Other investigators (66) have shown that patients with lone atrial fibrillation and a left atrial size greater than 4.5 cm were at increased risk of recurrence one month after cardioversion. Ewy and coworkers (67) found left atrial size to be predictive of success of medical cardioversion and helpful for electrical conversion.

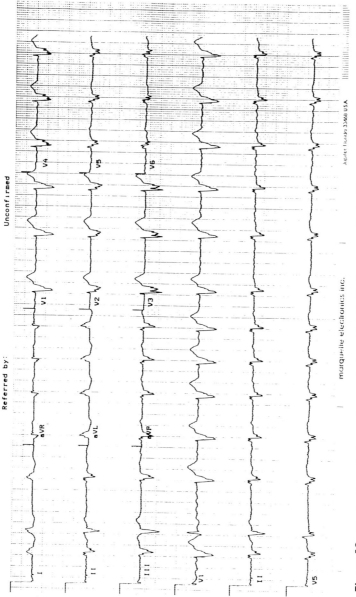

Figure 12 Twelve-lead electrocardiogram during atrial fibrillation in a patient with an accessory AV connection (Wolff-Parkinson-White syndrome). Note the variable, wide and bizarre QRS complexes, which result from activation of the ventricles over both the accessory connection and the normal specialized conduction system (via the AV node).

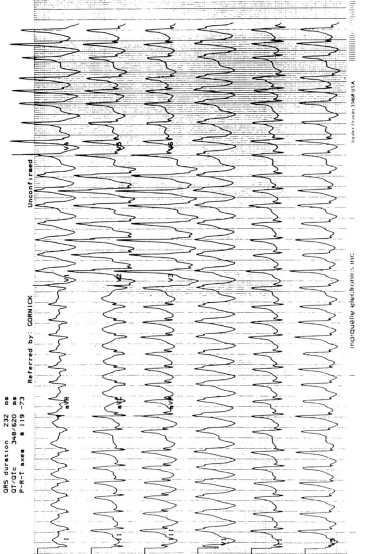

Figure 13 Twelve-lead electrocardiogram (ECG) that fortuitously captured the transition from an antidromic reentry tachycardia to atrial fibrillation. During the reentry tachycardia the QRS is wide secondary to accessory connection activation of the ventricles (left side of ECG). With the development of atrial fibrillation the QRS normalizes and the ventricular response becomes irregular.

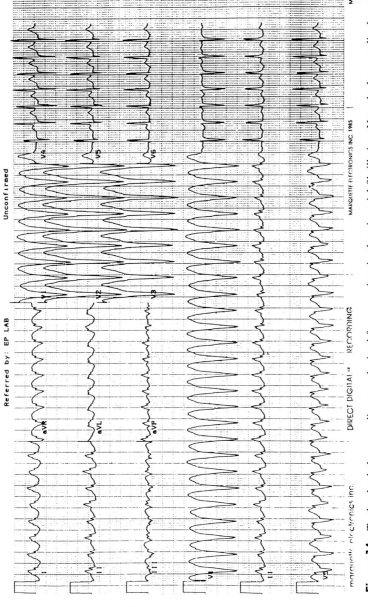

Figure 14   Twelve-lead electrocardiogram obtained from a patient in chronic atrial fibrillation. Note the low amplitude and variable undulation of the baseline secondary to the fibrillating atria. The abnormal QRS complexes are secondary to an intraventricular conduction abnormality.

The subject has become controversial. A retrospective analysis by Dittrich and coworkers (68) failed to show any predictive value of M-mode measurements of left atrial size or of two-dimensional echocardiographic measurements of atrial dimensions for either initial success or maintenance of sinus rhythm at 6 months. The best predictor of maintenance of sinus rhythm at 1 and 6 months, but not of successful cardioversion, was duration of atrial fibrillation. Patients with large atria as a result of mitral valve disease may not only remain in sinus rhythm but have evidence of atrial contraction, with visible "A" waves on the Doppler flow profile. Olsson et al. (69) reported spontaneous reversion of atrial fibrillation to sinus rhythm in 45 cases after periods ranging from 3 to 29 years. Echocardiographic left atrial size in some of these cases ranged from 6.0 to 7.0 cm. However, it was also shown that the left atrium did not exhibit mechanical activity in these cases.

Until the controversy is resolved, echocardiographically determined left atrial size should not be considered the sole criterion to determine whether to attempt cardioversion.

2. *Pharmacologic Cardioversion*

Acute cardioversion may be achieved either pharmacologically or electrically. Electrical cardioversion is preferred if the patient's condition is unstable. A variety of pharmacologic agents have been used. Although digoxin is commonly used, a controlled study demonstrated that digoxin is no more effective than placebo for the acute conversion of atrial fibrillation (70). Slow intravenous infusion of procainamide is effective (71). Type I antiarrhythmic agents such as procainamide should not be used in the absence of agents that slow AV conduction. Type I agents reduce concealed conduction within the AV node, which, combined with the vagolytic effects of these agents (tending to enhance AV conduction), can produce an increased rate of ventricular response to atrial fibrillation.

Drugs that slow conduction through the AV node can be useful, acutely, in controlling rapid rates associated with atrial fibrillation. Digitalis preparations have been used for this purpose. The disadvantage of digitalis preparations is the unpredictable and variable time course of response. Similarly, verapamil can be given in its intravenous form to control ventricular rate (72). Intravenous verapamil use, however, can result in significant hypotension and swings in heart rate as doses of the drug are increased. A second calcium-blocking agent that slows AV nodal conduction is diltiazem, which has been used to control the ventricular rate. Although hypotension remains a problem with this agent, diltiazem's use in a continuous intravenous infusion has advantages, including relatively smooth heart rate control (73), and its use clinically has been increasing. Finally intravenous beta-adrenergic blocking agents, particularly those with a short half life (e.g., esmolol), have been used successfully to control the ventricular response rate (74). Beta-adrenergic blocking agents may cause hypotension. Beta-blockers can, in selected patients with recent-onset atrial fibrillation, have the added advantage of converting a significant number of patients to sinus rhythm (74). Class IA agents (quinidine, procainamide, disopyramide) may be effective in converting atrial fibrillation to sinus rhythm. Quinidine is effective in up to 60% of patients (75). The newer class IC agents flecainide (75,76) and propafenone (77,78) are successful in 40–67% of cases. Amiodarone, a class III agent, restores and maintains sinus rhythm in up to 79% of cases in which other antiarrhythmic agents have failed (79). Low maintenance doses of amiodarone, less than 400 mg/day, may be sufficient. Amiodarone should be reserved for refractory cases because of the high incidence of potentially serious side effects. New agents have also been reported as effective in treatment of atrial fibrillation. These agents include ethmozine (very limited reported experience) and sotalol (80).

Drug therapy should be initiated while the patient is being monitored in the hospital, because of the potential proarrhythmic effects of type I agents, an effect that probably accounts for the early reports of quinidine syncope in patients being treated for atrial fibrillation (81).

Atrial fibrillation in the setting of ventricular preexcitation (Wolff-Parkinson-White syndrome) poses a particular problem. Agents used to slow the ventricular response rate by slowing AV conduction must be used with extreme caution. In these patients ventricular response rate can significantly increase as a result of preferential conduction over the accessory connection.

3. Electrical Cardioversion

Direct-current (DC) cardioversion is the safest and most reliable method of terminating acute episodes of atrial fibrillation. Pacing techniques are not useful in terminating atrial fibrillation. Optimum placement of the electrodes for elective transthoracic cardioversion of atrial fibrillation uses positions that are designed to place the heart in the center of the electrical field (82). The DC shock should be synchronized to the patient's QRS complex to reduce the likelihood of inducing ventricular arrhythmias. During cardioversion, an intravenous line must be placed for administration of anesthetic agents and other drugs as needed. The level of energy required to terminate atrial fibrillation is usually 100 J or greater. Therapy with digitalis preparations before cardioversion appears to be safe as long as the drug level is within the therapeutic range (83). In refractory cases, high-level transvenous intracavitary catheter cardioversion has been used (84). Low-level transvenous intracavitary catheter cardioversion has been used experimentally to terminate episodes of atrial fibrillation (85). However, the success rate was low, and therefore this technique has no clinical application at the present time. In patients with a slow ventricular rate on presentation (untreated), associated AV nodal disease, seen in 50% of those with a sick sinus syndrome, may be suspected. Placement of a temporary pacemaker or use of a standby external pacemaker should be considered as protection against unexpected asystole, occasionally seen after cardioversion in patients with sinus node dysfunction.

4. Maintenance of Sinus Rhythm Following Cardioversion

Chronic treatment of atrial fibrillation is undergoing change. Although cardioversion has an initial success rate of up to 90% (86), the incidence of recurrence is high (50–85%) (73,87–91). Factors associated with initial success include younger age and shorter duration of arrhythmia (92). Prediction of long-term maintenance of sinus rhythm has been correlated with a low New York Heart Association functional class and absence of rheumatic heart disease (92). Large left atrial size generally predicts long-term cardioversion failure (93–95). However, recent large studies have not found left atrial size useful in predicting long-term maintenance of sinus rhythm (68,92). Dethy et al., evaluating a new index in 50 patients, found that the return of atrial contractile function following cardioversion (assessed by Doppler) was a useful indicator of persistence of sinus rhythm at 6 months (96).

Table 2 summarizes currently available antiarrhythmic agents that are being used to maintain patients with atrial fibrillation in sinus rhythm.

A major concern in the treatment of atrial fibrillation is the known proarrhythmic effects of chronic pharmacologic therapy. A recent meta-analysis of studies using quinidine for the control of atrial fibrillation demonstrated an increased mortality in the quinidine treatment groups (54). However, some of these deaths were noncardiac, and the results of that study have been questioned. In patients being treated for ventricular arrhythmias after myocardial infarction, the Cardiac Arrhythmia Suppression Trial (CAST) demonstrated an

Table 2 Dosage and the Therapeutic Levels for Antiarrhythmic Drugs

Drug	Oral dose (mg)	Therapeutic level (mg/ml)	Major elimination route	Primary side effects
Quinidine	300–600 q6h	3–6	Liver	Diarrhea GI upset Cinchonism Proarrhythmia
Procainamide	750–1250 q6h	4–10	Kidneys	Lupus syndrome GI upset
Disopyramide	100–400 q6–8h	2–5	Kidneys	Urinary retention Dry mouth Congestive failure
Flecainide	100–200 q12h	0.2–1.0	Liver	Proarrhythmia CNS symptoms
Propafenone	150–300 q8–12h	0.2–3.0	Liver	Unusual taste GI upset Conduction disturbances CNS symptoms
Amiodarone	200–400 qd	0.5–1.5	Kidneys	Photosensitivity Liver/lung toxicity Thyroid abnormalities
Ethmozine	200–300 q8h	—	Liver	CNS symptoms GI upset Conduction disturbances
Sotalol	80–160 q12h	—	Liver	CNS symptoms Conduction disturbances Proarrhythmia

GI = gastrointestinal; CNS = central nervous system.

increase in mortality in patients treated with flecainide or encainide as compared with placebo (55). Furthermore, presumed proarrhythmic death not only occurred with the initiation of therapy but continued for the duration of therapy (55).

If atrial fibrillation persists with an excessive ventricular rate, consideration should be given to inducing iatrogenic permanent AV block. Catheter ablation in the electrophysiologic laboratory using either DC or, more recently, radiofrequency energy is successful in 80–90% of cases (97). In the remaining patients, although complete AV block is not achieved, catheter ablation can modify AV conduction and result in better control of heart rate in the absence of drugs or by the use of previously ineffective drugs. Following ablation, permanent cardiac pacing is required. Rate-responsive pacemakers can now be used to provide appropriate heart rate increases with exercise.

5. Surgical Cardioversion

Catheter or surgical ablation of the atrioventricular (AV) node effectively controls heart rate but does not provide normal atrial contraction. Consequently, patients treated with these methods are at increased risk for thromboembolism.

Experimental and clinical studies have documented the presence of reentrant circuits within the atrial myocardium of patients with atrial fibrillation. Cox and associates (98) devised a procedure in which the reentrant circuits are interrupted with surgical incisions placed to prevent the return of an electrical impulse to its point of origin. A path from the sinoatrial node to the AV node is created to preserve atrial contraction.

This new technique was applied to 22 patients refractory to all antiarrhythmic medications. Eleven patients had paroxysmal atrial fibrillation, nine had chronic atrial fibrillation, and two had paroxysmal atrial flutter. No operative deaths occurred. Perioperative atrial arrhythmias developed in eight patients, and one patient suffered a perioperative stroke. Echocardiography showed preservation of atrial transport function in all patients. High-intensity endocardial catheter stimulation failed to induce atrial fibrillation in any patient postoperatively, but atrial flutter was induced in four patients. Two patients required pacemaker insertion because of development of sinus node dysfunction. Cox and his colleagues concluded that this new operative procedure, when successful, preserved atrial function (98).

Several other surgical procedures have been proposed in an attempt to treat refractory cases of atrial fibrillation. The "corridor operation" creates an isolated strip of atrial tissue leading from the sinus node to the AV node, excluding most of the right and left atrium (99). Unfortunately this procedure, while useful for providing heart rate control, does not provide atrial transport function or prevent embolic problems, since the remainder of both atria continues to fibrillate. A new procedure, the "atrial maze operation," may provide similar success in heart rate control and is reported to preserve atrial transport function (98). It is noteworthy that following the atrial maze operation 41% of patients required insertion of rate-responsive dual-chambered pacemakers (99). To date, surgical procedures have been used in only a very small group of selected patients. Thus both their short-term and, particularly, their long-term success is unknown.

In patients with sinus node dysfunction, treatment with atrial pacing (coupled with ventricular pacing if required) can in some maintain a sinus/atrial paced rhythm. By preventing bradycardia, atrial pacing avoids establishing the milieu for recurrent atrial arrhythmias, including atrial fibrillation. Treatment with antiarrhythmic medications is often necessary in these patients. Furthermore, it has been reported that ventricular pacing alone, when used to treat sinus node dysfunction (symptomatic bradycardia), can result in a higher incidence of subsequent atrial fibrillation (100,101).

6.   *Thromboembolic Events Related to Cardioversion*

Embolic risk is independent of the mode of termination (DC or pharmacologic) of atrial fibrillation. The reported incidence is 1–3% (102). Although many studies report a decreased incidence of embolization in patients receiving anticoagulation therapy before cardioversion, they were all either nonrandomized or methodologically flawed. Despite the lack of definitive studies, the catastrophic consequences of cerebral emboli demand serious consideration of anticoagulation in all patients undergoing elective cardioversion. The risk of major hemorrhage with anticoagulation must be weighed against the potential benefit. If anticoagulation is used, the practice has been to initiate it 2 to 3 weeks before attempted cardioversion. In theory, this is to prevent the formation of new thrombi while allowing any old thrombi to organize. Anticoagulation should be continued for 2 to 3 weeks following cardioversion because of the occurrence of late embolic events. The latter may relate to a delay between return of atrial electrical activity (P waves on the electrocardiogram) and mechanical function or due to cardioversion failure (103). Direct evaluation of the left atrium by TEE for thrombi and/or SEC may eventually provide a more informed decision as to the need for anticoagulation before and after cardioversion. The role of TEE has not been systematically studied; however, Manning et al. reported that if TEE excludes left atrial thrombi, cardioversion can be performed safely. An important additional factor favoring anticoagulation after cardioversion is that these patients often develop paroxysmal or recurrent sustained atrial fibrillation, both of which predispose to systemic embolization.

Recently, left ventricular dysfunction and increased left atrial size detected echocardiographically were identified as independent predictors of increased thromboembolic risk in patients with nonrheumatic atrial fibrillation (104).

7. Overall Treatment Strategy for Cardioversion

In the past, attempts at cardioversion were made to improve hemodynamic status and prevent thromboembolic complications. Since anticoagulants can effectively reduce the risk of embolization, symptoms related to loss of atrial contraction remain the major indication for attempts at cardioversion and maintenance of sinus rhythm. In selected patients with significant symptoms, an aggressive staged approach to therapy can maintain sinus rhythm in over 60% (105).

The presence of symptoms that warrant attempts at restoring and maintaining sinus rhythm is related to the patient's age, underlying heart disease, and activity level. Lundstrom and Ryden (91) reported a series of 100 consecutive patients presenting with atrial fibrillation. At presentation 30% were asymptomatic. Furthermore, 53% were without symptoms when they returned for follow-up after cardioversion, despite reversion to atrial fibrillation.

Clearly, it would be desirable to maintain sinus rhythm, or a regularly paced atrial rhythm, in all patients who develop atrial fibrillation. New surgical techniques hold promise. Whether these will achieve the reported success rates with wider application or provide an adequate risk/benefit ratio is unknown. Pharmacologic agents (type IA and IC) that maintain sinus rhythm are associated with an increase in mortality, probably because of their proarrhythmic effect. Hence, at present aggressive attempts to convert atrial fibrillation and maintain sinus rhythm should be reserved for patients with significant symptoms or patients in whom anticoagulation is contraindicated.

E. Prophylaxis Against Systemic Embolization

1. Results of Placebo-Controlled Clinical Trials

A significant number of patients with either chronic, persistent, or paroxysmal atrial fibrillation do not have a reversible cause, and pharmacologic or electrical cardioversion is unsuccessful. In the mid 1980s several independently designed clinical studies were initiated with the objective of determining the most effective and safest approach to protect patients against embolic risk.

Each trial evaluated the efficacy of warfarin, in low (106–109) (PT ratio 1.2–1.5) to intermediate dose (110) (PT ratio of 1.7) ranges, in preventing systemic embolization in patients with atrial fibrillation. Two trials formally evaluated aspirin as an alternative treatment (106,110). Three considerations prompted these clinical trials. First, it was recognized that atrial fibrillation is an important predisposing factor for systemic embolization and stroke. Second, atrial fibrillation increases with aging, and with the aging of Western societies it will constitute an enormous health care problem. Last, and most important, was the demonstration that low-dose warfarin is as effective as conventional-dose warfarin for the treatment of patients with deep vein thrombosis but is associated with substantially fewer bleeding complications (111). The five trials were the Atrial Fibrillation,

Aspirin, Anticoagulation (AFASAK) study from Copenhagen, Denmark (110), the Stroke Prevention in Atrial Fibrillation (SPAF) study from the United States (106), the Boston Area Anticoagulation Trial for Atrial Fibrillation (BAATAF) (105), the Canadian Atrial Fibrillation Anticoagulation (CAFA) study (105), and the Stroke Prevention in Nonrheumatic Atrial Fibrillation (SPINAF) study (109). These trials have resolved, in a rigorous fashion, many issues regarding antithrombotic and antiplatelet therapy in patients with atrial fibrillation.

While these studies have major similarities, each provided important and unique information. All studies were placebo-controlled and randomized and were terminated early. The studies that evaluated aspirin used different doses; the Danish study (110) used 75 mg of aspirin per day, and the SPAF study (111) used 325 mg/day. The Boston study (107), which was not specifically designed to evaluate the role of aspirin, allowed patients in the placebo group to receive aspirin provided it was administered at a dose of 325 mg/day. The Boston and Danish studies were not blinded (107,110). The SPAF study was blinded for aspirin but not for warfarin therapy (112). The remaining two studies, the Canadian study (108) and the VA Cooperative Study (SPINAF) (109) specifically excluded use of aspirin or nonsteroidal anti-inflammatory agents. These last two studies were unique in that they were double-blinded. We believe these two trials were the first double-blinded studies of warfarin ever conducted. Each study used stroke or a variant thereof as their primary end point (Table 3). The characteristics of the patients in the nontreatment groups are shown in Table 4. In all studies hypertension, coronary artery disease, and heart failure were common and had

Table 3 End Points

	AFASAK	SPAF	BAATAF	CAN	SPINAF

Primary	Stroke
	TIA
	Systemic
	  embolism
		Ishemic
		  stroke
		Systemic
		  emboli
			Ischemic
			  stroke
				Ischemic stroke
				  (except
				  lacunar)
				Systemic
				  emboli
				Intracranial
				  hemorrhage
					Cerebral
					  infarction

Secondary	Death	Death
		Myocardial
		  infarction
		TIA
		Unstable
		  angina
			Intracerebral
			  hemorrhages
				TIA
				Lacunar
				  infarction
				Major bleed
				Minor bleed
				Death
					Cerebral
					  hemorrhage
					Death

Intercurrent
events
	Hemorrhages
	  major/
	  minor
			Minor
			  hemorrhages
					Noncerebral
					  major
					  hemorrhage
					Minor
					  hemorrhage
					TIA
					Myocardial
					  infarction
					Venous
					  thrombosis

TIA = transient ischemic attack.

Table 4 Baseline Characteristics of Patients

Characteristic	Control/Warfarin		Placebo/Aspirin	
	Control	Warfarin	Placebo	Aspirin
Total randomized	1236	1225	904	888
Age: (%)				
≤65	33	33	31	32
66–75	47	47	40	36
>75	20	20	29	31
Mean age	69	69	70	70
Gender (% male)	73	75	64	65
Race				
White	94	95	90	89
Black	3	2	4	3
Hispanic	2	2	5	7
Mean systolic BP	141	141	143	144
Mean diastolic BP	83	83	82	83
Hx of hypertension: (%)	46	45	44	46
Hx of diabetes: (%)	15	13	15	13
Hx of prior stroke/TIA: (%)	6	6	7	6
Hx of PVD: (%)	10	12	8	7
Hx of CHF: (%)	20	20	18	18
Hx of angina: (%)	22	23	11	0
Hx of MI: (%)	14	13	11	10
Current smoker: (%)	13	12	16	16
Carotid bruit: (%)				
Absent	97	96	96	97
Present	3	4	4	3

previously been noted to be associated with atrial fibrillation. Patients from the AFASAK study were older and more likely to have a history of heart failure. In the VA and AFASAK studies intermittent atrial fibrillation was an exclusion criterion. For all studies a major bleed was, in general, defined as one requiring a blood transfusion, hospitalization, or therapeutic intervention or occurring in a critical anatomic location, e.g., intracranially. The primary analysis was intention-to-treat for SPAF, BAATAF, and SPINAF. For the AFASAK study, events were counted until patients discontinued their study medication, and CAFA included all events that occurred within 28 days of permanent discontinuation of the study medication.

Each will be reviewed in the order in which the results were reported. Tables are provided to facilitate comparison between studies.

The Danish Study. In 1989 Dr. Palle Petersen and colleagues published the results of the Danish study, which randomized 1007 patients to receive warfarin, aspirin, or placebo (110). The characteristics of the patient population are provided in Table 4. The mean age of the patients was 74 years, greater by several years than in the other studies. An efficacy analysis found a highly statistically significant benefit afforded by warfarin as compared with both placebo and aspirin (Tables 5 and 6). Bleeding complications were equally divided among the three groups (Table 6). The results of this study were compelling. However, its unblinded

Table 5 Event Rates (%/pt-yr) Comparing Aspirin (A) with Placebo (P)

	AFASAK (n = 672)		SPAF (n = 1120)	
	A (n = 336)	P (n = 336)	A (n = 552)	P (n = 568)
Total pt-yr observation to death or end of study	422	417	742	767
Stroke	3.9	4.8	3.2	5.7
Systemic embolism	0.2	0.5	0.4	0.7
Intracerebral hemorrhage	0	0	0.1	0
Subdural hemorrhage	0	0	0.1	0.3
Subarachnoid hemorrhage	0	0	0	0
Transient ischemic attack	0.5	0.7	1.4	2.3
Death	5.7	6.5	5.3	6.5
Vascular	4.0	4.1	3.2	3.6
Nonvascular	1.2	1.9	2.0	2.1
Unknown	0.5	0.5	0	0.8
Myocardial infarction	NA	NA	0.9	1.6
Other bleeds	0.3	0	1.1	1.2

NA = Not recorded.

design and the fact that 38% of patients assigned to the warfarin group withdrew from this study, together with the fact that the analysis was an efficacy analysis, necessitated confirmation of these findings by other trials.

The SPAF Study.   The SPAF was the second to publish its results, which appeared in both a preliminary report (14) and a subsequent final paper (60). In SPAF, a determination was made whether eligible patients could safely be randomized to warfarin. Patients found to

Table 6 Event Rates (%/pt-yr) for Warfarin (W) in Each Study

	AFASAK (n = 671) W (n = 335)	BAATAF (n = 420) W (n = 212)	CAFA (n = 378) W (n = 187)	SPAF (n = 421) W (n = 210)	SPINAF (n = 525) W (n = 260)
Total pt-yr observation to death or end of study	423	487	239	271	456
Stroke	1.9	0.4	2.1	2.3	0.9
Systemic embolism	0	0	0.4	0	0.8
Intracerebral hemorrhage	0.2	0	0.4	0.4	0.2
Subdural hemorrhage	0	0.2	0	0.4	0
Subarachnoid hemorrhage	0	0	0	0	0
Transient ischemic attack	0.2	0.8	0.8	1.5	1.5
Death	4.7	2.3	4.2	2.2	3.3
Myocardial infarction	NA	0.8	NA	0.7	0.4
Major bleeds	0.3	1.0	1.7	0.4	1.5

NA = Not recorded.

be randomized to warfarin were then assigned to a warfarin, aspirin, or placebo group. Aspirin and placebo patients were blinded; warfarin patients were not. Patients who were otherwise eligible for the study but deemed not randomizable to warfarin were assigned, in a blinded manner, to either aspirin or placebo groups. At the meeting in November 1989 of the data-monitoring board overseeing this study, a decision was made to terminate the study because of a highly statistically significant benefit afforded by active treatment (either warfarin or aspirin) in comparison with placebo. Since these investigators planned a second phase of their study, involving a direct comparison between warfarin and aspirin therapy, the individual benefit of these two drugs was not revealed. The investigators reported that 52 patients with lone atrial fibrillation, which was strictly defined, had no cerebrovascular events in the short period of follow-up, and that in patients over the age of 75 aspirin was not of benefit. It is noteworthy that the event rate in the placebo group, 7.4% per year, was higher than the event rate reported in the other studies (Table 6).

The Canadian Study. In March 1990 the Canadian investigators terminated their study (108) without an interim analysis because they believed it was unethical to continue with a placebo group. Their study was a blinded comparison between warfarin and placebo and at the time of early termination had randomized 378 patients. Their analysis suggested a trend in favor of warfarin preventing systemic embolization, but this was not statistically significant. They also found that bleeding complications were fairly equally distributed between the two groups, although there were two deaths related to hemorrhages in the warfarin group.

The Boston Area Study (BAATAF). The BAATAF study (107) was an unblinded comparison between warfarin and placebo. Placebo patients were permitted aspirin at a dose of 325 mg/day. The study demonstrated a 86% benefit in favor of warfarin therapy in preventing both systemic embolization and stroke and a 35% reduction in mortality among patients with chronic atrial fibrillation. No benefit for aspirin was found.

The VA Cooperative Study (SPINAF). This study (109) was a double-blinded comparison of low-intensity anticoagulation with a prothrombin time ratio of 1.2 to 1.5 against placebo conducted under the auspices of the VA Cooperative Studies Program. Recruitment was initiated in July 1987 and terminated in June 1990. As mandated by protocol, an interim analysis was conducted in January 1991 from data that was current as of December 1, 1990. On the basis of this analysis and the results of other studies with similar goals (106–108,110), the study was terminated on March 1, 1991. Arm I of this study included patients without a previous stroke, and Arm II included patients who had had a stroke within the past month. A total of 525 patients were randomized to either placebo or warfarin in Arm I of the study. The mean age of the patient population was 67 years. Results of the study were as follows: 19 patients in the placebo group had a cerebral infarction as compared with four patients in the warfarin group, for a risk-benefit ratio of 79% (Fig. 15). There were 10 major hemorrhages, six in the warfarin group and four in the placebo group. One of these was fatal. All major hemorrhages were gastrointestinal in origin. There was one intracerebral hemorrhage in the warfarin group. Minor bleeding complications were more common in the warfarin group. In patients over the age of 70 a similar benefit was seen. These studies have provided guidance for important questions related to the treatment of patients with atrial fibrillation (109).

2. *Analysis of Pooled Data from Five Randomized Control Studies (134)*

Data on individual patients were pooled from the five recently conducted atrial fibrillation trials described above. For the pooled analysis, the mean age at the time of randomization was 69 years with a blood pressure of 142/82. Forty-six percent of the patients had

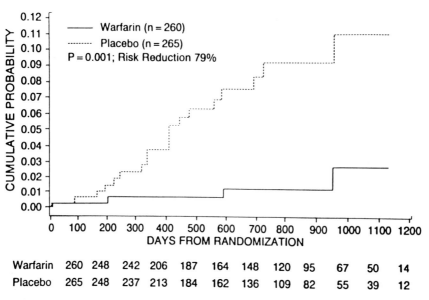

Figure 15 Cumulative probability of cerebral infarction. The numbers below the figure are the numbers of patients at risk for a cerebral infarction at each point. There was a significant reduction in risk in the warfarin group as compared with the placebo group (risk reduction, 0.79; p = 0.001). (From Ezekowitz MD et al., Warfarin in the prevention of stroke associated with nonrheumatic atrial fibrillation. N Engl J Med 1992; 327:1406–1412.)

hypertension, 6 a previous transient ischemic attack or stroke, and 14% had diabetes. For the warfarin control comparison there were 1889 patient years on warfarin and 1802 in the control group. For the aspirin/placebo comparison there were 1132 patient years on aspirin and 1133 on placebo. Using a multivariant analysis among the control patients increasing age, history of hypertension, previous transient ischemic attack or stroke and history of diabetes were independent risk factors for stroke. It was found that for patients under the age of 75 who had none of the above predictive factors (these constituted 15% of all patients) had an annual risk of stroke of 1% per year with 95% Confidence Intervals of 0.3 to 3.1%. The efficacy of warfarin was consistent across all studies and subgroups. The annual rate of stroke was 4.5% on control and 1.4% on warfarin with a 68% risk reduction, 95% Confidence Interval, 50–79% p < 0.01. The efficacy of aspirin was not consistent and has been described above. The annual rate of major hemorrhage was 1% in controls, 1% on aspirin, and 1.3% on warfarin and was not different. Thus, these five trials demonstrated that warfarin consistently decreases the risk of stroke with virtually no increase in the frequency of major bleeds. Patients with atrial fibrillation younger than 65 with none of the described risk factors, i.e., hypertension, previous stroke, or transient ischemic attack or diabetes were at very low risk for stroke, even when not treated. We, therefore, recommend that this group of patients not receive warfarin. This pooled analysis further confirms the need to clarify the role of aspirin in atrial fibrillation.

Which Is the Best Therapy for Prophylaxis Against Systemic Embolization; Warfarin or Aspirin? All studies found warfarin effective in protecting patients against systemic embolization (Figs. 16 and 17; Table 7). This was true for both chronic (103–107) and

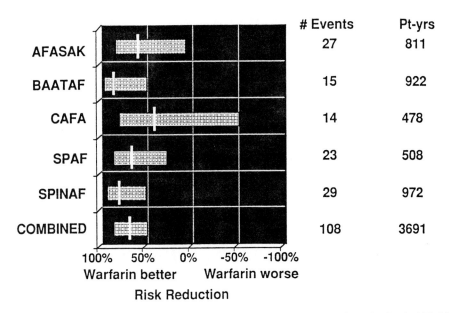

Figure 16   Risk reduction of stroke comparing aspirin with placebo. The reduction in AFASAK was 18%, which was not statistically significant. For the SPAF, the reduction was 44% (p <.02). The combined benefit was 36%.

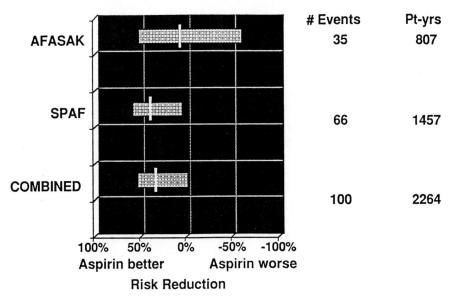

Figure 17   Risk reduction of stroke comparing warfarin with placebo. All studies except CAFA, which was stopped early, showed a benefit of warfarin. Overall benefit was 68%.

Table 7 Event Rates (%/pt-yr) for Placebo (P) in Each Study

	AFASAK (n = 671) P (n = 336)	BAATAF (n = 420) P (n = 208)	CAFA (n = 378) P (n = 191)	SPAF (n = 421) P (n = 211)	SPINAF (n = 525) P (n = 265)
Total pt-yr observation to death or end of study	417	435	251	259	440
Stroke	4.8	3.0	3.7	7.0	4.3
Systemic embolism	0.2	0	0.8	0.8	0.4
Intracerebral hemorrhage	0	0	0	0	0
Subdural hemorrhage	0	0	0	0.8	0
Subarachnoid hemorrhage	0	0	0	0	0
Transient ischemic attack	0.7	0.9	0.8	2.4	2.6
Death	6.5	6.0	3.2	3.1	5.0
Myocardial infarction	NA	0.7	NA	0.8	1.5
Major bleeds	0	1.9	0.8	0.8	0.9

NA = Not recorded.

intermittent (106–108) atrial fibrillation. The general similarity of baseline characteristics and the comparable risk reduction among the studies indicate that these results have wide application. In the three unblinded warfarin studies, the reduction in the risk of cerebral vascular events ranged from 67% to 86% (106,107,110). In SPINAF there was a 79% reduction of risk of cerebral infarction (109). The Canadian Atrial Fibrillation Study (106), the only other double-blind, placebo-controlled trial, was terminated early on the basis of data from the other trials and without consideration of its own interim data. That study showed a nonstatistically significant trend in favor of warfarin (108).

The risk of major hemorrhage as a result of low-intensity warfarin anticoagulation was similar for warfarin and placebo (108–110). Minor hemorrhages were more common in the warfarin group in the SPINAF study (109).

In contrast to the established efficacy of warfarin, the benefit of aspirin for the prevention of stroke remains controversial. The AFASAK study showed no benefit of aspirin compared with placebo (110). A preliminary report of the SPAF study (106) showed that patients over the age of 75 did not benefit from aspirin, whereas there was benefit for patients younger than 75 (2.2%/yr, risk reduction 65%) (Fig. 16). In the SPAF population overall (60), the incidence of ischemic stroke and systemic emboli for aspirin-treated patients was 3.6%/yr, as compared with the rate of 0.9%/yr for cerebral infarction alone among the warfarin-treated patients in the SPINAF study. Moreover, patients in the placebo group of the BAATAF study (105) were permitted to use aspirin, and no benefit was found.

Thus it is conclusively demonstrated that low-intensity anticoagulation with warfarin is effective in preventing cerebral infarction in patients with nonrheumatic atrial fibrillation and has minimal risk of major hemorrhage. The benefit persists in patients over the age of 70 (107). Considering all the studies, patients should be offered warfarin unless there is lone atrial fibrillation (see below) or a contraindication to warfarin therapy, in which case aspirin therapy should be considered.

What Is the Optimal Dose for Warfarin and Aspirin? The optimal dose for warfarin is the maintenance of a PT ratio in the range of 1.2 to 1.5, which translates in the VA Cooperative Study to an international normalized ratio (INR) of 1.38 to 2.5 (109). It is important to recognize that the lowest effective dose of warfarin has yet to be defined. Considerable controversy concerning the optimal dose of aspirin remains. A dose of 325 mg/day was shown in the SPAF study to be effective in patients under the age of 75 (106). If aspirin is to be administered for preventing systemic embolization in patients with chronic atrial fibrillation, our recommendation would be to use a dose of 325 mg/day, recognizing that a consistent benefit from aspirin has not been shown.

Are There Patient Groups in Which Low or High Risk of Systemic Embolization Can Be Identified? Identifying patients at high risk for cerebral infarction has proved difficult. Each of the studies has found different variables to predispose to stroke. The SPINAF study (109), together with BAATAF (107), identified active angina as a possible risk factor. There was a lack of unanimity with regard to mitral annular calcification (106,107), recent history of heart failure (105), left atrial size (105), or reduced left ventricular function (107).

Lone atrial fibrillators, i.e., patients without evidence of structural heart disease, hypertension, diabetes mellitus, or precipitating factors such as thyrotoxicosis, have a low incidence of systemic embolization. This group of patients, when strictly defined, constitutes 2–4% of the population with chronic atrial fibrillation (106–110). The risk of embolization in this group is low, 1.3–1.4%/yr (64,109,110), and not significantly different from the risk in the general population. The Framingham study described an increased stroke risk, but its population was not strictly defined and included patients older than 60 years as well as patients with hypertension and diabetes (2). None of the 18 patients in the SPINAF study with lone atrial fibrillation had a cerebral infarction. This is consistent with the SPAF study, which had 52 patients with lone atrial fibrillation, none of whom had cerebral events (14). Thus, lone atrial fibrillators would not require anticoagulation to reduce their risk of cerebral infarction but might benefit from aspirin, although this benefit is unproven. The pooled analysis has demonstrated that patients with atrial fibrillation <65 without hypertension, diabetes, or previous stroke are at very low risk and should not be anticoagulated. All other groups would benefit from warfarin.

What Is the Long-Term Benefit? All five of the atrial fibrillation studies were terminated early by their data monitoring boards (106–110), precluding the assessment of warfarin's long-term benefit. Each study demonstrates that cerebral infarction is a sporadic event in patients with chronic atrial fibrillation (Fig. 17) and that the risk of an event persists even with long-standing atrial fibrillation. Thus, chronicity of atrial fibrillation does not attenuate the indication for anticoagulation, and patients with long-standing atrial fibrillation would benefit from anticoagulation therapy.

The atrial fibrillation investigators, consisting of representatives from the five study groups, developed a common data base in an effort to answer questions that could not be addressed by the individual trials. Multivariate analysis showed that risk factors that predicted stroke in control patients were increased age, history of hypertension, previous transient ischemic attack or stroke, and diabetes. The 17% of all patients under the age of 65 who had none of the risk factors listed above had an annual risk of stroke of 1% per year, which was close to a level of risk exceeding that of comparable patients without atrial fibrillation. In this low-risk subgroup no benefit from warfarin therapy was found. However, in all the remaining patients a substantial benefit was afforded by warfarin. The pooled analysis further confirmed that the benefit of aspirin was less consistent than that shown for warfarin.

Mortality and Atrial Fibrillation. On the basis of the SPINAF study, it appears that mortality related to atrial fibrillation is not related to thromboembolic phenomena but rather, primarily, to sudden unexpected cardiac death (presumably arrhythmic). This may result from the association of atrial fibrillation with other clinical entities that provide a substrate for potentially lethal ventricular arrhythmias (e.g., cardiomyopathy) or to the concomitant use of drugs such as quinidine that may have a proarrhythmic effect and predispose to sudden death.

Role of Transesophageal Echocardiography and Other Techniques for the Diagnosis of Left Atrial Thrombi. It is clear that transesophageal echocardiography is an extremely useful technique for the identification of thrombi in both the left atrium and the left atrial appendage. However, the impact of these findings on the decision to treat patients with atrial fibrillation is unclear. Although the presence of SEC is an important marker for thrombus and embolic risk, there are no clear-cut studies to document a low embolic risk in patients without these finding. A test at a particular point in time may not be predictive of subsequent systemic embolization because thrombi may form and resolve as part of a continuous process that would be difficult to monitor by repeated TEE. At the present time it would be premature to recommend TEE to stratify risk for systemic embolization with nonrheumatic atrial fibrillation. If, however, an embolic etiology is being sought, TEE is a valuable and unique diagnostic test to identify a number of sources that cannot be imaged in other ways. These are discussed both here and in other chapters in this text.

What Is the Relative Risk in Patients with Intermittent Versus Chronic Atrial Fibrillation? Although patients with intermittent atrial fibrillation were excluded by protocol from the AFASAK and SPINAF studies (106–110), other studies (106–108) have reported that the risk of embolization is similar to that in patients with chronic atrial fibrillation. We believe that patients with intermittent atrial fibrillation should be treated similarly to those with chronic atrial fibrillation.

Which Patients Can Be Safely Anticoagulated? The exclusion criteria for the SPINAF trial are provided in Table 8. Since the major hemorrhagic rate was not different in the two groups, these exclusions, category C and selected exclusions under category D, should be used.

Secondary Prevention. The only study to address secondary prevention of stroke in atrial fibrillation in a prospective, randomized manner was Arm II of the SPINAF study (109). Unfortunately, recruitment to this arm of the study was far less than projected. However, it confirmed evidence available in the literature that the risk of a recurrent stroke in patients with nonvalvular atrial fibrillation and a previous stroke is higher than in patients who have nonvalvular atrial fibrillation without a previous stroke, this risk is estimated at between 13% and 32% in the first year (113–118). The risk is particularly high in the first 2 weeks after the stroke (53,113,115–117,119,120). It appears that previous stroke is also an independent predictor of subsequent stroke in the SPAF study. In the SPINAF study there appeared to be a benefit from warfarin, but this was not statistically significant because of the low numbers in that study. Thus, there is no long-term randomized trial evaluating anticoagulation for secondary prevention of stroke in nonvalvular atrial fibrillation. Such a study is under way in Europe. Enrollment should be complete in 1992 (121). From the results of the SPINAF study it appears that the risk of bleeding is comparable in this group to that seen in patients without prior stroke. Given the demonstrated efficacy of warfarin in primary prevention and the significant risk of recurrence, it seems appropriate to recommend anticoagulation for patients with nonvalvular atrial fibrillation and a previous stroke (122).

Rheumatic Heart Disease. The risk of stroke in patients with rheumatic mitral valve disease and atrial fibrillation is three times greater than in patients in atrial fibrillation without mitral stenosis (123). There are no randomized, controlled studies evaluating the

Table 8 Exclusion Criteria

A. Intermittent atrial fibrillation
B. Definite indication for anticoagulation/antiplatelet agents
    Rheumatic mitral valve disease
    Prosthetic heart valves
    Intracardiac thrombus
    Active thromboembolic disease
        Systemic embolus
        Myocardial infarction within 1 month
        Coronary artery bypass graft
C. Contraindication for anticoagulation
    Planned surgery or invasive procedure[a]
    Active bleeding
    History of gastrointestinal hemorrhage within 2 years[a]
        Documented peptic ulcer disease within 2 years.[a] Known esophageal varices, chronic
        alcoholism, history of intracranial hemorrhage
    Uncontrolled hypertension (>180/105 mm Hg)[a]
    Psychological or social condition
        Laboratory abnormalities:[a] HCT <32%, platelet count <100,000, SGOT, SGPT, alkaline
        phosphatase 2 times upper limit of normal, guaiac-positive stool and >5 red blood cells per
        high power field in urine
    Prothrombin time outside normal limit
    Atrial tumor
    Hemostasis disorder
    Coexisting medical disorder
    Bacterial endocarditis
D. Inappropriate for the study (administrative)
    Approved use of aspirin or nonsteroidal anti-inflammatory agents
    Patient did not undergo echocardiography
    Unstable angina and transient ischemic episodes within 5 years
    Limited life span or unwilling to complete follow-up
    Received anticoagulation within past 6 months for greater than 1 continuous month
    Reversible causes of atrial fibrillation
    Planned cardioversion
    Hyperthyroidism
    Refused consent

[a]Reversible

efficacy of antithrombotic therapy in patients with rheumatic heart disease in atrial fibrillation. Fukuda and Makamura followed patients with rheumatic valvular disease for a mean of 22 months (124). They found that the incidence of thromboembolism without anticoagulation was 5.5% per year and that this could be reduced to between 3% and 1% per year with warfarin therapy. In light of this evidence and the demonstrated efficacy of warfarin in nonrheumatic atrial fibrillation, long-term anticoagulation with warfarin is recommended for patients with rheumatic valvular disease in atrial fibrillation. Antiplatelet agents have not been adequately tested in this patient group.

Congenital Heart Disease. Among patients with congenital heart disease, those with atrial and ventricular septal defects, corrected transposition of the great vessels, and

Ebstein's anomaly are most likely to develop atrial fibrillation. There are insufficient data to determine whether long-term anticoagulant therapy is indicated for patients with congenital heart disease complicated by atrial fibrillation. However, given the benefit of warfarin in patients with nonvalvular atrial fibrillation, it would seem reasonable to anticoagulate these patients.

Thyrotoxic Heart Disease. Atrial fibrillation occurs in about 10–30% of thyrotoxic patients (125,126). Among 1212 patients with atrial fibrillation, Godtfredsen (127) found that in 2.5% fibrillation was due to thyrotoxicosis. A retrospective study that included 163 patients, with a mean follow-up of 34 months, found that the control of thyroid dysfunction alone resulted in spontaneous reversion to sinus rhythm in 101 patients. About three-fourths of those patients who converted spontaneously did so within 3 weeks of becoming euthyroid. The failure to revert spontaneously to sinus rhythm within 4 months usually mandates cardioversion (128). The frequency of systemic embolization in patients with atrial fibrillation due to thyrotoxicosis is not known but is at least as high as in those patients who are in atrial fibrillation and are euthyroid (129). Because the probability of embolization is high and warfarin is effective in nonrheumatic atrial fibrillation, it is recommended that patients with thyrotoxicosis who are in atrial fibrillation be anticoagulated. It is also recommended that after cardioversion, continuation of anticoagulation should be undertaken for 4 weeks after conversion to normal sinus rhythm (130–132). The rationale for this recommendation is based on the fact that the left atrium does not immediately return to its normal contractile state after reversion to sinus rhythm, and that patients may revert to either chronic or intermittent atrial fibrillation.

Recommendation. It is strongly recommended that long-term warfarin therapy (INR 1.5–3) be used in patients with nonrheumatic atrial fibrillation who are eligible for anticoagulation. Patients with lone atrial fibrillation, irrespective of age, should probably receive aspirin. Patients with atrial fibrillation who are younger than 65 and have no history of hypertension, previous stroke or transient ischemic attack, or diabetes are at low risk of stroke and should not be anticoagulated. Patients with thyrotoxicosis, rheumatic heart disease, or congenital heart disease should be anticoagulated. Patients who have a contraindication to warfarin therapy, but who otherwise could be treated with aspirin, should be treated at a dose of 325 mg daily because aspirin treatment is probably better than placebo. Its ultimate benefit requires further study.

REFERENCES

1. Beppu S, Nimura Y, Sakakibara, et al. Smoke-like echo in the left atrial cavity in mitral valve disease: its features and significance. J Am Coll Cardiol 1985; 6:744–9.
2. Suetsugu M, Matsuzaki M, Toma Y, et al. Detection of mural thrombi and analysis of blood flow velocities in the left atrial appendage using transesophageal two-dimensional echocardiography and pulsed Doppler flowmetry. J Cardiol 1988; 18:385–94.
3. Daniel WG, Nellessen U, Schroder E, et al. Left atrial spontaneous echo contrast in mitral valve disease: an indicator for an increased thromboembolic risk. J Am Coll Cardiol 1988; 11: 1204–11.
4. Black IW, Hopkins AP, Lee LCL, et al. Left atrial spontaneous echo contrast: a clinical and echocardiographic analysis. J Am Coll Cardiol 1991; 18:398–404.
5. Castello R, Pearson AC, Labovitz AJ. Prevalence and clinical implications of atrial spontaneous echo contrast in patients undergoing transesophageal echocardiography. Am J Cardiol 1990; 65:1149–53.

6. Obarski TP, Salcedo EE, Castle LW, Stewart WJ. Spontaneous echo contrast in the left atrium during paroxysmal atrial fibrillation. Am Heart J 1990; 120:988–90.

7. Hirabayashi T, Teranishi J, Mikami T. Spontaneous contrast echoes are associated with an increased incidence of cerebral infarction in patients with nonvalvular chronic atrial fibrillation (abstr). Circulation 1990; 82:III–108.

8. Zabalgoita M, Gandhi DK, McPherson DD, et al. Spontaneous echo contrast in severe left ventricular dysfunction: a risk factor for thromboembolism (abstr). Circulation 1990; 82:III109.

9. Sigel B, Coelho JCU, Spigos DG, et al. Ultrasonography of blood during stasis. Invest Radiol 1981; 16:71–6.

10. Turakia AK, Teague SM, Lawler B, et al. Echocardiographic "smoke" phenomenon: an in vitro simulation (abstr). Circulation 1991; 84 (suppl):II–692.

11. Chesebro JH, Fuster V, Halperin JL. Atrial fibrillation risk marker for stroke. N Engl J Med 1990; 323:1556–8.

12. Einthoven W. Le télécardiogramme. Arch Int Physiol 1906; 4:132–64.

13. Lewis T. Auricular fibrillation: a common clinical condition. Br Med J 1909; 2:1528.

14. Lewis T. Auricular fibrillation and its relationship to clinical irregularity of the heart. Heart 1909–10; 1:306–72.

15. Rothberger C, Winterberg H. Vorhofflimmern und arrhythmia perpetua. Wien Klin Wochenschr 1909; 22:839–44.

16. Rothberger C, Winterberg H. Ueber den pulsus irregularis perpetuus. Wien Klin Wochenschr 1909; 22:1792–5.

17. Gramiak R, Shah PM, Kramer DH. Ultrasound cardiography: contrast studies in anatomy and function. Radiology 1969; 92:939.

18. Meltzer RS, Lancee CT, Swart GR, et al. Spontaneous echocardiographic contrast on the right side of the heart. J Clin Ultrasound 1982; 10:240–2.

19. Schuchman H, Feigenbaum H, Dillon JC, Chang S. Intracavitary echoes in patients with mitral prosthetic valves. J Clin Ultrasound 1975; 3:107–10.

20. Panidis IP, Kotler MN, Mintz GS, et al. Intracavitary echoes in the aortic arch in type III aortic dissection. Am J Cardiol 1984; 54:1159–60.

21. Hjemdahl-Monsen CF, Daniels J, Kaufman D, et al. Spontaneous contrast in the inferior vena cava in a patient with constrictive pericarditis. J Am Coll Cardiol 1984; 4:165–7.

22. Mikell FL, Asinger RS, Eisperger KJ, et al. Regional stasis of blood in the dysfunctional left ventricle: echocardiographic detection and differentiation from early thrombosis. Circulation 1982; 66:755–63.

23. Maze SS, Kotler MN, Parry WR. Flow characteristics in the dilated left ventricle with thrombus: qualitative and quantitative Doppler analysis. J Am Coll Cardiol 1989; 13:873–81.

24. Doud DN, Jacobs WR, Moran JF, et al. The natural history of left ventricular spontaneous contrast. J Am Soc Echocardiog 1990; 3:465–70.

25. Castello R, Pearson AC, Fagan L, et al. Spontaneous echocardiographic contrast in the descending aorta. Am Heart J 1990; 120:915–9.

26. Mahony C, Ayappa IA, Brown LV, et al. Spontaneous contrast in the rabbit (abstr). Circulation 1991; 84 (suppl):II–692.

27. Mahony C, Sublett K, Harrison M. Resolution of spontaneous contrast with platelet disaggregatory therapy (trifluoperazine). Am J Cardiol 1989; 63:1009–10.

28. Archer SL, Kvernen LR, James K, et al. Does warfarin reduce the prevalence of left atrial thrombus in chronic atrial fibrillation? A double blind, placebo-controlled study (abstr). Circulation 1991; 84 (suppl):II–693.

29. Pollick C, Taylor D. Assessment of left atrial appendage function by transesophageal echocardiography: implications for the development of thrombus. Circulation 1991; 84:223–31.

30. Effert S, Domanig E. The diagnosis of intra-atrial tumor and thrombi by the ultrasonic echo method. Germ Med Meth 1959; 4:1.

31. Come PC, Riley MF, Markis JE, et al. Limitations of echocardiographic techniques in evaluation of left atrial masses. Am J Cardiol 1981; 48:947–53.

32. Nomeir A, Watts LE, Seagle R, et al. Intracardiac myxomas: twenty-year echocardiographic experience with review of the literature. J Am Soc Echocardiog 1989; 2:139–50.

33. Mugge A, Daniel WG, Haverich A, et al. Diagnosis of noninfective cardiac mass lesions by two dimensional echocardiography: comparison of transthoracic and transesophageal approaches. Circulation 1991; 83:70–8.

34. Alam M, Sun I. Transesophageal echocardiographic evaluation of left atrial mass lesions. J Am Soc Echocardiog 1991; 4:323–30.

35. Tomas AC, Mills PG, Giggs NM, et al. Secondary carcinoma of left atrium simulating myxoma. Br Heart J 1980; 44:541–4.

36. Mich RJ, Gillam LD, Weyman AE. Osteogenic sarcoma mimicking left atrial myxoma: clinical and two-dimensional echocardiographic features. J Am Coll Cardiol 1985; 1422–7.

36. Pearson AC, Labovitz AJ, Tatineni S, et al. Superiority of transesophageal echocardiography in detecting cardiac source of embolism in cerebral ischemia of uncertain origin. J Am Coll Cardiol 1991; 17:66–72.

37. Hanley PC, Tajik AJ, Hynes JK, et al. Diagnosis and classification of atrial septal aneurysm by two-dimensional echocardiography: report of 80 consecutive cases. J Am Coll Cardiol 1985; 6: 1370–82.

38. Belkin RN, Hurwitz BJ, Kisslo J. Atrial septal aneurysm: association with cerebrovascular and peripheral embolic events. Stroke 1987; 18:856–62.

39. Longhini C, Brunazzi C, Musacci G, et al. Atrial septal aneurysm—echopolycardiographic study. Am J Cardiol 1985; 56:653–66.

40. Gallet B, Malergue MC, Adamas C, et al. Atrial septal aneurysm—a potential cause of systemic embolization. An echocardiographic study. Br Heart J 1985; 53:292–7.

41. Belkin RN, Kisslo J. Atrial septal aneurysm: recognition and clinical relevance. Am Heart J 1990; 120:948–57.

42. Silver MD, Dorsey JS. Aneurysms of the septum primum in adults. Arch Pathol Lab Med 1978; 102:62–5.

43. Belkin RN, Waugh RA, Kisslo J. Interatrial shunting in atrial septal aneurysm. Am J Cardiol 1986; 57:310–2.

44. Wysham DG, McPherson DD, Kerber RE. Asymptomatic aneurysm of the interatrial septum. J Am Coll Cardiol 1984; 4:1311–4.

45. Barnett HJ, Boughner DR, Taylor DW, et al. Further evidence relating mitral-valve prolapse to cerebral ischemic events. N Engl J Med 1980; 302:139–44.

46. Sandok BA, Guiliani ER. Cerebral ischemic events in patients with mitral valve prolapse. Stroke 1982; 13:448–50.

47. Sharma AK, Ofili E, Castello R, et al. Effect of treatment on recurrent embolic events with atrial septal aneurysm and associated right to left shunting (abstr). J Am Soc Echocardiog 1991; 4:294.

48. Hiss RG, Lamb LE. Electrocardiographic findings in 122,043 individuals. Circulation 1962; 25:947–61.

49. Kopecky SL, Gersh BJ, McGoon MD, Whisnant JP, Holmes DR, Ilstrup DM, Frye RL. The natural history of lone atrial fibrillation. N Engl J Med 1987; 317:669–74.

50. Kannel WB, Abbott RD, Savage DD, McNamara PM. Epidemiologic features of chronic atrial fibrillation: The Framingham Study. N Engl J Med 1982; 306:1018–22.

51. Kitchin AH, Milne JS. Longitudinal survey of ischaemic heart disease in a randomly selected sample of older population. Br Heart J 1977; 39:889–93.

52. Phillips SJ, Whisnant JP, O'Fallon WM, Frye RL. Prevalence of cardiovascular disease and diabetes mellitus in residents of Rochester, Minnesota. Mayo Clin Proc 1990; 65:344–59.

53. Santamaria J, Graus F, Peres J. Cerebral embolism and anticoagulation. Neurology 1983; 33:1104.

54. Coplen S, Antman E, Berlin J, Hewitt P, Chalmers T. Efficacy and safety of quinidine therapy for maintenance of sinus rhythm after cardioversion. A meta-analysis of randomized control trials. Circulation 1990; 82:1106–16.

55. The Cardiac Arrhythmia Suppression Trial (CAST) Investigators. Preliminary report: effect of encainide and flecainide on mortality in a randomized trial of arrhythmia suppression after myocardial infarction. N Engl J Med 1989; 321:406–12.

56. Moe G, Abidskov J. Atrial fibrillation as a self-sustaining arrhythmia independent of focal discharge. Am Heart J 1959; 58:59–70.

57. Moe G. On the multiple wavelet hypothesis of atrial fibrillation. Arch Int Pharmacodyn Ther 1962; 140:183–8.

58. Kaseda S, Zipes D. Contraction-excitation feedback in the atria. A cause of changes in refractoriness. J Am Coll Cardiol 1988; 11:1327–36.

59. Corr P, Yamada K, Witkowski F. Mechanisms controlling cardiac autonomic function and their relation to arrhythmogenesis. In: Fozzard H et al., eds. The heart and cardiovascular system. New York: Raven Press, 1986:1343–1403.

60. Stroke Prevention in Atrial Fibrillation Investigators. Stroke Prevention in Atrial Fibrillation Study: final results. Circulation 1991; 84:527–39.

61. Kaplan B, Langendorf R, Lev M, Pick A. Tachycardia-bradycardia syndrome (so called "sick sinus syndrome"): pathology, mechanisms, and treatment. Am J Cardiol 1973; 31:497–508.

62. Takahashi N, Seki A, Imataka K. Clinical features of paroxysmal atrial fibrillation. An observation of 94 patients. Jpn Heart J 1981; 22:143–9.

63. Forfar J, Miller H, Toft A. Occult thyrotoxicosis: a correctable cause of "idiopathic" atrial fibrillation. Am J Cardiol 1979; 44:9–12.

64. Kopecky S, Gersh B, McGoon M, Whisnant J, Holmes D, Ilstrup D, Frye R. The natural history of long atrial fibrillation. N Engl J Med 1987; 317:669–74.

65. Henry WL, Morganroth J, Pearlman AS, Clark CE, Redwood DR, Itscoitz SB, Epstein SE. Relation between left atrial size and atrial fibrillation. Circulation 1976; 53:273–9.

66. Hoglund C, Rosenhamer G. Echocardiographic left atrial dimension as a predictor of maintaining sinus rhythm after cardioversion of atrial fibrillation. Acta Med Scand 1985; 217:411–5.

67. Ewy G, Ulfers L, Hager W, Rosenfeld A, Roeske W, Goldman S. Response of atrial fibrillation to therapy: role of etiology and left atrial diameter. J Electrocardiol 1980; 13:119–24.

68. Dittrich HC, Erickson JS, Schneiderman T, Blacky AR, Savides T, Nicod PH. Echocardiographic and clinical predictors for outcome of elective cardioversion of atrial fibrillation. Am J Cardiol 1989; 63:193–7.

69. Olsson SB, Orndahl G, Enestrom S, Eskilsson J, Persson S, Grennert M, Johansson B. Spontaneous reversion from long-lasting atrial fibrillation to sinus rhythm. Acta Med Scand 1980; 207:5–20.

70. Falk R, Knowlton A, Bernard S, Gotlieb N, Battinelli N. Digoxin for converting recent-onset atrial fibrillation to sinus rhythm. Ann Intern Med 1987; 106:503–6.

71. Fenster P, Comess K, March R, Katzenberg C, Hager W. Conversion of atrial fibrillation to sinus rhythm by acute intravenous procainamide infusion. Am Heart J 1983; 106:501–4.

72. Rinkenberger R, Prystowsky E, Heger J, Troup P, Jackman W, Zipes D. Effects of intravenous and chronic oral verapamil administration in patients with supraventricular tachyarrhythmias. Circulation 1980; 62:996–1009.

73. Ellenbogen K, Dias V, Plumb V, Heywood J, Mirvis D. A placebo-controlled trial of continuous intravenous diltiazem infusion for 24-hour heart rate control during atrial fibrillation and atrial flutter: a multicenter study. J Am Coll Cardiol 1991; 18:891–7.

74. Platia E, Michelson E, Porterfield J, Das G. Esmolol versus verapamil in the acute treatment of atrial fibrillation or atrial flutter. Am J Cardiol 1989; 63:925–9.

75. Borgeat A, Goy J, Maendly R, Kaufmann U, Grbic M, Sigwart U. Flecainide versus quinidine for conversion of atrial fibrillation to sinus rhythm. Am J Cardiol 1986; 58:496–8.

76. Van Gelder I, Crijns H, Van Gilst W, Van Wijk L, Hamer H, Lie K. Efficacy and safety of

flecainide acetate in the maintenance of sinus rhythm after electrical cardioversion of chronic atrial fibrillation or atrial flutter. Am J Cardiol 1989; 64:1317–21.

77. Antman E, Beamer A, Cantillion C, McGowan N, Goldman L, Friedman P. Long-term oral propafenone therapy for suppression of refractory symptomatic atrial fibrillation and atrial flutter. J Am Coll Cardiol 1988; 12:1005–11.

78. Antman E, Beamer A, Cantillon C, McGowan N, Friedman P. Therapy of refractory symptomatic atrial fibrillation and atrial flutter: a staged care approach with new antiarrhythmic drugs. J Am Coll Cardiol 1990; 15:698–707.

79. Gold R, Haffajee C, Charos G, Sloan K, Baker S, Alpert J. Amiodarone for refractory atrial fibrillation. Am J Cardiol 1986; 57:124–7.

80. Juul-Moller S, Edvardsson N, Rehnqvist-Ahlberg N. Sotalol versus quinidine for the maintenance of sinus rhythm after direct current conversion of atrial fibrillation. Circulation 1990; 82: 1932–9.

81. Selzer A, Wray HW. Quinidine syncope: paroxysmal ventricular fibrillation occurring during treatment of chronic atrial arrhythmias. Circulation 1964; 30:17–26.

82. Kerber R, Jensen S, Grayzel J, Kennedy J, Hoyt R. Elective cardioversion: influence of paddle-electrode location and size on success rates and energy requirements. N Engl J Med 1981; 305: 658–62.

83. Mann D, Maisel A, Atwood J, Engler R, LeWinter M. Absence of cardioversion-induced ventricular arrhythmias in patients with therapeutic digoxin levels. J Am Coll Cardiol 1985; 5: 882–8.

84. Levy A, Lacombe P, Cointe R, Bru P. High energy transcatheter cardioversion of chronic atrial fibrillation. J Am Coll Cardiol 1988; 12:514–8.

85. Benditt D, Kriett J, Tobler H, Benson DJ, Fetter J, Chevalier P. Cardioversion of atrial tachyarrhythmias by low energy transvenous technique. In: Cardiac pacing: proceedings of the Seventh World Symposium on Cardiac Pacing. 1983.

86. Lown B, Perlroth M, Kaidbey S, Abe Y, Harken D. Cardioversion of atrial fibrillation. N Engl J Med 1963; 269:325–31.

87. Morris J, Peter R, McIntosh H. Electrical conversion of atrial fibrillation. Immediate and long-term results and selection of patients. Ann Intern Med 1966; 65:216–31.

88. Radford M, Evans D. Long-term results of DC reversion of atrial fibrillation. Br Heart J 1968; 30:91–6.

89. McCarthy C, Varghese P, Barritt D. Prognosis of atrial arrhythmias treated by electrical counter shock therapy. Br Heart J 1969; 31:496–500.

90. Waris E, Kreus K, Salokannel J. Factors influencing persistence of sinus rhythm after DC shock treatment of atrial fibrillation. Acta Med Scand 1971; 189:161–6.

91. Lundstrom T, Ryden L. Chronic atrial fibrillation: longterm results of direct current conversion. Acta Med Scand 1988; 223:53–9.

92. Van Gelder I, Crijns H, Van Gilst W, Verwer R, Lie K. Prediction of uneventful cardioversion and maintenance of sinus rhythm from direct-current electrical cardioversion of chronic atrial fibrillation and flutter. Am J Cardiol 1991; 68:41–6.

93. Henry W, Morganroth J, Pearlman A, Clark C, Redwood D, Itscoitz S, Epstein S. Relation between echocardiographically determined left atrial size and atrial fibrillation. Circulation 1976; 53:273–9.

94. Halpern S, Ellrodt G, Singh B, Mandel W. Efficacy of intravenous procainamide infusion in converting atrial fibrillation to sinus rhythm: relation to left atrial size. Br Heart J 1980; 44:589–95.

95. Ewy G, Ulfers L, Hager W, Rosenfeld A, Roeske W, Goldman S. Response of atrial fibrillation to therapy: role of etiology and left atrial diameter. J Electrocardiol 1980; 13:119–24.

96. Dethy M, Chassat C, Roy D, Mercier L. Doppler echocardiographic predictors of recurrence of atrial fibrillation after cardioversion. Am J Cardiol 1988; 62:723–6.

97. Zipes D, Klein L, Miles W. Nonpharmacologic therapy: can it replace antiarrhythmic drug therapy? J Cardiovasc Electrophysiol 1991; 2:S225–72.

98. Cox J, Boineau J, Shuessler R, Ferguson B, Cain M, Lindsay B, Corr P, Kater K, Lappas D. Successful surgical treatment of atrial fibrillation. JAMA 1991; 266:1976–80.

99. Guiraudon G, Klein G, Sharma A, Yee R. Surgery for atrial flutter, atrial fibrillation, and atrial tachycardia, In: Zipes D, Jalife J, eds. Cardiac electrophysiology. From cell to bedside. Philadelphia: W.B. Saunders, 1990:915–20.

100. Rosenqvist M, Brandt J, Schuller H. Atrial versus ventricular pacing in sinus node disease: a treatment comparison study. Am Heart J 1986; 111:292–7.

101. Sutton R, Kenny R. The natural history of sick sinus syndrome. Pace 1986; 9:1110–4.

102. Mancini J, Goldberger A. Cardioversion of atrial fibrillation: consideration of embolization, anticoagulation, prophylactic pacemaker, and long-term success. Am Heart J 1982; 104:617–21.

103. Manning W, Leeman D, Gotch P, Come P. Pulsed Doppler evaluation of atrial mechanical function after electrical cardioversion of atrial fibrillation. J Am Coll Cardiol 1989; 13:617–23.

104. The Stroke Prevention in Atrial Fibrillation Investigators. Predictors of thromboembolism in atrial fibrillation: II. Echocardiographic features of patients at risk. Ann Intern Med 1992; 116:6–12.

105. Crijns H, Van Gelder I, Van Gilst W, Hillege H, Gosselink A, Lie K. Serial antiarrhythmic drug treatment to maintain sinus rhythm after electrical cardioversion for chronic atrial fibrillation or atrial flutter. Am J Cardiol 1991; 68:335–41.

106. Stroke Prevention in Atrial Fibrillation Investigators. Design of a multicenter randomized trial for the Stroke Prevention in Atrial Fibrillation Study. Stroke 1990; 21:538–45.

107. Boston Area Anticoagulation Trial for Atrial Fibrillation Investigators. The effect of low-dose warfarin on the risk of stroke in nonrheumatic atrial fibrillation. N Engl J Med 1990; 323: 1505–11.

108. Connolly SJ, Laupacis A, Gent M, et al. Canadian Atrial Fibrillation Anticoagulation (CAFA) Study. J Am Coll Cardiol 1991; 18:349–55.

109. Ezekowitz MD, Bridgers SL, James KE, Carliner NH, Colling CL, Gornick CC, et al. and SPINAF Investigators. Warfarin in the prevention of stroke associated with nonrheumatic atrial fibrillation. N Engl J Med 1992; 327:406–12.

110. Petersen P, Boysen G, Godtfredsen J, et al. Placebo-controlled, randomized trial of warfarin and aspirin for prevention of thromboembolic complications in chronic atrial fibrillation: The Copenhagen AFASAK Study. Lancet 1989; 1:175–9.

111. Hull R, Hirsh J, Jay R, et al. Different intensities of oral anticoagulant therapy in the treatment of proximal-vein thrombosis. N Engl J Med 1982; 307:1676–81.

112. Stroke Prevention in Atrial Fibrillation Study Group Investigators. Preliminary report of the Stroke Prevention in Atrial Fibrillation Study. N Engl J Med 1990; 322:863–8.

113. Sherman DG, Goldman L, Whiting RB, Jurgensen K, Kaste M, Easton JD. Thromboembolism in patients with atrial fibrillation. Arch Neurol 1984; 41:708–10.

114. Wolf PA, Kannel WB, McGee DL, Meeks SL, Bharucha NE, McNamara PM. Duration of atrial fibrillation and imminence of stroke: The Framingham Study. Stroke 1983; 14:699–693.

115. Fisher CM. Reducing risks of cerebral embolism. Geriatrics 1979; 34:59–66.

116. Sage JI, Van Uitert RL. Risk of recurrent stroke in patients with atrial fibrillation and non-valvular heart disease. Stroke 1984; 14:537–40.

117. Yamanouchi H, Shimada H, Tomonaga M, Matsushita S. Recurrence of embolic stroke in non-valvular atrial fibrillation (NVAF). An autopsy study. Acta Neurol Scand 1989; 80:123–9.

118. Darling RC, Austin WG, Linton RR. Arterial embolism. Surg Gynecol Obstet 1967; 124: 106–14.

119. Kelley RE, Berger JR, Alter M, Kovacs AG. Cerebral ischemia and atrial fibrillation: prospective study. Neurology 1985; 34:1285–91.

120. Hart RG, Coull BM, Hart D. Early recurrent embolism associated with nonvalvular atrial fibrillation: a retrospective study. Stroke 1983; 14:688–93.

121. Walker MD. Atrial fibrillation and anti-thrombotic prophylaxis: a prospective metaanalysis. Lancet 1989; 1:325–6.

122. Campbell A, Caird FI, Jackson TFM. Prevalence of abnormalities of electrocardiogram in old people. Br Heart J 1974; 36:1005–11.

123. Wolf PA, Dawber TR, Thomas HE, Kannel WB. Epidemiologic assessment of chronic atrial fibrillation and risk of stroke: The Framingham Study. Neurology 1978; 28:973–7.

124. Fukuda Y, Makamura K. The incidence of thromboembolism and the hemocoagulative background in patients with rheumatic heart disease. Jpn Circ J 1984; 48:59.

125. Barker PS, Bohning AL, Wilson FN. Auricular fibrillation in Grave's disease. Am Heart J 1932; 8:121–7.

126. Yuen RW, Gutteridge DH, Thompson PL, Robinson JS. Embolism in thyrotoxic atrial fibrillation. Med J Aust 1979; 1:630–1.

127. Godtfredsen J. Atrial fibrillation: etiology, course and prognosis: a follow-up study of 1,212 cases (thesis). Copenhagen: University of Copenhagen, 1975.

128. Nakazawa HK, Sakurai K, Hamada N, Momotani N, Ito K. Management of atrial fibrillation in the post-thyrotoxic state. Am J Med 1982; 72:903–6.

129. Presti CF, Hart RG. Thyrotoxicosis, atrial fibrillation and embolism. Am J Cardiol 1965; 16: 52–3.

130. Navab A, La Due JS. Postconversion systemic arterial embolism. Am J Cardiol 1965; 16:52–3.

131. Ikram H, Nixon PG, Arcan T. Left atrial function after electrical conversion to sinus rhythm. Br Heart J 1968; 30:80–3.

132. DeSilva RA, Lown B. Cardioversion for atrial fibrillation—indications and complications. In: Kulbertus HE, Olsson SB, Schlepper M, eds. Atrial fibrillation. Molndal, Sweden: AB Hassle, 1982:231–9.

133. Rose G, Baxter PJ, Reid DD, McCartney P. Prevalence and prognosis of electrocardiographic findings in middle-aged men. Br Heart J 1978; 40:636–43.

134. Atrial Fibrillation Investigators: Risk Factors for Stroke and Efficacy of Antithrombotic Therapy in Atrial Fibrillation: Analysis of Pooled Data from Five Randomized Controlled Trials. (Personal Communication)

Paradoxical Embolization: Diagnosis and Management

Eric K. Louie
Loyola University Medical Center, Stritch School of Medicine, Maywood, Illinois

Michael L. Dewar
Yale University School of Medicine, New Haven, Connecticut

Michael D. Ezekowitz
Yale University School of Medicine, West Haven Veterans Affairs, and Cardiovascular Thrombosis Research Laboratory, New Haven, Connecticut

I. INTRODUCTION

The preponderance of systemic emboli arise from sources in the left-sided cardiac chambers or from systemic arterial-to-arterial embolization (1,2). These common causes of systemic embolization are covered in other chapters of this book. Systemic embolization may also arise from the venous circulation or the right heart chambers, and this phenomenon is termed *paradoxical embolization* (2). The gist of the paradox lies in the fact that the embolized material is not filtered from the circulation by the pulmonary capillaries; instead it transits to the systemic arterial circulation by an occult (e.g., patent foramen ovale) or manifest (e.g., atrial septal defect, ventricular septal defect, patent ductus arteriosus, pulmonary arterio-venous malformation) right-to-left shunt (2–5). Such documentation of paradoxical embolization has been by either (1) definite pathologic demonstration (2,6) or (2) presumptive diagnosis based on a constellation of clinical observations and predisposing conditions (3–5,7,8).

Definitive evidence for paradoxical embolization across a patent foramen ovale has been provided at autopsy from patients who have elongated thrombi traversing the foramen ovale and extending into both atria in association with systemic venous thrombi, pulmonary emboli, and evidence for systemic arterial embolization (2,5) (Fig. 1). Evidence during life for paradoxical transit of venous thrombi has on rare occasion been obtained by echocardiography (9–11). Sustained systemic arterial oxygen desaturation in the absence of abnormalities in pulmonary gas exchange provides indirect evidence for a significant right-to-left shunt and the substrate for paradoxical embolization. Such shunting is persistent in cyanotic congenital heart diseases (Table 1). In patients with apparently normal hearts, saline contrast echocardiographic studies have provided visual evidence in vivo that the echogenic micro-

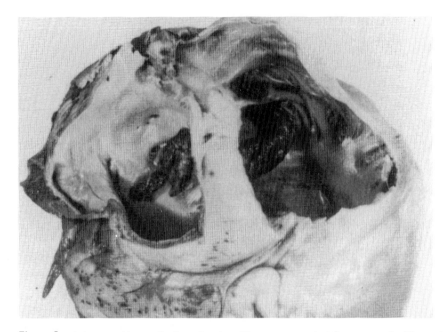

Figure 1 Autopsy evidence of a thrombus transiting across a patent foramen ovale. The postmortem specimen of the heart is viewed from its posterior aspect with both atria unroofed. An elongated thrombus extends from the right atrium, across a patent foramen ovale, into the left atrium in this 50-year-old man with bilateral pulmonary emboli and thrombosis of both femoral veins. (From Ref. 6.)

Table 1 Congenital Cardiac Conditions with Potential for Right-to-Left Shunting

I.	Interatrial communications
	a. Primum (partial atrioventricular canal defect) atrial septal defect
	b. Secundum atrial septal defect
	c. Sinus venosus atrial septal defect
	d. Patent foramen ovale
II.	Anomalous systemic venous drainage
	Left superior vena cava to left atrium
III.	Patent ductus arteriosus
IV.	Ventricular septal defects (with right ventricular systolic hypertension)
V.	Complete atrioventricular canal defects
VI.	Tetralogy of Fallot
VII.	Aortopulmonary window
VIII.	Postsurgical conditions
	a. Atrial septal defect with periprosthetic patch leak
	b. Ventricular septal defect with periprosthetic patch leak
	c. Fenestrated Fontan repair

cavitations in the right heart blood pool can intermittently traverse the atrial septum and enter the left heart blood pool, usually via a patent foramen ovale or a small atrial septal defect. Under the appropriate physiological circumstances (e.g., acute right ventricular hypertension due to pulmonary embolism), the right-to-left shunting may be sustained, resulting in systemic arterial desaturation (12–14). Under these conditions, when systemic arterial embolization occurs in association with manifest venous disease, it is possible that shunting across the foramen ovale represents the path of paradoxical embolization (10). Further support for this mechanism of systemic embolization is the demonstration of paradoxical systemic air embolism through a patent foramen ovale in patients undergoing neurosurgical procedures in the upright position (12). Venous air entrapment in the systemic venous circulation is a common accompaniment (30–40% prevalence of venous air embolism) of intracranial explorations performed in the seated position, and paradoxical air embolization of systemic arteries across a patent foramen ovale has been reported in two cases (15).

In most clinical circumstances there are insufficient data to make a definitive diagnosis of paradoxical systemic embolization. The clinician must make a presumptive diagnosis based on four cardinal findings (4,5): (1) an identifiable embolic source; (2) a potential or manifest communication between the systemic venous and systemic arterial circulations; (3) appropriate physiological conditions favoring right-to-left shunting across this communication, and (4) a systemic arterial embolic event (Table 2). An array of noninvasive and invasive tests are used to diagnose systemic arterial embolization, characterize manifest and potential intracardiac shunts, and identify systemic venous intravascular masses capable of paradoxical embolization. In patients with systemic embolism of obscure origin, paradoxical embolization from an occult venous thrombosis across an unrecognized patent foramen ovale becomes the major diagnostic consideration.

Table 2 Diagnostic Criteria for Clinical Diagnosis of Paradoxical Embolization

I. Embolic source
   a. Systemic venous thrombosis
   b. Intravascular systemic venous tumor (e.g., renal cell carcinoma, hepatocellular carcinoma)
   c. Thrombus or tumor (e.g., atrial myxoma) within the right heart chambers
   d. Vegetations of the right-sided cardiac valves
II. Communication between the right and left heart circulations that bypasses the pulmonary capillaries
   a. Manifest cardiac defects (e.g., atrial septal defect, ventricular septal defect, patent ductus arteriosus)
   b. Potential intracardiac shunt (e.g., patent foramen ovale)
   c. Pulmonary arteriovenous malformations (e.g., hereditary hemorrhagic telangiectasia syndrome)
III. Physiologic conditions predisposing to right-to-left shunting
   a. Chronic pulmonary hypertension
   b. Acute pulmonary hypertension (e.g., pulmonary embolism)
   c. Transient elevation of right heart pressures in excess of left heart pressures (e.g., Valsalva release, coughing
   d. Aberrant flow redirection across a patent foramen ovale
IV. Systemic arterial embolization

II. MECHANISMS OF PARADOXICAL EMBOLIZATION ACROSS A PATENT FORAMEN OVALE

Normally the flap valve of the foramen ovale formed by the septum primum closes during the early neonatal period as left atrial pressure rises above right atrial pressure, displacing the septum primum against the left atrial side of the septum secundum. In the majority of persons the septum primum fuses to the septum secundum, obliterating the foramen ovale. In a minority of persons the foramen ovale remains patent. One autopsy survey of 965 hearts, from patients ranging in age from 1 to 100 years, found the foramen ovale to be patent in 27.3% of patients (16). The incidence of anatomic patency of the foramen ovale declined progressively with age (34.3% for ages 1–29 years, 25.4% for ages 30–79 years, and 20.2% for ages 80–99 years). There was no sex predilection for patency of the foramen ovale in this series.

The mere presence of an anatomically patent foramen ovale is insufficient evidence to secure the diagnosis of paradoxical embolization across the defect. Several pathophysiologic conditions predispose to right-to-left shunting across the patent foramen ovale. Chronic pulmonary hypertension resulting from pulmonary disease can result in a persistent elevation in right atrial pressure, in excess of left atrial pressure, causing right-to-left shunting across an anatomically patent foramen ovale. Acute elevations in pulmonary artery pressure, such as may occur following hemodynamically compromising pulmonary embolism, may set the stage for right atrial hypertension and thus may result in right-to-left shunting across the patent foramen ovale (2–6,17). The simultaneous occurrence of a systemic and pulmonary embolus is particularly suggestive of paradoxical embolism. Venous thrombosis provides the potential source for both the systemic and the pulmonary emboli, and the pulmonary hypertension resulting from the pulmonary embolus establishes the physiological mechanism for right-to-left shunting.

Sustained elevations in right ventricular and right atrial pressure, however, are not required to cause right-to-left interatrial shunting across a patent foramen ovale. Transient increases in right atrial pressure above left atrial pressure can result in right-to-left shunting in patients with normal pulmonary artery pressures (13,16). Saline contrast echocardiographic techniques have demonstrated transient right-to-left interatrial shunting across the patent foramen ovale following respiratory maneuvers (Valsalva release, coughing, positive end-expiratory pressure ventilation) that temporarily increase right atrial pressure in excess of left atrial pressure in persons with normal pulmonary artery pressures (13–14,17–20). The pathophysiologic significance of these observations is heightened by the observation that the microcavitations noted by echocardiographic techniques may cross the interatrial septum and then subsequently produce characteristic auditory and spectral changes in the transcranial Doppler measurements of blood flow in the right middle cerebral artery (21). While "paradoxical embolization" of microbubbles may be insufficient to cause neurological sequelae (22–23), it does demonstrate the mechanism for larger emboli to cross the patent foramen ovale and occlude cerebral vessels. It is particularly worth noting that in the series of five patients with paradoxical embolization to the systemic circulation reported by Jones et al. (5), three patients experienced the onset of symptoms following straining while defecating. This maneuver presumably mimicked Valsalva release, permitting right-to-left interatrial shunting of embolic material across the patent foramen ovale in these patients.

During fetal life, venous return from the inferior vena cava preferentially streams across the patent foramen ovale (patency is obligatory for a normal fetal circulation), while venous return from the superior vena cava is directed across the tricuspid valve and out the right ventricular outflow tract. In the adult with a persistently patent foramen ovale (3) or an overt atrial septal defect (4), indicator dilution curves performed by selective injection into the two venae cavae demonstrate that when a transient right-to-left shunt occurs, it often originates from the inferior vena cava. Recently, we have reported the preferential streaming of superior vena cava flow across a patent foramen ovale caused by a right atrial mass that acted as a baffle (13) (Fig. 2). Venoarterial shunting across the patent foramen ovale in this patient resulted in sustained systemic oxygen desaturation and paradoxical embolization to the basilar artery of the brain (proven at autopsy) in the absence of pulmonary hypertension and despite mean right atrial pressures that were 4 mm Hg less than mean pulmonary capillary wedge pressures.

In summary, overt pulmonary hypertension, transient elevation of right atrial pressures with reversal of the normal transatrial septal pressure gradient, and preferential streaming of venous return can result in right-to-left shunting across a patent foramen ovale, providing a pathophysiological mechanism for venous thrombi to reach the systemic circulation and embolize to peripheral systemic arteries.

III. DIAGNOSIS OF PARADOXICAL EMBOLIZATION

As outlined in Table 2, in the absence of direct pathological or imaging evidence of emboli actually traversing a patent foramen ovale, the clinical diagnosis of paradoxical embolism is based on the demonstration of a source (e.g., deep venous thrombosis), a communication (e.g., anatomically patent foramen ovale), physiologic conditions favoring right-to-left shunting, and the documentation of a systemic embolic event. The greater the certainty of these diagnostic features, the higher the probability that the diagnosis of paradoxical embolism is correct. In this chapter we shall focus on the diagnosis of deep venous thrombosis as the most common source, and patent foramen ovale as the usual communication in adults free of manifest intracardiac communications.

A. Diagnosis of Deep Venous Thrombosis

The clinical diagnosis of deep venous thrombosis is unreliable, lacking both sensitivity and specificity (24,25). Therefore, the diagnosis should be confirmed by reliable objective tests. Historically, contrast venography (see Chap. 10) was recognized as the diagnostic standard, but limitations of this technique have led to the development of alternative tests. Venography is difficult to perform in critically ill patients; it is invasive and can be painful; and it is not suitable for repeated examinations. Rarely it can induce thrombosis and produce hypersensitivity reactions to the contrast material. In addition, technical difficulties can occur, even in the most experienced hands, and as a consequence approximately 10% of venograms are inadequate for interpretation (26). For this reason, a concerted effort has been made to develop alterative noninvasive diagnostic modalities (24,27–34). Of these noninvasive techniques, impedance plethysmography (IPG) and duplex ultrasound (DU) are commonly used, and platelet imaging and magnetic resonance imaging may play an adjunctive role in centers with this capability.

Blood flow through the lower extremity is dependent on the position of the limb and the degree of muscle activity. In the supine position the pressures in the venous system are

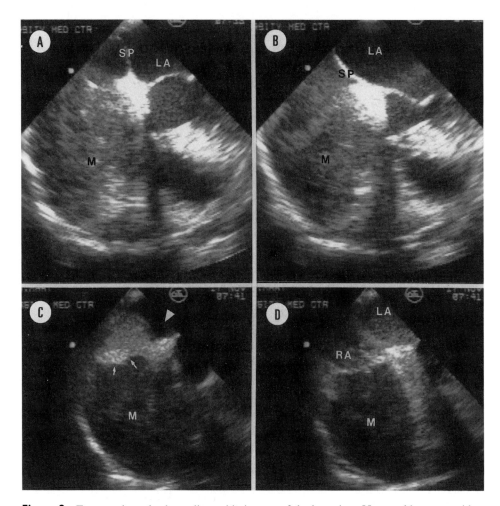

Figure 2 Transesophageal echocardiographic images of the heart in a 55-year-old woman with a right atrial mass. The patient suffered paradoxical embolization across a patent foramen ovale that resulted in a basilar artery occlusion confirmed at autopsy. (A) The septum primum (SP) of the fossa ovalis separates the left atrium (LA) from the right atrium, which contains a tumor mass (M) confirmed at autopsy. Throughout most of the cardiac cycle the septum primum was deflected toward the left atrium. (B) Transiently during each cardiac cycle, the septum primum returned to the plane of the interatrial septum (compare with panel A). (C) Following peripheral venous saline contrast administration, the right atrium is opacified, outlining (small arrows) the margin of the less echodense mass (M). Right-to-left shunting of saline contrast across the patent foramen ovale is evidenced by the presence of saline contrast within the left atrium (solid triangle). (D) In a stop-frame image that was obtained after that depicted in panel C, the left atrium becomes densely opacified by the systemic venous saline contrast injectate. Review of the entire video sequence in real time demonstrated that the stream of saline contrast from the superior vena cava was directed across the patent foramen ovale by the right atrial mass, resulting in opacification of the left atrium that was greater than that of the right ventricle. The redirection of superior vena caval flow across the atrial septum resulted in systemic arterial desaturation. Cerebral embolization subsequently resulted from dislodgement of a thrombus from the superior vena cava during positioning of a central venous catheter. Mean right atrial pressure was 4 mm Hg less than pulmonary capillary wedge pressure. There was no pressure gradient across the tricuspid valve. (From Ref. 13.)

slightly greater than that in the right atrium, and filling therefore is primarily hydraulic. Large volumes of blood are expelled from the deep venous system of the legs with each contraction of the muscles of the calf and thigh. Most flow is carried in the deep venous system, which is embedded in the muscles of the leg except in the area of the ankle, where the veins are superficial. The most distal part of the system is the plantar arch, which continues as the lateral plantar veins and is joined by the medial plantar veins. The anterior tibial veins and the peroneal veins all merge in the upper calf to form the popliteal vein, which continues as the superficial femoral vein and is later joined by the deep femoral vein in the proximal thigh. This ultimately forms the common femoral vein, which leads into the external iliac vein at the level of inguinal ligament. The normal venous anatomy of the lower limb can be divided into four categories: (1) the deep vein; (2) the deep muscle veins; (3) the superficial veins; and (4) the communicating or perforating veins. The superficial veins are found in the subcutaneous fascia and communicate with the deep system through the communicating or perforating veins. The veins contain valves that not only direct flow from the superficial to the deep system, but also facilitate flow centrally.

1. Impedance Plethysmography

Impedance plethysmography (see also Chap. 10) is a noninvasive bedside technique that has a high sensitivity for proximal thrombi and can be used to follow patients serially. The major disadvantages of this technique are that it is relatively insensitive for calf vein thrombi and that it requires considerable technical expertise. Sources of false-positive tests are (1) external compression; (2) poor patient positioning; (3) venous compression by pelvic masses; (4) muscle tensing; (5) arterial insufficiency; (6) increased venous pressures due to heart failure or constrictive pericarditis; and (7) vasoconstriction secondary to shock. False-negative results occur (1) when thrombi are nonocclusive; (2) when collateral circulation circumvents occlusive thrombi; or (3) when skin-stretching artifact is present.

2. Ultrasound

Venous ultrasonography (see also Chap. 7) is a noninvasive bedside test that requires minimal patient cooperation, is easily repeatable, and has high sensitivity and specificity for proximal vein thrombosis. It can be employed in amputees and patients who are in traction. The major disadvantages of the technique are that it is relatively insensitive for calf vein thrombosis and that interpretation requires observer expertise. False-positive studies may result from external venous compression, poor patient positioning, and evaluation of thrombi lodged in Hunter's canal. False-negative studies occur with nonocclusive thrombi, calf vein thrombi, abundant collateral circulation, and improper probe positioning.

3. Contrast Venography

Contrast venography (see also Chap. 10) is an accurate method for determining the presence of venous thrombosis (35–37). This is an invasive procedure that allows direct visualization of the radiographic patency of the venous system. The method generally used is that of Rabinov and Paulin (35), which involves positioning the patient in the semierect manner on a tilting fluoroscopic table. The patient supports himself on his unaffected leg, and the leg to be injected is left completely free. Injection is made through a small-caliber needle into the distal superficial dorsal vein. The injected dye is monitored fluoroscopically with multiple spot films and overhead radiographs taken over the entire leg. In a normal study all deep and superficial veins would be opacified. The most reliable signs of a deep venous thrombosis are the direct signs of venous thrombosis: a constant, sharply delineated filling defect on all films in different projections. Indirect signs are suggestive but not diagnostic of deep venous thrombosis. These indirect signs include abrupt termination of opacification of a vein, nonopacification of a vein, or the abnormal diversion of contrast through collateral flow. These indirect signs may also be caused by edema, cellulitis, muscle rupture, hematoma, or periarticular cysts. Chronic venous disease results in thin intraluminal streaky defects with irregular venous margins, the absence of venous valves, and the presence of large collaterals. False-positive venograms may also be caused by weight bearing or tensing of muscles during injection, causing incomplete filling of the deep venous system. Tourniquets, once proposed as an aid in filling the deep venous system, also may prevent their filling. Defects due to improper radiopaque dye mixing may occur and simulate clots. Severe systemic reactions after venography are fortunately rare (38–40). Muscle cramps may occur during venography, and the contrast agent may actually induce symptomatic deep venous thrombosis. Fortunately, the use of nonionic, low-osmolarity contrast material has decreased adverse reactions to dye.

4. Magnetic Resonance Imaging of Venous Thrombosis

It is possible to image patients from the right atrium to the ankle in 20 min using magnetic resonance imaging (see also Chap. 8) (41). The advantage of this technique is that it is highly accurate and, in our experience, provides a 100% correlation with venography. Not only is it possible to identify venous thrombi, but the technique may also identify conditions that enter into the differential diagnosis of venous thrombosis. The disadvantage of this technology is that it is expensive and that patients have to be moved to the instrument, precluding the bedside examination of the critically ill patient.

5. Platelet Scintigraphy

Platelet scintigraphy (see also Chap. 8) involves the intravenous injection of indium 111–labeled autologous platelets to patients suspected of an acute deep venous thrombosis. Platelet scintigraphy performed within 3 h of injection of labeled platelets is relatively insensitive (42), although specific, for the diagnosis of acute deep venous thrombosis, precluding its use as the sole diagnostic test in patients with clinically suspected venous thrombosis. These findings in *symptomatic* patients are in sharp contrast to the high sensitivity and specificity of platelet imaging as a screening test for asymptomatic venous thrombosis in patients who have hip surgery (28). The explanation for these apparently contradictory observations may reside in the fact that patients with symptomatic deep venous thrombosis may have older thrombi that are inactive (not actively incorporating platelets) at the time of diagnostic testing. False-positive tests are uncommon but occur when nonvenous thrombi are found in the imaging field. False-negative results are obtained predominantly from patients with old thrombi and anticoagulated patients.

6. Overview of Diagnostic Tests for Deep Venous Thrombosis

Both impedance plethysmography and duplex ultrasound are accurate methods for diagnosing venous thrombosis in symptomatic patients. The higher sensitivity of duplex ultrasound suggests that of the two tests, it is the noninvasive technique of choice. The specificity of duplex ultrasound is increased, without loss of sensitivity, if the region of Hunter's canal is excluded from the examination. Since neither duplex ultrasound nor impedance plethysmography detects calf vein thrombosis, a "negative" test should be followed with serial testing on days 3 and 7 to detect proximal extension of calf vein thrombosis and progression of initially nonocclusive proximal vein thrombosis (33,34,43–47). This recommendation is based on the observation that clinically important pulmonary embolism occurs rarely if the thrombus remains confined to the calf (48). On the other hand, approximately 20% of calf vein thrombi extend into the proximal venous segment, and these thrombi can be detected readily by serial testing (44). In hospitals where platelet imaging is available, sensitivity can be enhanced when the duplex ultrasound or impedance plethysmography examination is negative. Because of the long half-life of the isotope, surveillance is possible for the following 5 to 7 days without reinjection of labeled platelets. Where doubt exists regarding diagnosis, contrast venography should be performed if no contraindication exists. Magnetic resonance imaging is an accurate test that may also be useful when the diagnosis is in doubt.

B. Diagnosis of Patent Foramen Ovale

Transthoracic two-dimensional echocardiography can provide detailed images of the anatomy of the interatrial septum. Transesophageal echocardiography extends this capability to the many adult patients who have technically suboptimal transthoracic studies. Not only can overt atrial septal defects be identified (49–51) with these techniques, but it is also possible to routinely image the fossa ovalis as a central thinning of the atrial septum, comprising the septum primum acting as the flap valve to the foramen ovale. Normally, the septum primum is tightly applied to the left side of septum secundum, the limbus of the fossa ovalis (13,52,53) (Fig. 3). When the foramen ovale is patent, the septum primum is often redundant and has phasic deflections during the cardiac cycle (53). In the extreme situation, the protrusion of the septum primum beyond the plane of the atrial septum may be so exaggerated that the septum primum forms an actual atrial septum aneurysm (54,55).

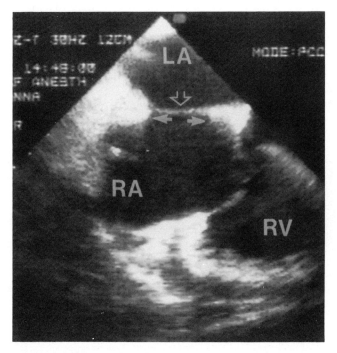

Figure 3 Stop-frame image from a transesophageal echocardiogram illustrating the anatomy of the fossa ovalis. The left atrium (LA) is in the near field. The right atrium (RA) and right ventricle (RV) are in the far field. The interatrial septum, which separates the two atria, has a central thinning represented by the septum primum (open arrow) which is the flap valve of the foramen ovale and when applied to the septum secundum forms the fossa ovalis (delimited by the pair of small arrows).

While it has been postulated that atrial septal aneurysms may serve as a source for left atrial thrombus formation and systemic embolization, atrial septal aneurysms are also associated with overt secundum atrial septal defects as well as patency of the foramen ovale (55,56) and may thus be associated with paradoxical embolization (57–61).

Evidence for patency of the foramen ovale and the potential for right-to-left interatrial shunting can be demonstrated by the intravenous administration of saline contrast during the echocardiographic examination of the atrial septum (20,52,53,62,63). A 0.9% normal saline solution is agitated between two interconnected 10 ml syringes. *Macroscopic* air entrapment is avoided. The resultant suspension of *microbubbles* is injected intravenously in a rapid bolus. This provides echodense opacification of the blood pool of the right atrium, which is imaged echocardiographically. In the presence of a patent foramen ovale microbubbles can be imaged crossing the atrial septum either spontaneously or following maneuvers such as Valsalva release (63) or coughing (20). Even the transient elevation of right atrial pressure above left atrial pressure by such maneuvers can induce right-to-left atrial shunting of saline contrast (Fig. 4). In general, "hand-agitated" saline solutions produce relatively large microbubbles (diameter = 24–180 μ) that cannot pass through the pulmonary capillaries (64,65). Thus the appearance of saline contrast in the left heart chambers must result from venoarterial shunting. To distinguish transatrial septal passage of saline contrast from intrapulmonary shunting (as may occur via pulmonary arteriovenous malformations), microbubbles should be imaged by echocardiography as they traverse the atrial septum, and they should appear in the left atrium within three cardiac cycles of full opacification of the right atrium (21,66). By contrast, intrapulmonary shunting will result in a significant delay in the appearance of microbubbles in the left atrium (66), and they will be detected initially in the pulmonary veins, not at the fossa ovalis. Use of more viscous echocardiographic blood pool contrast agents (e.g., 70% dextrose or an admixture of saline and autologous blood) (21,64) or mechanical ultrasonication techniques (64) results in smaller, more uniform

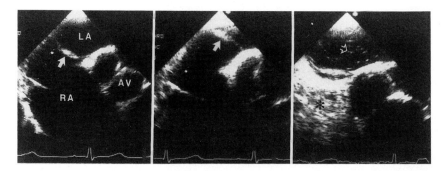

Figure 4 A series of stop-frame images from a transesophageal echocardiographic study of the interatrial septum illustrating mobility of the septum primum of the fossa ovalis and right-to-left shunting of systemic venous saline contrast across a patent foramen ovale. All three panels show comparable views of the left atrium (LA), right atrium (RA), and aortic valve (AV). Left panel. The septum primum (solid arrow) bows slightly toward the right atrium, reflecting left atrial pressures that are higher than right atrial pressures. Middle panel. In a stop frame following that illustrated in the left panel, the septum primum (solid arrow) is noted to be mobile and to deflect toward the left atrium. The curvature of the septum primum is now convex with respect to the left atrium (which contrasts with the situation illustrated in the left panel), indicating that right atrial pressure now exceeds left atrial pressure. Right panel. Systemic venous saline contrast administration fully opacifies the right atrium (asterisk) and traverses the patent foramen ovale to enter the left atrium (open arrow).

microbubbles with the capability of transpulmonary passage through the pulmonary capillaries. Thus, these techniques are less suited for identifying right-to-left shunting across a patent foramen ovale.

Employing saline contrast techniques in conjunction with transthoracic echocardiography in a relatively young (mean age 27 years) population of healthy volunteers, Lynch et al. (63) found an 18% prevalence of interatrial right-to-left shunting presumably due to patency of the foramen ovale. This prevalence of *functional* right-to-left shunting is substantially lower than the prevalence of *anatomic* patency of the foramen ovale found in autopsy series (16). The discrepancy may relate to the inability of some individuals to reverse the trans–atrial septal pressure gradient with respiratory maneuvers. This may be a frequent occurrence in patients with left heart disease and abnormally elevated left atrial pressures (67), but it is generally not a problem in cooperative subjects without apparent heart disease. In any event, the demonstration of the *potential for right-to-left atrial shunting* may be more relevant than the demonstration of *anatomic* patency of the foramen ovale for predicting risk for paradoxical embolization. Another reason for the relatively low rate of detection of right-to-left atrial shunting by transthoracic echocardiography may be related to technical considerations. In adults, transesophageal echocardiography provides superior anatomic imaging of the atrial septum and higher detection rates of patent foramen ovale as compared with transthoracic echocardiography, even when echocardiographic contrast techniques are used (14,68–71). Recently we have examined the prevalence of patent foramen ovale in an adult population undergoing cardiac surgery using intraoperative saline contrast transesophageal echocardiography. Positive airway pressure release was used to mimic Valsalva release (53). In this population of patients (mean age 62 years), without prior history of stroke, there was a 22% prevalence of right-to-left interatrial shunting through a patent foramen ovale. This is slightly lower than the 25.4% prevalence of anatomic patency of the foramen ovale in persons of comparable age reported at autopsy (16).

There are recent reports using color-flow Doppler, in conjunction with transthoracic and transesophageal echocardiography, as a means of detecting interatrial shunting across the patent foramen ovale (72). Defects in the fossa ovalis created by transseptal catheter passage during percutaneous mitral valvuloplasty have also been detected using this approach (14,73). Color Doppler is useful for detecting both right-to-left and left-to-right shunting across a patent foramen ovale, and it may help to localize the anatomic discontinuity in the fossa ovalis. In persons with apparently normal hearts, the trans–atrial septal pressure gradient across a patent foramen ovale is usually small. Hence the low flow velocities across the patent foramen ovale may be difficult to detect and differentiate from *normal* low-velocity blood flow in the vicinity of the fossa ovalis. In addition, color-flow imaging may be disrupted by provocative maneuvers (e.g., coughing or Valsalva release) that are used to elevate right atrial pressure over left atrial pressure (72), whereas saline contrast imaging is less disrupted during such provocative maneuvers. On the other hand, color Doppler imaging may be the preferred technique for detecting left-to-right interatrial shunts, since the negative saline contrast effect (contrast-free left atrial blood displacing contrast opacification in the right atrium) may be difficult to identify if the shunt is small.

C. Masses in the Right Heart as Sources for Paradoxical Embolization

Masses on the right side of the heart, apart from tricuspid endocarditis, are quite rare but represent potential sources for paradoxical embolization. Examples are thrombi, primary and secondary tumors, and masses related to heart valves. Right-sided thrombi usually originate in the venous system and transit through the heart. However, thrombi may also form de novo in patients with dilated right atria, atrial fibrillation, or depressed right ventricular systolic function.

Tumors of the heart are uncommon but may present in protean ways. Cardiac myxomas are by far the most common cardiac tumors and may occur infrequently on the right side of the heart as opposed to their more common location in the left atrium. Myxomas in the right atrial cavity constitute about 20% of all myxomas (74). If they produce tricuspid valve obstruction the resulting elevation in right atrial pressure will favor paradoxical embolization across a patent foramen ovale. Atrial myxomas may pass through the foramen ovale, and in these rare instances will be shaped like a dumbbell (75). Discreet myxomas may also coexist in each atrium (76). Malignant tumors of the heart are fortunately quite rare. Primary malignant tumors are almost always sarcomas. Angiosarcomas usually originate in the right atrium or pericardium and are intensely vascular (77). Rhabdomyosarcomas are the next most frequent primary sarcomas of the heart and may occur in any chamber (78,79). Secondary malignant tumors of the heart are 20 to 40 times more common than primary tumors (80,81). Secondary spread to the heart occurs by direct contiguous growth from adjacent structures, lymphatic spread, or direct growth along or inside the venae cavae or pulmonary veins. Carcinoid tumors rarely metastasize to the heart and pericardium and produce distinctive endocardial and valvular lesions involving the right side of the heart, with the propensity for atrial dilation and clot formation (82). Hypernephromas arising from the kidney and hepatocellular carcinoma arising from the liver may spread in the inferior vena cava and produce a mass effect in the right side of the heart.

To pose an embolic threat, secondary malignant tumors of the heart must involve or extend through the endocardial surface of the heart and be sufficiently friable for tumor emboli to break off. In decreasing order of frequency, the parietal pericardium and epicardium, the myocardium, and the endocardium are sites of malignant metastases (83). Breast and lung carcinoma commonly metastasize to the pericardium and epicardium by regional lymphatic invasion, whereas malignant melanoma and lymphomas metastasize to the myocardium by hematogenous spread (83). Direct metastases to the endocardium are uncommon, but when they occur the tumor is most often hematologic (83).

All of these mass lesions are well characterized by echocardiographic techniques, particularly if the masses are small and mobile. Transesophageal echocardiography is particularly useful (83–87) in the patient with suboptimal transthoracic acoustic windows. In addition, transesophageal echocardiography allows anatomical definition of the venous return to both atria, which may be important for defining the path of intravascular spread of malignant tumors to the heart. Other tomographic techniques such as ultrafast computed tomography and cine magnetic resonance imaging also are useful for imaging intracardiac masses, although the superior temporal resolution of echocardiography favors its use in the detection of small, highly mobile masses. The strength of x-ray computed tomography and magnetic resonance imaging lies in the ability to relate intracardiac masses to other extracardiac thoracic or abdominal structures. This is particularly valuable in the evaluation of local tumor invasion and the propagation of venous thrombi.

IV. IS PARADOXICAL EMBOLISM MORE COMMON THAN IS RECOGNIZED IN CLINICAL PRACTICE?

The incidence of paradoxical embolization as the mechanism responsible for systemic arterial embolism is difficult to quantify, because a definitive diagnosis is uncommon.

Satisfaction of the criteria for a presumptive diagnosis does not preclude the coexistence of alternative mechanisms for systemic embolism. In addition, anatomical patency of the foramen ovale is a relatively common morphologic variant, occurring in as many as 27.5% of autopsied patients (16), and occult deep venous thrombosis is a not infrequent occurrence in elderly, hospitalized, or ill patients. Thus, the identification of a patent foramen ovale in an elderly hospitalized patient does not establish it as the cause for systemic embolism, and a search for other sources of embolization must be made.

Investigators have focused their attention on younger patients with nonhemorrhagic stroke who are free of overt cardiac or arterial sources of systemic embolism, in order to define the prevalence of patent foramen ovale (and hence the risk for paradoxical embolization) relative to control populations (10,14). Using saline contrast transthoracic echocardiography, Harvey et al. (88) found evidence for right-to-left interatrial shunting in 8 of 11 consecutive patients (under the age of 50) who had suffered an embolic stroke but were free of clinical evidence of cardiac disease. Subsequent cardiac catheterization demonstrated that five of these patients had atrial septal defects. This surprisingly high incidence of clinically silent atrial septal defects with normal resting hemodynamics suggested that paradoxical embolization through small interatrial communications might be a significant cause for systemic embolism in young patients without overt clinical evidence for cardiac disease. Webster et al. (89) performed an age- and sex-matched controlled study of the incidence of right-to-left interatrial shunting, defined by transthoracic saline contrast echocardiography with the Valsalva maneuver, in 40 patients (less than 40 years of age) with nonhemorrhagic stroke or transient ischemic attacks. The 50% prevalence of right-to-left interatrial shunting (presumed due to a patent foramen ovale) in these young patients with stroke or transient ischemic attacks was significantly greater than the 15% prevalence ($p < 0.001$) found in controls. Among this select group of young patients, who were not expected to have arterial vascular disease as the etiology for their neurologic symptoms, it seems likely that paradoxical embolism through a patent foramen ovale may be an important mechanism for nonhemorrhagic stroke and transient ischemic attacks. Using transthoracic saline contrast echocardiography with the Valsalva maneuver, Lechat et al. (90) compared the incidence of right-to-left interatrial shunting in 60 patients (less than 55 years of age) with ischemic strokes with that in 100 age-matched control subjects undergoing routine contrast echocardiography before posterior fossa surgery (for routine determination of the risk for systemic air embolism). The stroke patients had a significantly higher incidence of right-to-left interatrial shunting (40% versus 10%, $p < 0.001$) than did controls. The patients with stroke but without other identifiable causes for stroke (n = 26) had the highest prevalence of right-to-left interatrial shunting (54%). These results suggest that paradoxical embolization, via a patent foramen ovale, may be a common mechanism for cerebral embolism among relatively young patients who do not have clinical evidence for alternative sources of systemic embolization. These observations have been extended to more elderly patients by a recent cross-sectional study employing nested case-control analysis of patients with cryptogenic stroke (91). Patients who had nonhemorrhagic stroke with cryptogenic source (n = 45) were compared with patients having determined sources (n = 101) with respect to the prevalence of patent foramen ovale, defined by transthoracic saline contrast echocardiography and the Valsalva maneuver. The prevalence of patent foramen ovale was higher in patients with cryptogenic stroke for those less than 55 years of age (48% versus 4%, $p < 0.001$). Multiple logistic regression analysis identified patent foramen ovale as a risk factor for cryptogenic stroke *irrespective of patient age* after correction for recognized risk factors for stroke.

Transesophageal saline contrast echocardiography now provides a highly sensitive means of detecting patent foramen ovale (53). Preliminary communications of data obtained with this technique have conflicted with regard to the prevalence of patent foramen ovale in patients with cryptogenic nonhemorrhagic stroke. A recently published report from de Belder et al. (92) does suggest that the prevalence of patent foramen ovale, defined by transesophageal echocardiography is higher (26%) in patients with cryptogenic stroke or peripheral arterial emboli than in patients with recognized risk factors for embolism or stroke (14%) or subjects undergoing transesophageal echocardiography (3.2%) for unrelated reasons. Implicit in such an analysis is the assumption that selection biases incurred in defining the subgroups for analysis did not influence the results. The authors acknowledge that their overall detection rate for patent foramen ovale was unusually low (3.2% for "control" subjects), relative to the 22% prevalence defined in other relatively nonselective series (53). In another study, Hausmann et al. (93), using transesophageal echocardiographic techniques, detected a patent foramen ovale in 50% of young patients ($<$ 40 years of age) with otherwise unexplained ischemic stroke, a significantly higher percentage than the 22% prevalence among control subjects. Obviously, future studies will require blinded analyses of carefully matched control subjects to assess the value of transesophageal echocardiography in identifying patent foramen ovale as a risk factor for embolic stroke.

V. TREATMENT

The assessment of paradoxical embolization as a potential mechanism for systemic embolization demands a diligent search for systemic venous and right heart chamber sources for embolic material. While occult venous thrombosis is probably the most common source, the possibility of intravascular or intracardiac tumor or vegetations should not be overlooked. The latter possibility should be particularly sought in patients with an indwelling intravascular prosthetic device (e.g., pacemaker lead, chronic venous access, etc.). Therapy is directed toward the primary source of the embolus as well as the communication through which it has passed. In the case of deep venous thrombosis, anticoagulation with intravenous heparin followed subsequently by oral warfarin is the treatment of choice (10,90). In 1980 a National Institutes of Health consensus panel suggested that thrombolytic therapy was not being used often in patients with thromboembolic disease (94). In the treatment of deep venous thrombosis, thrombolytic therapy may prevent venous valve damage and subsequent venous stasis as well as effect rapid clearance of the clot. Clinical trials comparing streptokinase with heparin (95–100) were of insufficient size to determine both efficacy and safety. Pooled analyses by Goldhaber (101) found that streptokinase was more efficient than heparin but that major bleeding complications were more frequent with streptokinase than with heparin. There is also evidence that tissue plasminogen activator may hold promise for the treatment of venous thrombosis. If anticoagulation or thrombolysis is not possible or is unsuccessful, consideration should be given to caval filtration to prevent recurrent embolization, with the understanding that this may not be a complete solution if collateral venous channels develop or thrombus develops proximal to the filtration device. Since occult pulmonary embolism concurrent with systemic embolism is always a risk, and may be a contributing factor to the mechanism for paradoxical embolization, diagnostic studies (e.g., radionuclide ventilation-perfusion lung scanning) to exclude pulmonary embolism are appropriate in most patients. Primary closure of the cardiac defect should be considered, particularly if it is hemodynamically significant. This is unfortunately not possible when the defect is complicated by severe fixed pulmonary hypertension. In unusual circumstances where an intracardiac thrombus is identified traversing the interatrial septum (10–12) consideration should be given to prompt surgical removal. Where communications of a more complex nature exist, the feasibility of surgical correction may be governed by the underlying pathophysiology and anatomy.

VI. PREVENTION

In patients in whom a substrate for a paradoxical embolism exists (i.e., a communication between the right and left sides of the heart and a high risk for venous thrombosis), prophylactic measures to prevent venous thrombosis should be employed while the patient is at bed rest. Nonpharmacological prophylaxis against deep venous thrombosis includes stockings, electrical stimulation of calf muscles, and intermittent compression of the calf muscles using an external compressor. Favorable effects have been seen with all these measures (101–104). Pharmacological approaches that have been used include fixed low-dose heparin, adjusted low-dose heparin, dextran, aspirin, and warfarin. Success has been demonstrated with all these agents, but the optimal prophylaxis against deep venous thrombosis remains an unresolved issue. Many physicians rely on early ambulation and graded-compression stockings to prevent deep venous thrombosis, and it is reasonable to combine fixed low-dose subcutaneous heparin with graded-compression stockings to prevent deep venous thrombosis. For patients at greater risk of venous thrombosis, higher-dose heparin therapy (or full anticoagulation) and intermittent calf compression may be appropriate.

REFERENCES

1. Edwards EA, Tilney N, Lindquist RR. Causes of peripheral embolism and their significance. JAMA 1966; 196:119–38.
2. Thompson T, Evans W. Paradoxical embolism. Quart J Med 1930; 23:135–50.
3. Gazzaniga AB, Dalen JE. Paradoxical embolism: its pathophysiology and clinical recognition. Ann Surg 1970; 171:137–42.
4. Meister SG, Grossman W, Dexter L, Dalen JE. Paradoxical embolism, diagnosis during life. Am J Med 1972; 53:292–8.
5. Jones HR Jr, Caplan LR, Come PC, Swinton NW Jr, Breslin DJ. Cerebral emboli of paradoxical origin. Ann Neurol 1983; 13:314–9.
6. Corrin B. Paradoxical embolism. Br Heart J 1964; 26:549–53.
7. Poole-Wilson PA, May ARL, Taube D. Paradoxical embolism complicating massive pulmonary embolus. Thorax 1976; 31:354–5.
8. Richey WA, Jaques PF. Paradoxical embolism in morbidly obese patients. Radiology 1977; 123:43–6.
9. Nellessen V, Daniel WG, Matheis G, Oelert H, Depping K, Lichtten PR. Impending paradoxical embolism from atrial thrombus: correct diagnosis by transesophageal echocardiography and prevention by surgery. J Am Coll Cardiol 1985; 5:1002–4.
10. Loscalzo J. Paradoxical embolism: clinical presentation, diagnostic strategies, and therapeutic options. Am Heart J 1986; 112:141–5.
11. Gin KG, Thompson CR, Jue J, Ling H. Embolic occlusion of a patent foramen ovale: a cause of false negative contrast echocardiogram. J Am Soc Echocardiog 1992; 5:444–6.
12. Shenoy MM, Vijaykumar PM, Friedman SA, Grief E. Atrial septal aneurysm associated with systemic embolism and interatrial right to left shunt. Arch Intern Med 1987; 147:605–6.
13. Langholz D, Louie EK, Konstadt SN, Rao TLK, Scanlon PJ. Transesophageal echocardiographic demonstration of distinct mechanisms for right to left shunting across a patent foramen ovale in the absence of pulmonary hypertension. J Am Coll Cardiol 1991; 18:1112–7.

14. Movsowitz C, Podolsky LA, Meyerowitz CB, Jacobs LE, Kotler MN. Patent foramen ovale: a nonfunctional embryological remnant or a potential cause of significant pathology. J Am Soc Echocardiog 1992; 5:259–70.

15. Gronert BA, Messick JM Jr, Cucchiara RF, Michenfelder JD. Paradoxical air embolism from a patent foramen ovale. Anesthesiology 1979; 50:548–9.

16. Hagen PT, Scholz DG, Edwards WD. Incidence and size of patent foramen ovale during the first 10 decades of life: an autopsy study of 965 normal hearts. Mayo Clin Proc 1984; 59:17–20.

17. Shaw RC, Ludbrook PA, Weiss AN, Weldon CS. Massive pulmonary embolism permitting paradoxical systemic arterial embolism: successful surgical management. Ann Thorac Surg 1976; 22:293–5.

18. Cheng TO. Paradoxical embolism, a diagnostic challenge and its detection during life. Circulation 1976; 53:565–8.

19. Kronik G, Mosslacher H. Positive contrast echocardiography in patients with patent foramen ovale and normal right heart hemodynamics. Am J Cardiol 1982; 49:1806–9.

20. Dubourg O, Bourdarias JP, Farcot JC, Gueret P, Terdjman M, Ferrier A, Rigaud M, Bardet JC. Contrast echocardiographic visualization of cough-induced right to left shunt through a patent foramen ovale. J Am Coll Cardiol 1984; 4:587–94.

21. Nemec JJ, Marwick TH, Lorig RJ, Davison MB, Chimowitz MI, Litowitz H, Salcedo EE. Comparison of transcranial Doppler ultrasound and transesophageal contrast echocardiography in the detection of interatrial right to left shunts. Am J Cardiol 1991; 68:1498–1502.

22. Bommer WJ, Shah PM, Allen H, Meltzer R, Kisslo J. The safety of contrast echocardiography: report of the committee on contrast echocardiography for the American Society of Echocardiography. J Am Coll Cardiol 1984; 3:6–13.

23. Gillam LD, Kaul S, Fallon JT, Levine RA, Hedley-Whyte T, Guerrero JL, Weyman AE. Functional and pathologic effects of multiple echocardiographic contrast injections on the myocardium, brain and kidney. J Am Coll Cardiol 1985; 6:687–94.

24. Hull R, Hirsh J, Sackett DL, et al. Replacement of venography in suspected venous thrombosis by impedance plethysmography and I-125 fibrinogen leg scanning. A less invasive approach. Ann Intern Med 1981; 94:12–15.

25. Wheeler HB, Anderson FA. Diagnostic approaches for deep vein thrombosis. Chest 1986; 89: 407S–412S.

26. Rabinov K, Paulin S. Roentgen diagnosis of venous thrombosis in the leg. Arch Surg 1972; 104: 133–44.

27. Heaton WA, Davis HH, Welch MJ, et al. Indium 111: a new radionuclide label for studying human platelet kinetics. Br J Haematol 1979; 42:613–22.

28. Ezekowitz MD, Pope CF, Sostman HD, et al. Indium-111 platelet scintigraphy for the diagnosis of acute venous thrombosis. Circulation 1986; 73:668–74.

29. Langsfeld M, Hershey FB, Thorpe L. Duplex B-mode imaging for the diagnosis of deep venous thrombosis. Arch Surg 1987; 122:587–91.

30. Lensing AW, Prandoni P, Brandjes D, et al. Detection of deep-vein thrombosis by real-time B mode ultrasonography. N Engl J Med 1989; 320:342–5.

31. White RH, McGahan JP, Daschbach MM, Hartling RP. Diagnosis of deep-vein thrombosis using duplex ultrasound. Ann Intern Med 1989; 111:297–304.

32. Hull RD, Van Aken WG, Hirsh J, et al. Impedance plethysmography using the occlusive cuff technique in the diagnosis of venous thrombosis. Circulation 1976; 53:696–700.

33. Vogel P, Laing FC, Jeffrey RB Jr, et al. Deep venous thrombosis of the lower extremity: US evaluation. Radiology 1987; 163:747–51.

34. Rosner NH, Doris PE. Diagnosis of femoropopliteal venous thrombosis: comparison of duplex sonography and plethysmography. Am J Radiol 1988; 150:623–7.

35. Rabinov K, Paulin S. Roentgen diagnosis of venous thrombosis of the leg. Arch Surg 1972; 104:134.

36. Hull R, Hirsh J, Sackett DL, et al. Cost-effectiveness of clinical diagnosis venography and non-

invasive testing in patients with symptomatic deep-vein thrombosis. N Engl J Med 1981; 304:1561.

37. Hull R. Current approach to diagnosis of deep vein thrombosis. Mod Con Cardiovasc Dis 1982; 51:129.

38. Bettmann MA, Paulin S. Leg phlebography: the incidence, nature and modification of undesirable side effects. Radiology 1977; 122:101.

39. Coel MN, Dodge W. Complication rate with supine phlebography. Am J Radiol 1978; 131:821.

40. Thomas ML, McAllister V, Tonge K. Simplified phlebography in deep venous thrombosis. Clin Radiol 1971; 22:490.

41. Pope CF, Dietz MJ, Ezekowitz MD, Gore JC. Technical variables influencing the detection of acute deep vein thrombosis by magnetic resonance imaging. Magn Reson Imag 1990; 9:3.

42. Farlow DC, Ezekowitz MD, Ran Rao S, et al. The value of early image acquisition after administration of indium-111 platelets in patients with suspected acute deep venous thrombosis. Am J Cardiol 1989; 64:363–8.

43. Appelman PT, De Jong TE, Lampmann LE. Deep venous thrombosis of the leg: US findings. Radiology 1987; 163:743–6.

44. Philbrick JT, Becker DM. Calf deep vein thrombosis. A wolf in sheep's clothing? Arch Intern Med 1988; 148:2131–8.

45. Cronan JJ, Dorfman GS, Grusmark J. Lower extremity deep venous thrombosis: further experience with and refinements of US assessment. Radiology 1988; 168:101–7.

46. Barnes RW, Nix ML, Barnes CL, et al. Perioperative asymptomatic venous thrombosis: role of duplex scanning versus venography. J Vasc Surg 1989; 9:251–60.

47. Foley DW, Middleton WD, Lawson TL, et al. Color Doppler ultrasound imaging of lower-extremity venous disease. Am J Radiol 1989; 152:371–6.

48. Hull RD, Raskob GE, Coates G, et al. A new noninvasive management strategy for patients with suspected pulmonary embolism. Arch Intern Med 1989; 149:2549–55.

49. Hanrath P, Schluter M, Langenstein BA, Polster J, Engel S, Kremer P, Krebber H-J. Detection of ostium secundum atrial septal defects by transesophageal cross-sectional echocardiography. Br Heart J 1983; 49:350–8.

50. Morimoto K, Matsuzaki M, Tohma Y, Ono S, Tanaka N, Michishige H, Murata K, Anno Y, Kusukawa R. Diagnosis and quantitative evaluation of secundum-type atrial septal defect by transesophageal Doppler echocardiography. Am J Cardiol 1990; 66:85–91.

51. Kronzon I, Tunick PA, Goldfarb A, Freedberg RS, Chinitz L, Slater J, Schwinger ME, Gindea AJ, Glassman E, Daniel WG. Echocardiographic and hemodynamic characteristics of atrial septal defects created by percutaneous valvuloplasty. J Am Soc Echocardiog 1990; 3:64–71.

52. Konstadt SN, Louie EK, Black S, Rao TLK, Scanlon P. Intraoperative detection of patent foramen ovale by transesophageal echocardiography. Anesthesiology 1991; 74:212–6.

53. Louie EK, Konstadt SN, Rao TLK, Scanlon PJ. Transesophageal echocardiographic diagnosis of potential interatrial shunting across the foramen ovale in adults without prior stroke. J Am Coll Cardiol 1993; 21:1231–7.

54. Silver MD, Dorsey JS. Aneurysms of the septum primum in adults. Arch Pathol Lab Med 1978; 102:62–5.

55. Hanley PC, Tajik AJ, Hynes JK, Edwards WD, Reeder GS, Hagler DJ, Seward JB. Diagnosis and classification of atrial septal aneurysm by two-dimensional echocardiography: report of 80 consecutive cases. J Am Coll Cardiol 1985; 6:1370–82.

56. Belkin RN, Waugh RA, Kisslo J. Interatrial shunting in atrial septal aneurysm. Am J Cardiol 1986; 57:310–2.

57. Gallet B, Malergue MC, Adams C, Saudemont JP, Collot AMC, Druon MC, Hiltgen M. Atrial septal aneurysm—a potential cause of systemic embolism. Br Heart J 1985; 53:292–7.

58. Belkin RN, Hurwitz BJ, Kisslo J. Atrial septal aneurysm: association with cerebrovascular and peripheral embolic events. Stroke 1987; 18:856–62.

59. Zabalgoitia-Reyes M, Herrera C, Gandhi DK, Mehlman DJ, McPherson DD, Talano JV. A

possible mechanism for neurologic ischemic events in patients with atrial septal aneurysm. Am J Cardiol 1990; 66:761–4.

60. Schneider B, Hanrath P, Vogel P, Meinertz T. Improved morphologic characterization of atrial septal aneurysm by transesophageal echocardiography: relation to cerebrovascular events. J Am Coll Cardiol 1990; 16:1000–9.

61. Pearson AC, Nagelhout D, Castello R, Gomez CR, Labovitz AJ. Atrial septal aneurysm and stroke: a transesophageal echocardiographic study. J Am Coll Cardiol 1991; 18:1223–9.

62. Fraker TD Jr, Harris PJ, Behar VS, Kisslo JA. Detection and exclusion of interatrial shunts by two-dimensional echocardiography and peripheral venous injection. Circulation 1979; 59:379–84.

63. Lynch JJ, Schuchard GH, Gross CM, Wann LS. Prevalence of right to left atrial shunting in a healthy population: detection by Valsalva maneuver contrast echocardiography. Am J Cardiol 1984; 53:1478–80.

64. Feinstein SB, Ten Cate FJ, Zwehl W, Ong K, Maurer G, Tei C, Shah PM, Meerbaum S, Corday E. Two-dimensional contrast echocardiography. I. In vitro development and quantitative analysis of echo contrast agents. J Am Coll Cardiol 1984; 3:14–20.

65. Teague SM, Sharma MK. Detection of paradoxical cerebral echo contrast embolization by transcranial Doppler ultrasound. Stroke 1991; 22:740–5.

66. Barzilai B, Waggoner AD, Spessert C, Picus D, Goodenberger D. Two-dimensional echocardiography in the detection and follow-up of congenital pulmonary arteriovenous malformations. Am J Cardiol 1991; 68:1507–10.

67. Siostrzonek P, Lang W, Zangeneh M, Gossinger H, Stumpflen A, Rosenmayr G, Heinz G, Schwarz M, Zeiler K, Mosslacher H. Significance of left sided heart disease for the detection of patent foramen ovale by transesophageal contrast echocardiography. J Am Coll Cardiol 1992; 19:1192–6.

68. Pearson AC, Laboritz AJ, Tatineni S, Gomez CR. Superiority of transesophageal echocardiography in detecting cardiac source of embolism in patients with cerebral ischemia of uncertain etiology. J Am Coll Cardiol 1991; 17:66–72.

69. Siostrzonek P, Zangeneh M, Gossinger H, Lang W, Rosenmayr G, Heinz G, Strumpflen A, Zeiler K, Schwarz K, Mosslacher H. Comparison of transesophageal and transthoracic contrast echocardiography for detection of a patent foramen ovale. Am J Cardiol 1991; 68:1247–9.

70. Cujec B, Polasek P, Voll C, Schuaib A. Transesophageal echocardiography in the detection of potential cardiac source of embolism in stroke patients. Stroke 1991; 22:727–33.

71. Lee RJ, Bartzokis T, Yeoh T-K, Grogin HR, Choi D, Schnittger I. Enhanced detection of intra-ardiac sources of cerebral emboli by transesophageal echocardiography. Stroke 1991; 22:734–9.

72. Brickner ME, Grayburn PA, Fadel B, Carry MM, Eichhorn EJ, Lange RA, Taylor AL. Detection of patent foramen ovale by Doppler color flow mapping in patients undergoing cardiac catheterization. Am J Cardiol 1991; 68:125–9.

73. Yoshida K, Yoshikawa J, Akasaka T, Yamaura Y, Shakudo M, Hozumi T, Fukaya T. Assessment of left to right atrial shunting after percutaneous mitral valvuloplasty by transesophageal color Doppler flow mapping. Circulation 1989; 80:1521–6.

74. O'Neil MB Jr, Grehl TM, Hurley EH. Cardial myxomas: a clinical diagnostic challenge. Am J Surg 1979; 138:68.

75. Dashkoff N, Boersma RB, Nanda NC, Gramiak R, Anderson MN, Subramanian S. Bilateral atrial myxomas: echocardiographic considerations. Am J Med 1977; 62:792.

76. Fitteret JD, Spicer MJ, Nelson WP. Echocardiographic demonstration of bilateral atrial myxomas. Chest 1976; 70:282.

77. Bjerregaard P, Baandrup U. Haemangioendotheliosarcoma of the heart: diagnosis and treatment. Br Heart J 1979; 42:734.

78. Van Bruggen HW, de Koning J. Pulmonic stenosis caused by a malignant tumor of the heart. Am Heart J 1968; 76:526.

79. Schmaltz AA, Apitz J. Primary rhabdomyosarcoma of the heart. Pediatr Cardiol 1982; 2:73.

80. Prichard RW. Tumors of the heart: review of the subject and report of one hundred and fifty cases. Arch Pathol 1951; 51:98.

81. DeLoach JF, Haynes JW. Secondary tumors of heart and pericardium: review of the subject and report of one hundred thirty-seven cases. Arch Intern Med 1953; 92:224.

82. Strickman NE, Rossi PA, Massumkhani GA, Hall RJ. Carcinoid heart disease: a clinical, pathologic, and therapeutic update. Curr Probl Cardiol 1982; 6:1.

83. Rutherford JD, Sgroi DC. A 75 year old man with carcinoma of the colon and a right ventricular mass. N Engl J Med 1992; 327:1442–8.

84. Panidis IP, Kotler MN, Mintz GS, Ross J. Clinical and echocardiographic features of right atrial masses. Am Heart J 1984; 107:745–8.

85. Obeid AI, Marvasti M, Parker F, Rosenberg J. Comparison of transthoracic and transesophageal echocardiography in diagnosis of left atrial myxoma. Am J Cardiol 1989; 63:1006–8.

86. Mugge A, Daniel WG, Haverich A, Lichtlen PR. Diagnosis of noninfective cardiac mass lesions by two-dimensional echocardiography. Comparison of the transthoracic and trans-esophageal approaches. Circulation 1991; 83:70–8.

87. Edwards LC III, Louie EK. Transthoracic and transesophageal echocardiography for the evaluation of cardiac tumors, thrombi and valvular vegetations. Am J Cardiac Imag 1993; 7:(in press).

88. Harvey JR, Teague SM, Anderson JL, Voyles WF, Thadani U. Clinically silent atrial septal defects with evidence for cerebral embolization. Ann Intern Med 1986; 105:695–7.

89. Webster WI, Chancellor AM, Smith HJ, Swift DL, Sharpe DN, Bass NM, Glasgow GL. Patent foramen ovale in young stroke patients. Lancet 1988; 2:11–12.

90. Lechat P, Mas JL, Lascault G, Loron P, Theard M, Klimczac M, Drobinski G, Thomas D, Grosgogeat Y. Prevalence of patent foramen ovale in patients with stroke. N Engl J Med 1988; 318:1148–52.

91. Di Tullio M, Sacco RL, Gopal A, Mohr JR, Homma S. Patent foramen ovale as a risk factor for cryptogenic stroke. Ann Intern Med 1992; 117:461–5.

92. De Belder MA, Tourikis L, Leech G, Camm AJ. Risk of patent foramen ovale for thrombo-embolic events in all age groups. Am J Cardiol 1992; 69:1316–20.

93. Hausmann D, Mugge A, Becht I, Daniel WG. Diagnosis of patent foramen ovale by trans-esophageal echocardiography and association with cerebral and peripheral embolic events. Am J Cardiol 1992; 70:668–72.

94. Thrombolytic therapy in thrombosis: A National Institutes of Health consensus development conference. Ann Intern Med 1980; 93:141.

95. Robertson BR, Nilsson IM, Nylander G. Value of streptokinase and heparin in treatment of acute deep venous thrombosis: a coded investigation. Acta Chir Scand 1968; 134:203.

96. Kakkar VV, Flanc C, Howe CT. Treatment of deep vein thrombosis. A trial of heparin, streptokinase, and Arvin. Br Med J 1969; 1:806.

97. Robertson BR, Nilsson IM, Nylander G. Thrombolytic effect of streptokinase as evaluated by phlebography of deep venous thrombi of the leg. Acta Chir Scand 1970; 136:173.

98. Tsapogas MJ, Peabody RA, Wu KT, et al. Controlled study of thrombolytic therapy in deep vein thrombosis. Surgery 1973; 74:973.

99. Porter JM, Seaman AJ, Common HH, et al. Comparison of heparin and streptokinase in the treatment of venous thrombosis. Ann Surg 1975; 41:511.

100. Elliot MS, Immelman EJ, Jeffrey P, et al. A comparative randomized trial of heparin versus streptokinase in the treatment of acute proximal venous thrombosis. An interim report of a prospective trial. Br J Surg 1979; 66:838.

101. Goldhaber SZ, ed. Pulmonary embolism and deep venous thrombosis. Philadelphia: W.B. Saunders, 1985, pp. 121–133.

102. Wilkins RW, Mixter G Jr, Stanton JR, et al. Elastic stockings in the prevention of pulmonary embolism: a preliminary report. New Engl J Med 1952; 246:360.

103. Wilkins RW, Stanton JR. Elastic stockings in the prevention of pulmonary embolism. New Engl J Med 1953; 248:1087.

104. Makin GS. A clinical trial of "Turbigrip" to prevent deep venous thrombosis. Br J Surg 1969; 56:373.

The Aorta and the Carotid Arteries

Terence L. Chen
*Diablo Neurosurgery Medical Group, Inc.,
Walnut Creek, California*

Douglas Chyatte
Northwestern University Medical School, Chicago, Illinois

I. INTRODUCTION

The understanding of the etiology and management of extracranial cerebrovascular disease has undergone continuous evolution since ancient times. Head injuries resulting in hemiplegia and aphasia and the existence of a set of great arteries connecting the body to the head were described in the Edwin Smith Papyrus, which documented the general state of medical science in the Pyramidal Age (3000–2500 B.C.) (1). The truncal viscera were considered the locus of thought until the Greeks, and specifically Hippocrates, in the fourth and fifth century B.C. described apoplexy and were the first to theorize that the brain, and not the heart, directed the body (2). The influence of the Greek school of medicine is evident even today: the contralateral relationship between brain injury and paralysis was recognized by the Greeks, and the word "carotid" is derived from a Greek word meaning to stupefy or render into a deep sleep. The ancient Greeks were well aware of the significance of these arteries to maintaining consciousness.

Classical Greek paradigms were not challenged until centuries later, when Renaissance scholars and anatomists such as Variolus, Dryander, Berengarius, Da Vinci, Vesalius, and Fallopius advanced our knowledge of cerebral anatomy by studying dissected specimens (3). In the 17th century obstructive vascular disease involving the circle of Willis and carotid and vertebral arteries were described by Johann Wepfer, a contemporary of Thomas Willis. It was not until the late eighteenth and early nineteenth centuries that the two types of stroke, occlusive and hemorrhagic, were differentiated from other types of neurological diseases (4). The latter half of the 19th century saw further refinements in the understanding of cerebrovascular anatomy through the efforts of scientists such as Huebner, Charcot, Duret, Gowers, and Beevor.

These developments occurred concurrently with attempts at surgery on the extracranial carotid arteries. In 1808, Astley Cooper, a student of John Hunter, was the first to successfully ligate the carotid artery for treatment of a carotid aneurysm. This case was reported in the first volume of the Guy's Hospital Report of 1836. By the mid–19th century over 200 carotid artery ligations had been performed (5). The syndrome of ipsilateral blindness and contralateral weakness as a consequence of carotid artery thrombosis was first described by Ramsay Hunt in 1913 in an address to the American Neurological Association (6). Moniz, in the next decade, pioneered cerebral angiography and helped focus attention on the pathology of the carotid arteries (7). Much of the present-day understanding of cerebrovascular disease is based on the original contributions of Fisher and Adams (8,9).

The 1950s saw the birth of modern carotid surgery. In 1955 Carrea and his colleagues reported that 4 years earlier they had successfully resected a stenosed internal carotid artery and had reconstructed it using an end-to-end anastomosis with the proximal external carotid artery (10). In 1953 Strully and colleagues in New York reported an unsuccessful attempt at endarterectomy for a completely occluded carotid artery. The operation was aborted and the internal carotid artery was ligated when it became clear that the thrombus extended beyond reach and no backflow could be established (11). In the same year, on August 7, DeBakey and his colleagues in Houston performed a successful endarterectomy on an occluded carotid artery and were able to establish backflow (12). In the same paper they reported the fatal postoperative outcome of three patients. All were comatose and densely hemiplegic before the procedure. This was the first recognition that an important contraindication to endarterectomy is the presence of a recent major completed stroke. In 1954 in England, Eastcott and colleagues reported the successful reconstruction of an angiographically demonstrated stenotic internal carotid artery. The stenotic lesion was resected under hypothermia. The artery was reconstructed with an end-to-end anastomosis between the internal and common carotid arteries. The patient's transient monocular and hemispheric ischemia resolved without complication, and the patient lived another twenty years (13). In 1956, Cooley reported a successful carotid endarterectomy in a patient with an angiographically demonstrated stenosis of the common carotid artery that was located immediately below the bifurcation. This report also described the use of a temporary arterial shunt (14).

With these pioneering efforts, the prevention of stroke with an extracranial revascularization procedure became a reality. Significant complications remained. Perioperative stroke is always a risk of the procedure. Because the risks of angiography and surgery are significant, the appropriate selection of patients for operation is critical. One factor that makes this decision difficult is the lack of reliable natural history data for occlusive cerebrovascular disease.

II. ANATOMY AND PATHOPHYSIOLOGY

Extracranial cerebral arteries extend from the aortic arch to the sites of entry into the skull at the cranial base. The origins of the left common carotid artery and the brachiocephalic trunk are variable (15). The bifurcation of the common carotid artery usually occurs at the C4 vertebral body level and is a region particularly prone to the development of atherosclerotic plaques (16). Within the fork of the bifurcation lies the carotid sinus nerve complex. From the bifurcation, the cervical segment of the internal carotid artery extends to the foramen lacerum. In this region, the artery is relatively immobile and slightly anterior to the lateral mass of the atlas, where it is prone to injury. Distally, the internal carotid artery traverses the petrous temporal bone (17). The internal carotid artery then traverses the cavernous sinus, where it gives off the meningohypophyseal, semilunar, and meningeal arteries. The ophthalmic artery also arises from the cavernous carotid in 8% of the population (18). Most commonly it originates from the supraclinoid segment of the internal carotid.

The curious vulnerability of the carotid bifurcation to plaque formation has been ascribed to the local dynamics of flow. Flow studies of model bifurcations have demonstrated heterogeneous regions of high and low flow velocity, high and low shear stress, boundary layer separation, stagnation points, and secondary flow motions such as vortex and eddy formations (19,20). The specific characteristic(s) of flowing pulsating blood that potentiate(s) plaque formation is controversial. Most investigators believe that carotid lesions tend to localize in regions of low flow velocity, low shear stress, disordered flow patterns, and flow separation (21). This corresponds to the outer wall of the carotid sinus, opposite the flow divider. Regions of high-velocity laminar flow and high shear stress are the apex of the bifurcation, the inner wall of the sinus, and the distal internal carotid artery (22). Most flow studies fail to take into account the complexity of blood flow in a biological system. Blood is not a Newtonian fluid, arteries are elastic, not rigid conduits, and blood flow is pulsatile. These factors are thought to make only small differences (23,24). The pathogenesis of atherosclerosis and thrombus formation is ubiquitous within the vasculature and not believed to be unique to the carotid artery. The endothelium may play a pivotal role. Aging and short-term exercise may increase permeability (25,26), but the relationship of these findings to atherosclerosis is not known. Studies in cell-to-cell interactions, platelets, vasoactive substances, endothelial metabolism, and growth factors have advanced the field enormously and are too broad for the scope of this book.

A comprehensive understanding of cerebrovascular disease requires knowledge of the collateral circulations. There are two families of collateral vessels: those that are preexisting and able to immediately supply blood flow in the event of an acute occlusion, and those that develop over time in response to gradual vessel occlusion and tissue metabolic demands. To a certain extent the distinction is artificial, since vessels of the first group can also be developed and vessels of the second group must also be preexisting. Examples of extracranial collateral pathways are the inferior thyroid branch connecting with the superior thyroid branch of the external carotid artery; the ascending cervical artery connecting with the descending branch of the occipital artery; the occipital artery connecting with the vertebral artery via muscular branches; branches of thyrocervical and costocervical trunks that anastomose with their contralateral counterparts; and branches of the external carotid artery that communicate with their contralateral counterpart (27). Extracranial vessels form connections with intracranial vessels. Superficial temporal and occipital arteries connect with the cortical circulation via leptomeningeal branches. The ophthalmic artery forms a variety of collaterals with the external carotid circulation via leptomeningeal, lacrimal, ethmoidal, supratrochlear, and supraorbital branches. The best-known example of cerebrovascular collateral circulation is the circle of Willis. The functional importance of the circle is difficult to determine in any given person because of the wide variations in anatomy (28), but it is generally believed that anomalies of the circle of Willis contribute to a decrease in the tolerance of ischemia (29). Of little known significance is the presence of the primitive carotid-vertebrobasilar anastomoses such as the persistent trigeminal, acoustic, and hypoglossal arteries. These occur in about three of 1000 of the population (30).

III. CLINICAL ASPECTS

Stroke is the third most frequent cause of death in the United States, after heart disease and neoplasms. An estimated 400,000 to 500,000 new strokes occur each year (31). The fatality rate is between 30% and 40%. Of the survivors, only 10% will be unimpaired. Forty percent live with mild residual disability that interferes with activities of daily life, employment, and social function. Fully half of the survivors require special care or are institutionalized. About 16% of the residents of nursing facilities are stroke victims (32). The best treatment of stroke is prevention. This is achieved by education and the control of risk factors. These include hypertension, atheromatous disease, atrial fibrillation, congestive heart failure, smoking, hypercholesterolemia, diabetes mellitus, polycythemia, blood dyscrasias, and a previous transient ischemic attack (TIA) (33). Known risk factors that are uncontrollable are age, male sex, and race. It has been estimated that 70,000 new patients per year suffer TIAs in the United States. Half of these patients will have diagnostic studies demonstrating carotid atherosclerosis. Between 10% and 50% of stroke patients have had a warning TIA preceding the stroke (34,35). Several mechanisms may produce cerebral ischemia. Emboli are generally believed to cause most focal ischemic events including TIAs. Hemodynamic hypoperfusion is thought to be less common than emboli and responsible for events in which ischemia is diffuse or in watershed regions (36). In some cases, both mechanisms may coexist. In rare cases, investigators even postulate the existence of an intracranial steal phenomenon, though this is controversial (37).

A. Diagnosis

Symptoms of cerebral ischemia are categorized as transient ischemic attacks, reversible ischemic neurological deficits (RINDs), and cerebrovascular accidents (CVAs). Transient ischemic attacks are defined as focal ischemic neurological deficits that completely resolve within 24 h. Most TIAs actually last less than an hour. Transient ischemia of the retina producing temporary monocular blindness (amaurosis fugax) is considered a specific form of TIA (38). Clusters of TIAs in which the frequency dramatically increases are referred to as crescendo TIAs and are believed to represent an unstable cerebrovascular state. Reversible ischemic neurological deficits are neurological deficits that completely resolve but take more than 24 h. Irreversible neurological deficits are strokes or CVAs. "Stroke in evolution" refers to slow progressive cerebral ischemia manifesting over several hours to days and finally culminating in a completed stroke. The clinical manifestations of cerebral ischemia can vary widely, depending upon the particular territory of ischemic brain. Localization of the symptoms require a thorough and detailed clinical history, physical, and neurological examination.

Emboli generally arise from thrombus formation on the irregular surface of ulcerated plaques. Ulceration and severe stenosis both favor platelet adhesion (39). Emboli are usually platelet aggregates in a fibrin mesh (40). Occasionally a plaque may liberate atheromatous fragments and cholesterol emboli (41). Besides the carotid bifurcation, other extracranial arterial sources of emboli include the brachiocephalic trunk, the origin of the left common carotid artery, and the superior wall of the aortic arch (42).

Historically, the aorta has received little attention as a possible source of unexplained embolic stroke or other embolic phenomena. The aortic arch is usually not visualized in detail during routine transthoracic echocardiography, although with the introduction of transesophageal echocardiography it can now be seen with high resolution. By means of this technique, large, protrusive plaques in the aortic arch and descending aorta, which have mobile projections that move freely with the blood flow, have been identified in patients with embolic events (43). In a large series of patients with stroke, TIA, or peripheral emboli, the presence of protruding atheromas of the thoracic aorta was strongly related to the occurrence of embolic symptoms even when other known risk factors were considered. Protruding atheroma in the thoracic aorta can be detected by transesophageal echocardiography and should be considered as a cause of stroke, TIA, and peripheral emboli (44). Additionally, the stump of an occluded extracranial artery may generate emboli (45). Intracranial vessels rarely embolize. The exception is intracranial aneurysms, which often contain intraluminal clot (46).

It is postulated that an intraplaque hemorrhage frequently initiates the onset of symptoms in patients with carotid artery disease (47). Atheromatous emboli stream with the blood flow and often lodge at the bifurcation of arteries. They may undergo subsequent fragmentation, fibrinolysis, and molding that reduces their size and allows passage to smaller distal vessels (48). Ultimately, many atheromatous emboli lodge in small arteries with diameters of 100 μm or less. These are found in the retina or cerebral cortex (49). Ulceration of a carotid plaque may be accompanied by an abnormal computed tomography CT scan of the brain, even when cerebral infarction is not clinically apparent (50). The majority of carotid emboli lodge in tributaries of the middle cerebral artery (51). This propensity is believed to be due to the direct course of the middle cerebral artery with the intracranial internal carotid artery. The middle cerebral artery is also the largest derivative of the internal carotid artery with the highest volume of blood flow.

1. *Diagnostic Tests*

The most popular noninvasive test used to study the carotid arteries is ultrasonography, which is discussed in detail in Chapter 7 (52). Contemporary machines use two modes, Doppler and B-mode imaging, and are thus referred to as duplex. This method uses B-mode ultrasound to visualize the anatomy (53,54), and the reflected ultrasound signals are displayed in two dimensions. Arteries are differentiated from veins by their pulsatile nature. Views of the vessels in longitudinal and cross-sectional orientations can be obtained and dimensions measured. Ultrasound may be used to determine the extent of stenosis and also whether the vessel is occluded, ulcerated, calcified, and/or thrombosed (55). The velocity of blood flow can be measured at several points along the course of the artery, and stenotic lesions can be qualified (56,57). Technical difficulties are a limitation of this technique and are related to the size of the patient's neck, high bifurcation out of range of the transducer, tortuosity, anatomical variation, and calcific deposit. Technical difficulties are experienced in about 15% of patients.

A recent advance has been the development of the transcranial Doppler technique. This technology, using ocular and temporal windows, allows flow velocity analysis of the larger intracranial arteries in the region around the circle of Willis. This approach allows differentiation between internal carotid and middle cerebral artery disease and is able to determine direction of flow in the major intracranial arteries and thus to clarify collateral flow patterns (58).

Magnetic resonance angiography (MRA) is an alternative noninvasive technique for the study of carotid pathology. This modality may become a screening test for carotid disease. It is equally suited for investigating intracranial vascular pathology and extracranial carotid and vertebral disease (59). Unlike conventional x-ray contrast angiography which provides anatomic detail, MRA reflects anatomy as well as blood flows. Its accuracy often exceeds that of duplex ultrasonography, but it has not replaced conventional angiography as the reference standard. Magnetic resonance angiography may overestimate the degree of vessel stenosis, because turbulent blood flow causes signal dropout (60). The disadvantages of this technique are long scan times, claustrophobia, and disqualification of patients with implanted metallic devices.

Digital subtraction angiography (DSA) can be performed via either venous or arterial routes. A mask image is obtained and then stored digitally. A contrast agent is injected, and a series of images are digitally acquired and stored. The mask image is subtracted, producing a computer-processed angiogram of the vasculature (61). Arterial DSA yields much higher resolution of arterial anatomy than venous DSA. It is slightly inferior in image quality compared with standard cut film angiography. Advantages include lower contrast dye requirements and the convenience of manipulating digitally acquired images. It has many of the disadvantages of standard angiography, including contrast agent hypersensitivity reactions, renal complications, and in the case of arterial DSA, catheter-related complications (62). The standard for evaluating carotid and intracranial vascular disease is cut film angiography. The most serious risks from this procedure are cerebrovascular complications, principally embolization from the catheter, arising especially when the length of the procedure exceeds 80 minutes. In major institutions, the incidence of complications ranges from 1.5% to 5%, with a less than 1% risk of persistent neurological deficit.

B. Management

Medical management in symptomatic carotid disease is derived from contemporary understanding of the pathophysiology of the disease process. Treatment ranges from risk factor management to platelet antiaggregation therapy to systemic anticoagulation, and thrombolytic therapy. Modification of risk factors alone is appropriate only for asymptomatic patients who fall into high-risk categories. Once symptoms develop, modification of risk factors should be combined with other measures.

1. Antiplatelet Agents

Aspirin, which inhibits platelet aggregation by irreversibly binding to cyclooxygenase, is the standard pharmacological agent used for stroke prevention. Two large studies have evaluated the value of aspirin in preventing vascular events in asymptomatic persons without overt evidence of vascular disease (Table 1). In one study, more than 5000 male physicians received either aspirin (500 mg/day) or placebo. No difference in vascular mortality was found between the two groups (63). In another study of 22,071 physicians, aspirin (325 mg qOD) was compared with placebo in the prevention of cardiovascular mortality and stroke. Myocardial infarction was reduced by 44% in the aspirin-treated group, but the study was inconclusive regarding the effect of aspirin on stroke. The aspirin-treated group showed a trend toward an increased incidence of severe hemorrhagic strokes although this was not statistically significant (64).

There have been many studies evaluating the use of aspirin and other antiplatelet agents

Table 1 Aspirin in Primary Prevention of Cerebral Ischemia

Study	No. of patients	Groups	Results
United Kingdom (63)	5139	ASA (500 mg/day) Placebo	No significant difference in vascular mortality between the two groups
American Physicians' Health Study (64)	22,071	ASA (325 mg qod) Placebo	MI reduced by 44% in ASA-treated group; effect on stroke inconclusive

ASA = aspirin; MI = myocardial infarction.

for the secondary prevention of cerebral infarction after cerebral ischemic events. These studies are summarized in Table 2 (65–78). Of the seven randomized, controlled trials comparing aspirin with placebo, only two (the AICLA and Canadian Cooperative trials) showed a significant reduction of the number of strokes among aspirin-treated patients. The Canadian study evaluated 585 patients (69% men, 31% women) with cerebral or retinal TIAs or minor stroke. Aspirin reduced the risk of stroke or death by 31%; however, if stroke alone was considered there was little overall benefit. There was a difference in the effect of aspirin between men and women, with a 48% reduction of risk of stroke or death among men and no significant risk reduction among women. No beneficial effect was noted with sulfinpyrazone alone or in combination with aspirin (67). The AICLA trial studied 604 French patients with TIAs or strokes and found fewer strokes among the aspirin-treated patients. No added benefit was noted with dipyridamole. This particular study has been criticized because the exceptionally long period between ischemic symptoms and study entry (1 year) may have biased the results to a more favorable outcome (73).

The dose of aspirin required to show a beneficial effect is controversial. One recent study failed to show a therapeutic difference between low-dose (325 mg/day) and high-dose (1300 mg/day) aspirin. A higher incidence of side effects was seen with the high dose (77).

Ticlopidine hydrochloride is a newly developed potent platelet antiaggregant that acts primarily by irreversibly inhibiting the adenosine diphosphate pathways of the platelet membrane. It is reported to reduce plasma fibrinogen levels and increase erythrocyte deformability. Two large multicenter trials were recently completed measuring the clinical efficacy of ticlopidine versus placebo and aspirin in symptomatic patients (Table 3) (79–84). Ticlopidine was found to be more effective than aspirin in preventing strokes in both sexes. The 3-year rate for nonfatal strokes or death from any cause was 17% for ticlopidine and 19% for aspirin. The 3-year rate for all strokes was 10% for ticlopidine and 13% for aspirin. Ticlopidine was associated with a much higher incidence of side effects, mostly diarrhea (20%) and skin rash (14%), than aspirin, although it was associated with a lower incidence of serious gastrointestinal bleeding. A significant increase in total serum cholesterol level was also found with ticlopidine (9%) versus aspirin (2%). The most serious potential side effect of ticlopidine is a severe, reversible neutropenia that occurs in fewer than 1% of patients (79,80).

2. Anticoagulation and Thrombolytic Therapy

Long-term systemic anticoagulation with warfarin may reduce the incidence of stroke. This is controversial and has not been definitively demonstrated in controlled, randomized trials (85,86). This therapy is also associated with a high rate (2–22%) of complications, especially intracranial hemorrhages (87). It may still be appropriate for occasional cooperative patients who do not respond to aspirin therapy and are not surgical candidates. Similarly, the use of thrombolytic agents in thromboembolic strokes is as yet an investigational therapy. Published reports tend to include few patients, and the results are difficult to interpret (88).

3. Surgery

Carotid endarterectomy was introduced in the 1950s. By the mid-1980s it had become the second most frequently performed operation, after coronary artery bypass grafting (89). The operation carries a risk of a few per hundred of stroke, an outcome it was designed to prevent. Diagnostic angiography adds a small increment of risk (90). Risks of iatrogenic morbidity and mortality must be measured against the natural history of the disease and the

Table 2 Studies of Aspirin in Secondary Prevention of Cerebral Ischemia

Study	No. of patients	Diagnosis	Timing of entry	Groups	Follow-Up	Results
ASA-USA (65)	178	Carotid TIA	<3 months	ASA (1300 mg/day) Placebo	2 years	Favorable outcome in 81% ASA vs. 56% placebo at 6 months. No statistically significant benefit of ASA in outcomes of death, or cerebral or retinal infarction except with frequent, multiple TIAs, carotid stenosis >50%, or ulceration.
Reuther, Dorndorf (66)	58	TIA RIND	<3 months	ASA (1500 mg/day) Placebo	2 years	No significant differences.
Canadian Cooperative (67)	585	TIA, minor stroke	<3 months	ASA (1300 mg/day) SPZ (800 mg/day) ASA + SPZ Placebo	26 months (average)	Number of major strokes similar in both groups. ASA decreased stroke and death by 48% in men. No benefit in women.
Argentinian CooperativeZ (68)	66	TIA	<30 days	ASA (1050 mg/day) + DIP (150 mg/day) PTXF (1200 mg/day)	1 year	ASA + DIP had higher number of recurrent TIAs (28%) than PTXF (10%).
Argentinian Cooperative (69)	125	TIA	30 days	ASA (1050 mg/day) + DIP (150 mg/day) PTXF (1200 mg/day)	6 months	Fewer nonfatal strokes (6%) with PTXF than with ASA + DIP (3%). ASA + DIP had higher number or recurrent TIAs (28%) than PTXF (12%).
ATIAIS (70)	124	TIA	<3 months	ASA (100 mg/day) SPZ (800 mg/day)	1 year	ASA had 53% reduction in further cerebral and cardiac events in men. SPZ no better than ASA.
Guiraud-Chaumeil et al (71)	440	TIA	?	ASA (900 mg/day) + (DHE (4.5 mg/day) ASA (900 mg/day) + DIP (150 mg/day) + DHE (4.5 mg/day) DHE (4.5 mg/day)	3 years	No differences in outcome between groups.

Study	n				Results
Danish (72)	203	TIA RIND	<1 month	ASA (1000 mg/day) Placebo	25 months	No benefit of ASA in preventing death or disabling stroke.
AICLA (73)	604	TIA Stroke	1 year	ASA (1000 mg/day) ASA + DIP (225 mg/day) Placebo	3 years	Fewer strokes with ASA (9%) than with placebo (15%). No sex difference in the efficacy of aspirin. No additional benefit of DIP.
American-Canadian Cooperative Study (74)	390	Carotid TIA	<3 months	ASA (1300 mg/day) + placebo ASA + DIP (225 mg/day)	25 months	No difference between the groups.
ESPS (75)	1861	TIA RIND Strokes	<3 months	ASA (975 mg/day) + DIP (225 mg/day) Placebo	2 years	Beneficial effect in preventing stroke or death of any cause in the treated group.
Swedish (76)	505	Stroke	1–3 weeks	ASA (1500 mg/day) Placebo	2 years	No difference in TIA or recurrent stroke between groups.
United Kingdom (77)	2435	TIA Minor stroke	<3 months	ASA (1200 mg/day) ASA (300mg/day) Placebo	4 years	Number of disabling strokes the same in all groups. ASA decreased risk of combined MI, major stroke, or death by 18% and disabling stroke or vascular death by 7%. Benefits restricted to men. Less gastric toxicity with smaller dose ASA.
Spain (78)	264	TIA RIND Stroke	1 year	ASA (250 mg/day) + Nicardipine (60 mg/day) ASA (250 mg/day)	1 year	Fewer recurrent ischemic events in the ASA-NIC group (12%) compared with ASA (19%).

TIA = transient ischemic attack; RIND = reversible ischemic neurological deficit; ASA = aspirin; SPZ = sulfinpyrazone; PTXF = pentoxifylline; DHE = dihydroergotamine; DIP = dipyridamole; ATIAIS = Anturane TIA Italian Study; AICLA = Accidents Ischémiques Cérébraux Liés a l'Athérosclérose; ESPS = European Stroke Prevention Study; NIC = nicardipine.

Table 3 Trials Evaluating the Efficacy of Ticlopidine in Cerebrovascular Disease

Study	No. of patients	Diagnosis	Timing of entry	Groups	Follow-Up	Results
CATS (79)	1053	Stroke (atherothrombo-embolic)	<17 weeks	Ticlopidine (500 mg/day) Placebo	1 year	Ticlopidine had a 23–30% risk reduction in recurrent stroke, MI, or vascular death. Benefit applied equally to men and women.
TASS (80)	3069	TIA RIND Minor stroke	<3 months	ASA (1300 mg/day) Ticlopidine (500 mg/day)	3 years	Ticlopidine had a 21% risk reduction in fatal and nonfatal stroke. Greater risk reductions of stroke in women (27%) compared with men (11%).
Murakami (81)	113	TIA RIND Minor stroke	<12 months	ASA (500 mg/day) Ticlopidine (200 mg/day)	44 months	Decreased incidence of stroke with ticlopidine (10.2%) versus ASA (20.3%).
Ticlopidine-pentoxifylline combination (82)	79	TIA stroke	?	Ticlopidine (500 mg/day) + pentoxifylline (1200 mg/day) Aspirin (300 mg/day) + dipyridamole (300 mg/day) + buflomedil (1350 mg/day) Buflomedil (1350 mg/day) + placebo	24 months	Decreased incidence of recurrent cerebral ischemia with ticlopidine plus pentoxifylline (13.5%) vs. aspirin plus dipyridamole plus buflomedil (28%) and buflomedil plus placebo (41%).
Ticlopidine-postacute ischemic stroke (83)	30	Ischemic stroke	12 hours	Ticlopidine (500 mg/day) Placebo	3 weeks	Slight improvement on neurological outcome (Hachinski scale) and hemorheologic parameters in the ticlopidine group.
Ticlopidine-aspirin combination (84)	64	TIA Stroke	?	ASA (300 mg/day) Ticlopidine (200 mg/day) ASA (81 mg/day) + TIC (100 mg/day)		Potent platelet antiaggregation with ASA + TIC combination. Increased risk of hemorrhagic complications with ASA + TIC combination (8) vs TIC (3) and ASA (2).

TIA = transient ischemic attack; RIND = reversible ischemic neurological deficit; ASA = aspirin; SPZ = sulfinpyrazone; PTXF = pentoxifylline; DHE = dihydroergotamine; DIP = dipyridamole; TIC = ticlopidine

Table 4 Trials Comparing Surgery with Medical Treatment in Carotid Stenosis

Study	No. of patients	Diagnosis	Degree of stenosis	Timing of entry	Groups	Results
NASCET (93)	659	TIA Small stroke	70–99%	<120 days	CEA + ASA ASA	CEA highly beneficial.
ECST (94)	2200	TIA Small stroke	30–99%	<120 days	CEA + ASA ASA	CEA highly beneficial for severe (70–99%) stenosis. Uncertain benefit for lesser stenoses.
VA (95)	189	TIA Small stroke	50–99%	<120 days	CEA + ASA ASA	CEA beneficial. Benefit more profound in patients with stenoses >70%.

TIA = transient ischemic attack; CEA = carotid endarterectomy; ASA = aspirin.

results of medical treatment. Skepticism regarding the efficacy of the procedure in the era of improving medical treatment and declining stroke fatality rate was amplified by the report that the extracranial-intracranial bypass procedure was ineffective in preventing strokes (91,92). Several trials were designed to study the effectiveness of this procedure in both symptomatic and asymptomatic patient populations. The results of two large trials involving the former group are now available. Studies involving the latter are ongoing (Table 4).

The North American study found that carotid endarterectomy was highly beneficial in patients with recent hemispheric TIAs, retinal TIAs, or nondisabling strokes and ipsilateral high-grade carotid stenosis (≥70%) when compared with aspirin therapy (93). The 2-year overall stroke rate was 26% for medically treated patients and 9% for surgical patients. The 2-year rate of major or fatal stroke was 13.1% for medical and 2.5% for surgical patients. The early disadvantage related to operative mortality and morbidity among the surgically treated patients was reversed at about 3 months after operation. The beneficial effects of surgery persisted for at least 30 months (length of the study). The medical branch of this study also highlighted the "malignant" nature of symptomatic carotid artery disease. The European Carotid Surgery Trial demonstrated similar results (94). At 3 years, surgery provided a six- to eightfold reduction in the stroke rate among patients with high-grade stenosis when compared with medical therapy. Both studies showed a clear short-term (3-year) advantage to carotid artery surgery in this population. Whether carotid endarterectomy will compare favorably with medical treatment in the long term is unknown, since the data are not available. In terms of human productivity and suffering, even a short-term advantage appears to justify the procedure as worthwhile and "cost-effective." These data do not address questions concerning symptomatic patients with moderate-grade carotid stenosis. Both studies are continuing to recruit and randomize these patients for comparison. Parallel asymptomatic carotid trials are also in progress (96).

IV. AORTIC DISSECTION

While aortic dissection does not constitute a "thromboembolic" disease, it occasionally enters the differential diagnosis of cerebral or, more commonly, peripheral ischemia. Acute proximal aortic dissection, if untreated, is almost invariably lethal. Although management continues to improve, many patients die despite modern diagnosis and therapy. A high index of clinical suspicion coupled with immediate referral to a cardiovascular surgeon has resulted in a decrease of morbidity and mortality.

Aortic dissections occur when a tear in the intima of the thoracic aorta allows blood to track within the aortic wall. This usually causes sudden severe chest or interscapular pain. Unlike myocardial infarction, the pain is worst at the onset and the blood pressure is normal or increased despite the shock-like state. Hypertension, Marfan's syndrome, pregnancy, congenital bicuspid aortic valve, and coarctation are all risk factors, and the presence of one of these conditions should increase the clinical suspicion. There may also be evidence of acute aortic valvular insufficiency, a difference in blood pressure between the two arms, or signs of ischemia in the territory of the coronary, carotid, spinal, visceral, renal, or iliac arteries as a result of branch occlusion by the dissection. An electrocardiogram may be helpful if it fails to show evidence of a recent myocardial infarction. Chest radiographs are abnormal in about 80% of cases, commonly showing mediastinal widening and a left pleural effusion.

Drug therapy should be started if the diagnosis is suspected, and a cardiovascular surgeon should be consulted. Left ventricular ejection velocity and systemic arterial pressure are the two most important factors related to progressive dissection. These should be controlled with nitroprusside and propranolol. Labetolol, which has both alpha- and beta-blocking actions, may be slightly easier to regulate than a combination of agents.

Although magnetic resonance imaging, transesophageal echocardiography, and computer tomography may be useful diagnostic tools, thoracic aortography remains the most widely accepted method of definitive diagnosis. Noninvasive techniques, however, may be more useful in postsurgical follow-up. Aortograms may show splitting, distortion of the contrast column, abnormal flow patterns, lack of filling of major aortic branches, or aortic valvular insufficiency. It is important to determine if the ascending aorta is affected, since untreated dissections of this segment have an especially high early mortality, chiefly from rupture of the false channel.

Ascending dissections are treated by immediate surgery. The goal of surgery is to replace the ascending aorta with a prosthetic segment and to obliterate entry into the false channel. The dissected aorta is very fragile, and buttressing the suture lines with a felt collar and use of pledget-backed sutures are usually required. Resuspension of the aortic valve is necessary if the valve is involved. Severe damage is treated by valve replacement. Coronary reimplantation may then be required.

Traditionally, dissections that do not involve the ascending aorta are treated by drug therapy alone unless complications occur or medical therapy fails to arrest dissection progression. Surgery may be considered with persistent or recurrent pain, progressive branch occlusion, impending rupture indicated by an enlarging aortic shadow or blood in the pleural cavity, poor blood pressure control, or major aortic branch occlusion (97).

REFERENCES

1. Breasted JH. The Edwin Smith surgical papyrus: published in facsimile and hieroglyphic transliteration with translation and commentary in two volumes. Vol. 1. Chicago: The University of Chicago Press, 1930.
2. Castiglioni A. A history of medicine. New York: Alfred A. Knopf, 1941.
3. Lord RSA. Surgery of occlusive cerebrovascular disease. St. Louis: C. V. Mosby, 1986.
4. Abercrombie J. Pathological and practical researches on diseases of the brain and the spinal cord. Edinburgh: Waugh and Innes, 1828.

5. Willius FA, Dry TJ. A history of the heart and the circulation. Philadelphia: W. B. Saunders, 1948.

6. Hunt JR. The role of carotid arteries in the causation of vascular lesions of the brain, with remarks on certain special features of the symptomatology. Am J Med Sci 1913; 147:704.

7. Moniz E. L'encéphalographie artérielle: son importance dans la localisation des tumeurs cérébrales. Rev Neurol 1927; 34:72.

8. Fisher CM. Occlusion of the internal carotid artery. Arch Neurol Psychiat 1951; 65:346.

9. Fisher CM, Adams RD. Observations on brain embolism with special reference to the mechanism of hemorrhagic infarction. J Neuropathol Exp Neurol 1951; 10:92.

10. Carrea R, Mollins M, Murphy G. Surgical treatment of spontaneous thrombosis of the internal carotid artery in the neck: carotid-carotideal anastomosis; report of a case. Acta Neurol Latinoam 1955; 1:71.

11. Strully KJ, Hurwitt ES, Blankenberg HW. Thromboendarterectomy for thrombosis of the internal carotid artery in the neck. J Neurosurg 1953; 10:474.

12. Crawford ES, DeBakey ME, Fields WS, et al. Surgical treatment of arterial occlusive lesions in patients with cerebral artery insufficiency. Circulation 1959; 20:168.

13. Eastcott HHG, Pickering GW, Robb CG. Reconstruction of internal carotid artery in a patient with intermittent attacks of hemiplegia. Lancet 1954; 2:994.

14. Cooley DA, Al-Naaman YD, Carton CA. Surgical treatment of arteriosclerotic occlusion of common carotid artery. J Neurosurg 1956; 13:500.

15. McDonald JJ, Anson BJ. Variations in origin of arteries derived from aortic arch, in American whites and Negroes. Am J Phys. Anthropol 1940; 27:91.

16. Schwartz CJ, Mitchell JRA. Observations on localization of arterial plaques. Circulation Res 1962; 11:63.

17. Paullus WS, Pait TG, Rhoton AL Jr. Microsurgical exposure of the petrous portion of the carotid artery. J Neurosurg 1977; 47:713.

18. Harris FS, Rhoton AL Jr. Anatomy of the cavernous sinus: a microsurgical study. J Neurosurg 1976; 45:169.

19. Nicholls SC, Phillips DJ, Primozich JF, et al. Diagnostic significance of flow separation in the carotid bulb. Stroke 1989; 20:175–82.

20. Caro CG, Pedley TJ, Schroter RC, Seed WA. The mechanics of the circulation. New York: Oxford University Press, 1978.

21. Zarins CK, Giddens DP, Balasubramanian K, et al. Carotid plaques localize in regions of low flow velocity and shear stress. Circulation 1981; 64(suppl 4):44.

22. Heath D, Smith P, Harris P, et al. The atherosclerotic human carotid sinus. J Pathol 1973; 110:49.

23. LoGerfo FW, Nowak MD, Quist WC, et al. Flow studies in a model carotid bifurcation. Arteriosclerosis 1981; 1:235.

24. Bergan JJ, Yao JST. Cerebrovascular insufficiency. New York: Grune & Stratton, 1983.

25. Ezekowitz MD, Parker KH, Salpidoru N, Oxenham RCK. Effect of aging on permeability of cockerel aorta to 125-I-albumin. Am J Physiol 1980; 239:H642–50.

26. Ezekowitz MD, Morgan MA, Kelley JL, Parker DE, Stone HL. Effect of short duration constant exercise on permeability of cockerel aorta to 125-I-albumin. J Appl Physiol 1985; 59:985–9.

27. Fields WS, Bruetman H, Weibel J. Collateral circulation of the brain. Monogr Surg Sci 1965; 2:183.

28. Yasargil MG. Microneurosurgery. Vol. 1. New York: Thieme-Stratton, 1984.

29. Alpers BJ, Berry RG. Circle of Willis in cerebral vascular disorders. Arch Neurol 1963; 8:398.

30. Ramsey RG. Neuroradiology with computed tomography. Philadelphia: W.B. Saunders, 1981.

31. Bernstein EF, Dilley RB. Late results after carotid endarterectomy for amaurosis fugax. J Vasc Surg 1987; 6:333.

32. Department of Health and Human Services. Arteriosclerosis. V. Working group on arteriosclerosis of National Heart, Lung and Blood Institute. NIH Pub 81–2034, 1981.

33. Shaper AG, Phillips AN, Pocock SJ, et al. Risk factors for stroke in middle aged British men. Br Med J 1991; 302.

34. Whisnant JP, Sandok BA, Sundt TM Jr. Carotid endarterectomy for unilateral carotid system transient cerebral ischemia. Mayo Clin Proc 1983; 58:171.

35. Sundt TM Jr. Occlusive cerebrovascular disease: diagnosis and surgical management. Philadelphia: W. B. Saunders, 1987.

36. Wodarz R. Watershed infarctions and computed tomography: a topographical study in cases with stenosis or occlusion of the carotid artery. Neurol Radiol 1980; 29:245.

37. Sloan MA, Haley EC Jr. The syndrome of bilateral hemispheric border zone ischemia. Stroke 1990; 21:1668.

38. The Amaurosis Fugax Study Group. Current management of amaurosis fugax. Stroke 1990; 21:201.

39. Isaka Y, et al. Platelet accumulation in carotid atherosclerotic lesions: semiquantitative analysis with indium-111 platelets and technetium-99M human serum albumin. J Nucl Med 1984; 25:556.

40. Eisenberg RL, Nemzek WR, Moore WS, et al. Relationship of transient ischemic attacks and angiographically demonstrable lesions of carotid artery. Stroke 1977; 8:483.

41. Hollenhorst RW. Significance of bright plaques in the retinal arterioles. JAMA 1961; 178:23.

42. Lord RSA, Berry NA. Atherosclerotic ulceration of the brachiocephalic artery. Aust NZ J Surg 1975; 44:370.

43. Tunick PA, Kronzon I. Protruding atherosclerotic plaque in the aortic arch of patients with systemic embolization: a new finding seen by transesophageal echocardiography. Am Heart J 1990; 120:658.

44. Tunick PA, Perex JL, Kronzon I. Protruding atheroma in the thoracic aorta and systemic embolization. Ann Intern Med 1991; 115:432.

45. Barnett HJM. Delayed cerebral ischemic episodes distal to occlusion of major cerebral arteries. Neurology 1978; 28:769.

46. Antunes JL, Correll LW. Cerebral emboli from intracranial aneurysms. Surg Neurol 1976; 6:7.

47. Lusby JR, Ferrell LD, Ehrenfeld WK, et al. Carotid plaque hemorrhage. Its role in production of cerebral ischemia. Arch Surg 1982; 117:1479.

48. Fisher CM. Transient monocular blindness associated with hemiplegia. Arch Ophthalmol 1952; 47:167.

49. Sturgill BC, Netsky MG. Cerebral infarction by atheromatous emboli: report of a case and review of literature. Arch Pathol 1963; 76:189.

50. Zukowski AJ, et al. The correlation between carotid plaque ulceration and cerebral infarction seen on the CT scan. J Vasc Surg 1984; 1:782.

51. Yates PO, Hutchinson PC. Cerebral infarction: the role of stenosis of the extracranial cerebral vessels. Med Res Counc Spec Rep 1961; 300:1.

52. Feussner JR, Matchar DB. When and how to study the carotid arteries. Ann Intern Med 1988; 109:805.

53. Ricotta JJ. Plaque characterization by B-mode scan. Surg Clin NA 1990; 70:191.

54. Cooperberg PL, Robertson WD, Fry P, Sweeney V. High resolution real-time ultrasound of the carotid bifurcation. J Clin Ultrasound 1979; 7:13.

55. Zwiebel WJ, Austin CW, Sackett JF, Strother CM. Correlation of high-resolution B-mode and continuous wave Doppler sonography with arteriography in the diagnosis of carotid stenosis. Radiology 1983; 149:523.

56. Blackwell E, Merory J, Toole JF, MacKinney W. Doppler ultrasound scanning of the carotid bifurcation. Arch Neurol 1977; 34:145.

57. Lewis RR, Beasley MG, Hyams DE, Gosling RG. Imaging of the carotid bifurcation using continuous-wave Doppler-shift ultrasound and spectral analysis. Stroke 1978; 9:465.

58. Mattle H, Grolimund P, Huber P, et al. Transcranial Doppler sonographic findings in middle cerebral artery disease. Arch Neurol 1988; 45:289.

59. Ross JS, Masaryk TJ, Modic MT, et al. Magnetic resonance angiography of the extracranial carotid arteries and intracranial vessels: a review. Neurology 1989; 39:1369.

60. Mattle HP, Kent KC, Edelman RR, et al. Evaluation of the extracranial carotid arteries: correlation of magnetic resonance angiography, duplex ultrasonography, and conventional angiography. J Vasc Surg 1991; 13:838.

61. Earnest F IV, Houser OW, Forbes GS, et al. The accuracy and limitations of digital subtraction angiography in the evaluation of atherosclerotic cerebrovascular disease. Angiographic and surgical correlation. Mayo Clin Proc 1983; 58:735.

62. Mani RL, Eisenberg RL, McDonald EJ, et al. Complications of catheter angiography. Analysis of 5000 procedures. I. Criteria and incidence. Am J Radiol 1978; 131:861.

63. Peto R, Gray R, Collins R, et al. Randomized trial of prophylactic daily aspirin in British male doctors. Br Med J 1988; 296:313.

64. Steering committee on the Physicians' Health Study Research Group. Preliminary report findings from the aspirin component of the ongoing Physicians' Health Study. N Engl J Med 1988; 318:262.

65. Fields WS, Lemak NA, Frankowski RF, et al. Controlled trial of aspirin in cerebral ischemia. Stroke 1977; 8:301.

66. Reuther R, Dorndorf W. Aspirin in patients with cerebral ischemia and normal angiograms or nonsurgical lesions. In: Breddin K, Dorndorf W, Loew D, eds. Acetylsalicylic acid in cerebral ischemia and coronary heart disease. Stuttgart: F.K. Shattaver Verlag, 1978:97.

67. Canadian Cooperative Study Group. A randomized trial of aspirin and sulfinpyrazone in threatened stroke. N Engl J Med 1978; 299:53.

68. Herskovits E, Vazques A, Famulari A, et al. Randomized trial of pentoxifylline versus acetylsalicylic acid plus dipyridamole in preventing transient ischemic attacks. Lancet 1981; 1:966.

69. Herskovits E, Famulari A, Tamaroff L, et al. Preventive treatment of cerebral transient ischemia. Comparative randomized trial of pentoxifylline versus conventional antiaggregants. Eur Neurol 1985; 24:73.

70. Candelise L, Handi G, Perrone P, et al. A randomized trial of aspirin and sulfinpyrazone in patients with TIA. Stroke 1982; 13:175.

71. Guirand-Chaumeil B, Rascol A, David J, et al. Prevention des récidives des accidents vasculaires cérébraux ischémiques par les anti-aggréants plaquettaires. Résultats d'un essai thérapeutique controlé de 3 ans. Rev Neurol (Paris) 1982; 138:367.

72. Sorensen PS, Pedersen H, Marquardsen J, et al. Acetylsalicylic acid in the prevention of stroke in patients with reversible cerebral ischemic attacks. A Danish Cooperative Study. Stroke 14:15.

73. Bousser MG, Eschwege E, Haguenau M, et al. "AICLA" controlled trial of aspirin and dipyridamole in the secondary prevention of athero-thrombotic cerebral ischemia. Stroke 1983; 14:7.

74. The American-Canadian Cooperative Study Group. Persantine Aspirin Trial in Cerebral Ischemia. Part II: End point results. Stroke 1985; 16:406.

75. The ESPS Group. The European Stroke Prevention Study (ESPS). Principal end-points. Lancet 1987; 2:1351.

76. High-dose acetylsalicylic acid after cerebral infarction: A Swedish cooperative study. Stroke 1987; 18:325.

77. United Kingdom Transient Ischemic Attack (UK-TIA) Study Group. Aspirin trial: interim results. Br Med J 1988; 296:316.

78. Marti-Masso JF, Lozano R. Nicardipine in the prevention of cerebral infarction. Clin Ther 1990; 12:344.

79. Gent M, Blakely JA, Easton JD, et al. The Canadian American Ticlopidine Study (CATS) in thromboembolic stroke. Lancet 1989; 333:1215.

80. Hass WK, Easton JD, Adams HP Jr, et al. A randomized trial comparing ticlopidine hydrochloride with aspirin for the prevention of stroke in high-risk patients. Ticlopidine Aspirin Stroke Study Group. N Engl J Med 1989; 321:501.

81. Murakami G. Effects of aspirin and ticlopidine on transient ischemic attacks. Shindan To Chiryo 1986; 74:2255.

82. Appollonio A, Castgnani P, Margrini L, Angeletti R. Ticlopidine pentoxifylline combination in the treatment of atherosclerosis and the prevention of cerebrovascular accidents. Int Med Res 1989; 17:28.

83. Ciuffetti G, Aisa G, Mercuri M, et al. Effects of ticlopidine on the neurologic outcome and the hemorheologic pattern in the postacute phase of ischemic stroke: A pilot study. Angiology 1990; 41:505.

84. Uchiyama S, Sone R, Nagayama T, et al. Combination therapy with low-dose aspirin and ticlopidine in cerebral ischemia. Stroke 1989; 20:1643.

85. Baker RN, Schwartz W, Rose AS. Transient ischemic attacks—a report of a study of anti-coagulant treatment. Neurology 1966; 16:841.

86. Veterans Administration Cooperative Study of Atherosclerosis, Neurology Section. An evalua-tion of anticoagulant therapy in the treatment of cerebrovascular disease. Neurology 1961; 11:132.

87. Levine M, Hirsch J. Hemorrhagic complications of long-term anticoagulant therapy for ischemic cerebral vascular disease. Stroke 1986; 17:111.

88. Herderschee D, Limburg M, van Royen EA, et al. Thrombolysis with recombinant tissue plasminogen activator in acute ischemic stroke: evaluation with rCBF-SPECT. Acta Neurol Scand 1991; 83:317.

89. Pokras R, Dyken ML. Dramatic changes in the performance of endarterectomy for diseases of the extracranial arteries of the head. Stroke 1988; 19:1289.

90. Hankey GJ, Warlow CP, Sellar RJ. Cerebral angiographic risk in mild cerebrovascular disease. Stroke 1990; 21:209.

91. Scheinberg P. Controversies in management of cerebral vascular disease. Neurology 1988; 38:1609.

92. The EC/IC Bypass Study Group. Failure of extracranial-intracranial arterial bypass to reduce the risk of ischemic stroke: results of an international randomized trial. N Engl J Med 1985; 313:1191.

93. North American Symptomatic Carotid Endarterectomy Trial Collaborators. Beneficial effect of carotid endarterectomy in symptomatic patients with high-grade carotid stenosis. N Engl J Med 1991; 325:445.

94. European Carotid Surgery Trialists' Collaborative Group. MRC European Carotid Surgery Trial: interim results for symptomatic patients with severe (70–99%) or with mild (0–29%) carotid stenosis. Lancet 1991; 337:1235.

95. Mayberg MR, Wilson E, Yatsu F, Weiss DG, et al. Carotid endarterectomy and prevention of cerebral ischemia in symptomatic carotid stenosis. JAMA 1991; 266:3289.

96. Callow AD, Caplan LR, Correll JW, et al. Carotid endarterectomy: What is its current status? Am J Med 1988; 85:835.

97. Nienaber CA, Spielmann RP, Von Kodolitsch Y, Siglow V, Piepho A, Javp T, Nicholas V, Weber P, Triebel HJ, Bleifield W. Diagnosis of thoracic aortic dissection: Magnetic resonance imaging versus transesophageal echocardiography. Circulation 1992; 85:434–47.

17

Ventricular Assist Devices and the Total Artificial Heart: Clinical Uses and Thromboembolic Complications

Robert S. D. Higgins
Henry Ford Hospital, Detroit, Michigan

Kenneth L. Franco
Yale University School of Medicine, New Haven, Connecticut

I. INTRODUCTION

In 1982, a pneumatically driven Jarvik-7 total artificial heart was implanted in a 61-year-old man with congestive heart failure secondary to idiopathic cardiomyopathy (1). This historic implantation was the first of its kind in humans, and it represented the culmination of years of intensive research in an effort to assist the failing heart. The artificial heart functioned for 112 days without mechanical failure, but the patient's postoperative course was complicated by acute renal failure, seizures, pulmonary insufficiency, complications of anticoagulation therapy, and sepsis, which eventually led to his death.

This case was typical of the early experience with ventricular assist devices (VADs) and the total artificial heart (TAH), and thrombosis and thromboembolic events have been the major limiting factor in the development and application of these devices in more extensive clinical trials. Strategies to assist the failing heart involve the temporary use of these devices until the native heart recovers after cardiac surgery, or until an appropriate donor organ becomes available for cardiac transplantation. Continued progress in this field requires a delicate balance between adequate suppression of the body's normal reaction to foreign substances at the blood-device interface and the risk of excessive anticoagulation leading to bleeding complications that may preclude subsequent orthotopic transplantation. In this review, the major cardiac assist devices and their use in clinical practice will be discussed, as well as the incidence of thromboembolic complications and strategies to prevent these catastrophic events (Table 1).

II. ETIOLOGY OF SYSTEMIC EMBOLIZATION

The major sources of thromboemboli in cardiac assist devices are the suture lines between the device and native tissue, inflow and outflow conduits, mechanical valves and their

Table 1 Cardiac Assist Devices, Clinical Uses and Thromboembolic Complications

Device	Class	Blood-contacting surface	Thrombotic prophylaxis	Bleeding complications	Thromboembolic complications
Ventricular assist devices					
Biomedicus					
Bolman et al. (10) Park et al. (9)	Centrifugal pump	Polyurethane	Heparin IV infusion using ACT (150–200 s)	None	1/9 pts (11%)
Thoratec					
Pennington et al. (11)	Heterotopic pneumatic pulsatile	Polyurethane	Heparin IV infusion at implantation	Mediastinal bleeding requiring reoperation in 18/30 pts.	+ thrombus in VAD 3/30 pts. 2/30 pts. CVA
Termuhlen et al. (12)	Heterotopic	Polyurethane		Generalized bleeding	+ thrombus in VAD 9/41 (support >4 h) + 4/9 embolic events 2 CVAs, 2 peripheral emboli
Farrar et al. (3)	Heterotopic	Polyurethane	Dextran postop. Heparin during weaning Warfarin/dipyridamole in transplant bridge pts.	Bleeding required reoperation 16/72 pts.	+ CVA 6/72 pts.
Novacor					
Portner et al. (17)	Heterotopic pusher plate electric	Polyurethane	Low-dose Heparin using PTT (1.5 × ml) LMW dextran Warfarin/dipyridamole	+ bleeding 8/20 pts. required reoperation	+ CVA 2/20 pts. TIA 1 pt.

Thermedics					
Nakatoni (15)	Heterotopic	Textured polyurethane	Low-dose Heparin LMW Dextran	Postop. bleeding 2/13 pts.	No thromboembolic complications
Hemopump					
Frazier and Cooley (16)	Axial flow pump	Stainless steel	Heparin using ACT (150–200 s)	None	No thromboembolic complications
Total artificial heart					
Jarvik					
Griffith (20)	Orthotopic dual-chamber	Polyurethane	Heparin IV 500 U/hr using PTT 2–2.5 × normal Dipyridamole 75 mg t.i.d.	Postop. bleeding 33%, reoperation in 33%	1 pt. thrombus at valve-housing interface
Muneretto et al. (21)	Orthotopic dual-chamber	Polyurethane	Heparin IV 1000–5000 U/day Dipyridamole/aspirin Aprotinin/pentoxifylline Anastomotic "GRF" glue	No postop. bleeding	No thromboembolic complications

IV = intravenous; ACT = activated clotting time; VAD = ventricular assist device; CVA = cerebrovascular accident; PTT = partial thromboplastin time; TIA = transient ischemic attack; LMW = low-molecular-weight; GRF = gelatin resorcine formal.

fittings, and the blood-contacting surface of the pumping chamber. In order to understand why these surfaces are thrombogenic, it is important to appreciate the thromboresistant characteristics of the endothelium (Fig. 1). Normal endothelium prevents intravascular thrombosis by several mechanisms, including the production and secretion of prostaglandins that inhibit platelet aggregation; the release of a potent thrombolytic agent, tissue plasminogen activator; and the expression on the endothelial surface of heparin, which binds antithrombin III to inhibit the coagulation enzymes (2). These functions are contingent on adequate flow within the lumen without stasis. The endocardium and cardiac valves do not generate thrombi unless the endothelium is damaged or dysfunctional.

In contrast, when blood makes contact with a foreign material, proteins adhere to the surface and create an environment to which platelets and leukocytes adhere (2). The pseudointima that forms traps cellular elements, and mediators released by these elements further promote the accumulation of the protein matrix, resulting in further cellular entrapment (Fig. 2). The absence of a normal endothelium allows this process to proceed without inhibition.

These early observations led to the development of several biocompatible surfaces for blood pumps over the past 25 years. The most commonly used material today is a segmented polyurethane (Biomer) developed by DuPont. This material has been found to be sturdy, flexible, and relatively antithrombogenic. The surface is seam-free and smooth. This material has been modified by adding a copolymer, BPS-215M (Thoratec Corp., Berkeley, California), that improves the thromboresistance of the bulk material (3). The copolymer migrates to the blood-contacting surface during the fabrication process to reduce surface tension at the interface. This material is now used in the Pierce-Donachy VAD and serves as the current clinical standard for biocompatible surfaces.

An alternative approach to improving these blood-contacting surfaces has been the

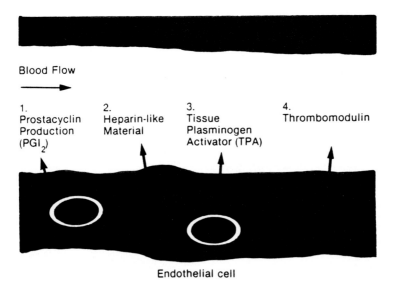

Figure 1 Schematic diagram of endothelial cell–derived factor inhibition of thrombosis in normal blood vessels. (From Hill JD. In: Chin R, ed. Transformed muscle for cardiac assist and repair. Mount Kisco, New York: Futura, 1990:293.)

Blood Flow

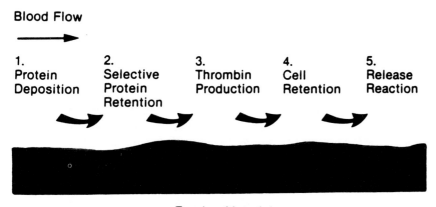

Foreign Material

Figure 2 Schematic representation of foreign materials in contact with blood elements leading to development of a pseudointima. (From Hill JD. In: Chin R, ed. Transformed muscle for cardiac assist and repair. Mount Kisco, New York: Futura, 1990:294.)

development of textured surfaces in VAD (Figs. 3a and 3b). The Thermedics pneumatic VAD is at this time the only device in clinical trials that employs this technology (4). The "integrally textured polyurethane" is designed to encourage the formation and adherence of a pseudointimal biological lining. This membrane is antithrombogenic and functions as a permanent biocompatible blood contacting surface.

Heparin-bonded materials have been developed to prevent thrombosis at the blood-surface interface in experimental assist devices (5). Heparin binds to circulating antithrombin III at the interface, thereby inhibiting thrombin formation. While this approach has been

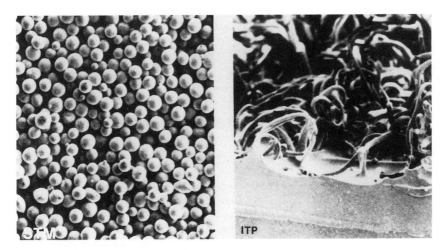

Figure 3 Textured blood-contacting surfaces used in the Thermedics VAD. (Courtesy of Thermedics, Inc., Berkeley, California)

applied to extracorporeal circuits, it has not been employed in cardiac assist devices. It does, however, offer an important option in the development of future devices.

Another important source is heart valves and connectors used to allow unidirectional flow. The Thoratec VAD and Jarvik TAH use Bjork-Shiley monostrut tilting-disc valves. These valves and their housings were recognized as sites of thrombus formation, despite adequate anticoagulation (6) (Fig. 4). More recently, VADs such as the Novacor and Thermedics devices have used either pericardial or porcine tissue valves. These valves do not require long-term anticoagulation. While tissue valves have been shown to be less durable in the long term as compared with mechanical valves, their durability in cardiac assist devices has yet to be tested. Most VADS are implanted for relatively short periods. In general, the materials used in current VAD devices require pharmacologic inhibitors of thrombogenesis for safe use. These include heparin and warfarin together with antiplatelet drugs such as aspirin. Dextran, a partially hydrolized polymer of glucose, has also been

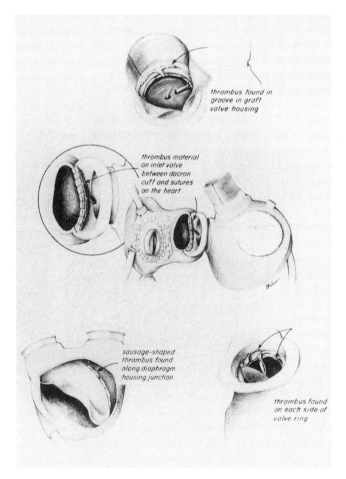

Figure 4   Thrombus formation on prosthetic valves in early implantations of the Jarvik heart. (From Unger F, ed. Assisted circulation. Berlin: Springer-Verlag 1989.)

used. It prolongs the bleeding time by interfering with the polymerization of fibrin and inhibits platelet aggregation. The most common complication is postoperative bleeding.

III. CLINICAL APPLICATIONS

It has been estimated that circulatory support is needed for fewer than 1% of all patients undergoing cardiopulmonary bypass (7). Demand will increase as the number of critically ill patients requiring surgery increases. The indications for left ventricular circulatory support include postoperative cardiac failure resulting in dependency on cardiopulmonary bypass despite pharmacologic and/or IABP support; cardiac failure due to cardiomyopathy or acute viral myocarditis; cardiogenic shock complicating acute myocardial infarction; failed donor heart after transplantation; and use as a bridge to transplantation (8). Assist devices for right ventricular failure are indicated in cases of isolated acute right ventricular failure alone or in association with left ventricular failure.

The numerous devices under development fall into two types, orthotopic and heterotopic prosthetic ventricles (2). The orthotopic ventricles are generally dual-chambered devices that function in place of the native right and left ventricle. They are positioned in the mediastinum after attachment to the right and left atrial cuffs. The heterotopic ventricles are attached to the native heart by Dacron cannulae and are positioned in the abdomen.

The most commonly implanted devices will be reviewed with respect to thrombosis prophylaxis, bleeding complications, and the incidence of thromboembolic complications.

IV. VENTRICULAR ASSIST DEVICES

A. The Centrifugal Pump—Biomedicus

Centrifugal pumps generate pressure by spinning blood as a vortex within a rigid chamber (Fig. 5). Blood leaves the chamber through the exit cannula and enters through a central inlet port. The majority of VADs use the left atrium, left ventricle, or pulmonary veins to provide adequate inflow for the device. The ascending aorta usually receives the outflow from these devices.

The Biomedicus pump (Minneapolis, Minnesota) is the only centrifugal pump available for use as a VAD at this time. It is used primarily to support patients with postcardiotomy myocardial failure. In 1986, Park et al. reported their experience with 41 patients who required mechanical ventricular assist utilizing the Biomedicus pump (9). Patients were assisted for a mean of 41 h (range 2–186 h). Thirteen patients (32%) were successfully weaned from the device and were discharged from the hospital. Another eight patients were weaned from the device but died within 30 days of surgery. The remaining 20 patients could not be weaned from ventricular assist. In this study, the patients were not anticoagulated if blood flow was maintained at more than 2 L/min. Minimal heparinization (10,000–20,000 U/24 h) was employed when the flow was less than 2 L/min and was adjusted to maintain an activated clotting time of 150 s. While there were no bleeding or thromboembolic complications, small blood clots were found in a number of devices.

The centrifugal pump has also been used successfully as a bridge to cardiac transplantation. In one series, seven of nine patients underwent successful transplantation after an average of 1.6 days of circulatory support (range 0.5–3 days) (10). A continuous heparin infusion was instituted in all patients after mediastinal drainage had decreased. Activated

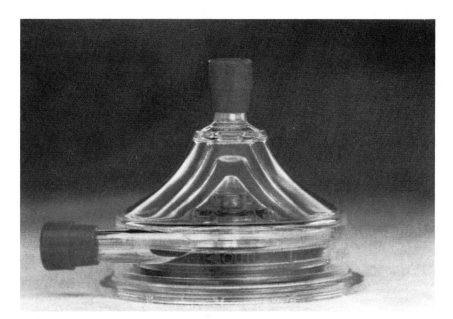

Figure 5   The Biomedicus centrifugal pump. (Courtesy of Biomedicus Inc., Minneapolis, Minnesota.)

clotting times were maintained between 150 and 200 s. One patient sustained a cerebrovascular accident leading to brain death before a donor could be located.

B. Thoratec (Pierce Donachy) VAD

The pneumatic pulsatile VAD is a heterotopic prosthetic ventricle that relies on an external console to pump compressed carbon dioxide. The compressed CO_2 displaces a flexible diaphragm that ejects blood from the sac. The Thoratec (Pierce-Donachy) VAD developed at Pennsylvania State University is the most commonly used pump of this type (11). The blood-contacting surface is composed of a flexible, smooth, segmented polyurethane blood sac and diaphragm that lies within a rigid case (Fig. 6). This VAD employs Bjork-Shiley monostrut tilting-disc inlet and outlet valves. Cannulation usually involve the left atrial appendage and ascending aorta. The cannulae exit the skin below the left costal margin to enter the device on the anterior abdominal wall.

In 1989, Pennington et al. reported their experience with the Thoratec VAD in patients with cardiogenic shock after cardiac surgery (11). Thirty patients were supported for a mean 3.6 days (range 3 h to 22 days). In all patients, heparin was used for anticoagulation during cardiopulmonary bypass. When the patients were weaned from bypass with the VAD, heparin was reversed with protamine. Heparin was not used again until the patients were weaned from the VAD. An additional 22 patients received low-molecular-weight dextran (25 ml/h) in the postoperative period. Sixteen patients (53%) had improvements in cardiac function, 15 were weaned from the device (50%), and 11 (37%) were eventually discharged from the hospital. Eighteen of the 30 patients required reoperation for bleeding. The authors conclude that leaving the sternum open with the device in place during their early experience

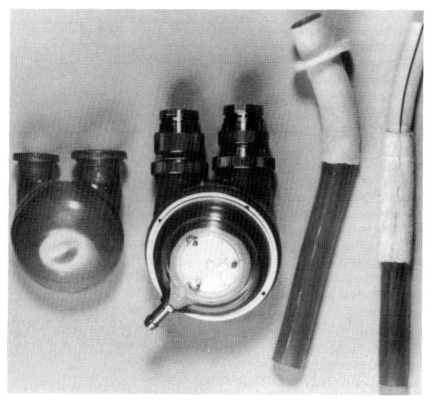

Figure 6 The Thoratec Pierce-Donachy VAD with polyurethane blood sac, rigid case, and Dacron cannulae (left to right). (From Baumgartner W, ed. Heart and heart-lung transplantation. Philadelphia: W.B. Saunders, 1990.)

contributed to bleeding complications. In later implantations, the sternum was routinely closed and significantly reducing bleeding complications. In the series of Pennington et al., thrombus was found in three VAD sacs. In one patient the thrombus may have formed when the right VAD cannula was intermittently clamped to perform cardiac output measurements. There were two cerebrovascular accidents during the perioperative period, both occurring during low-flow states. There was no evidence of thrombus formation in either device at the time of explantation. One patient succumbed to multiple complications including a stroke, while the other patient regained full function and was discharged from the hospital.

This series from the Saint Louis University Medical Center has recently been updated with respect to thromboembolic complications (12). Fifty-four patients were supported for 3 h to 81 days. All patients received low-molecular-weight dextran and heparin during the weaning phase of VAD support. Patients in whom the VAD was implanted as a bridge to transplantation received oral dipyridamole and warfarin after extubation. For the 27 patients supported for less than 4 days, there were no visible thrombi in the VAD at the time of explantation. Nine of 27 patients supported for longer than 4 days had visible thrombi. Of the nine patients who had thrombi in the VAD, four had cerebral or peripheral emboli at autopsy. In addition, one patient without thrombi in the VAD sustained a stroke while being weaned from the device. There were no statistically significant differences in the degree of anticoagulation, time of support, or average device flow between those patients who had thrombi and those who did not. Four patients with thrombi had mechanical problems leading to periods of decreased blood flow. The overall incidence of thrombus formation was 17%, with an incidence of embolization of 4–8%.

C. Novacor

The Novacor ventricular assist device is a heterotopic prosthetic ventricle that was designed for long-term support. It is an implantable pump that consists of a seamless polyurethane sac bonded to dual symmetrically opposed pusher plates in a lightweight housing (13) (Fig. 7). The pump has a smooth blood-surface interface and pericardial tissue valves with custom silicone flanges. The dual pusher plate system is coupled to a pulsed solenoid energy converter and connected to the control console by leads that are contained in a percutaneous vent tube. The pump drive unit is positioned in the anterior abdominal wall of the left upper quadrant. Dacron inflow and outflow conduits pass through the diaphragm to connect the pump to the left ventricular apex and the ascending aorta. Patients receive low-dose intravenous heparin after mediastinal drainage has decreased. The partial thromboplastin time is maintained at 1.5 times normal. In patients with extended support, low-molecular-weight dextran is combined with heparin and later replaced by warfarin and dipyridamole.

Since 1984, the Novacor device has been implanted as a bridge to heart transplantation.

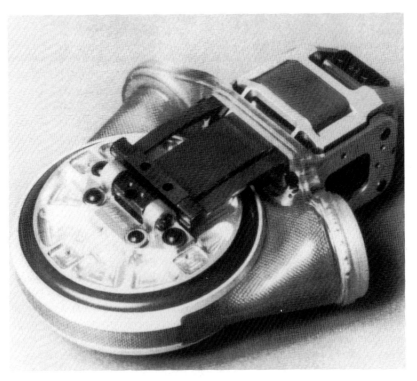

Figure 7   The Novacor VAD. (From Baumgartner W, ed. Heart and heart-lung transplantation. Philadelphia: W.B. Saunders, 1990.)

Portner et al. reported the largest series, including 20 patients who required circulatory support (14). Ten patients (50%) underwent cardiac transplantation after implants whose duration ranged from 2 to 90 days (mean 30 days). Eight of these patients (40%) were eventually discharged from the hospital. Serious complications occurred in 16 patients and precluded transplantation in 10. Bleeding was the most common complication and was found in eight patients with reoperation needed in four. Two patients had a fatal perioperative cerebrovascular accident. In one patient embolization occurred from a left ventricular mural thrombus, and the other had an air embolus. A third patient had two focal neurological events that were probably embolic in origin.

D. Thermedics (Heartmate)

The Thermedics VAD is a pusher plate blood pump that is pneumatically powered by an external control system (15). The pump bladder and metal components are covered by a textured membrane composed of prosthetic polyester fibrils that facilitate the formation of a pseudointimal biologic lining (Fig. 8). Inflow and outflow conduits are made of Dacron. These are attached to the left ventricular apex and the ascending aorta. Each conduit contains a glutaraldehyde-preserved porcine tissue valve. The patients receive heparin, low-molecular-weight dextran, dipyridamole, and aspirin for intermittent periods after implantation.

At the Texas Heart Institute, 13 patients have been supported with the Thermedics VAD as a bridge to transplantation (16). Five patients were supported for extended periods longer than 30 days (range 35 to 135 days), and all underwent successful cardiac transplantation. Device-related complications included postoperative bleeding in two patients, both

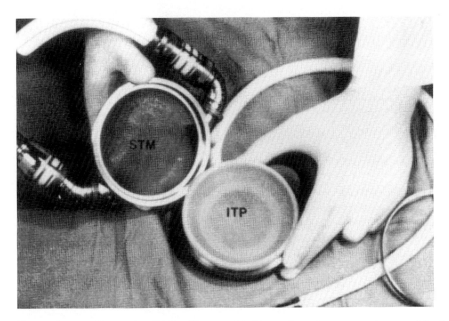

Figure 8   The Thermedics VAD with pump bladder and metal components covered by textured membrane. (Courtesy of Thermedics, Inc., Berkeley, California.)

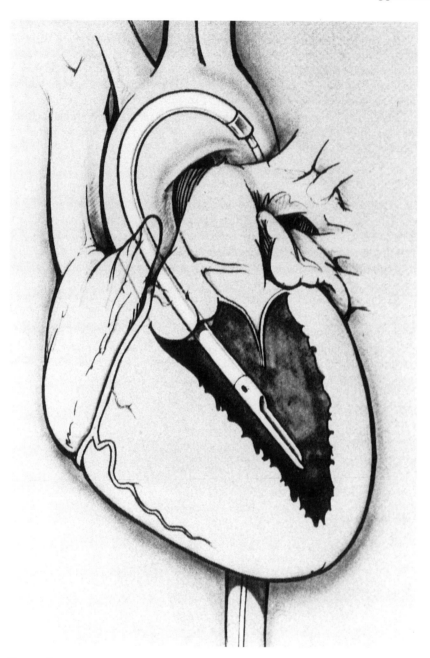

Figure 9 The Nimbus hemopump left ventricular assist device. (From Ref. 17.)

required reoperation. There was no evidence of mineralization or thrombus formation. There have been no thromboembolic events to date.

E. Hemopump (Nimbus)

The Hemopump left ventricular assist device is an axial-flow pump (17). The device is implanted through the femoral artery or ascending aorta and positioned in the apex of the left ventricle (Fig. 9). The pump consists of an inlet cannula, which is made of flexible silicone rubber. The inlet cannula is connected to the thromboresistant stainless steel blood pump housing. The axial-flow pump, which is located within the housing, is connected to the external power source by a flexible drive shaft enclosed in a polymeric sheath (Fig. 10). When the pump is activated, the impeller spins at 15,000 to 27,000 rpm, providing unidirectional, nonpulsatile flow. Blood is drawn from the left ventricle and propelled into the aorta to achieve a maximum flow of approximately 4 L/min.

This device has been used in seven patients suffering from cardiogenic shock, with successful circulatory support seen in all patients. Heparin was administered to maintain an activated clotting time of 1.5 to 2 times control. Anticoagulation therapy was withheld until adequate hemostasis was achieved postoperatively. The patients were supported for 26 to 113 h (mean 66 h) without evidence of valvular damage or vascular injury. There were no thromboembolic events. Five patients had evidence of intravascular hemolysis, which was mild to moderate as demonstrated by serial plasma free hemoglobin levels. In all but one patient, plasma free hemoglobin levels returned to normal within 24 h after device removal. Five of the seven patients were alive more than 30 days after device insertion. The two remaining patients died of biventricular failure and arrhythmias after the device had been removed.

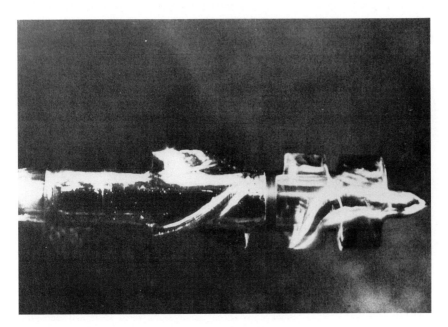

Figure 10 The Nimbus axial-flow pump. (From Ref. 17.)

V.   TOTAL ARTIFICIAL HEART (TAH)

The ultimate goal of mechanical circulatory assist devices is the safe and effective replacement of the human heart. Since the first implantation of a TAH, technologic advancements have provided artificial hearts with smaller, more efficient power sources. Additional refinements include the development of prosthetic ventricles that can be attached to fabric cuffs sewn to the native atria.

Widespread use of total artificial hearts for permanent replacement has been limited by persistent problems related to infection and thromboembolic events. In 1982, DeVries electively implanted a pneumatically driven Jarvik-7 heart (1). The Jarvik-7 heart consists of two separate prosthetic ventricles constructed of a flexible diaphragm and a smooth blood surface fabricated of segmented polyurethane (Fig. 11). Compressed air is delivered by a percutaneous drive line to displace the diaphragm and empty the blood sac. The cardiac valves were Bjork-Shiley monostrut tilting-disc prostheses. Dacron prosthetic grafts were used to connect the device to the pulmonary artery and the aorta. The patients were anticoagulated with heparin and warfarin. Antiplatelet therapy was used intermittently. As noted earlier, the initial postoperative course was complicated by renal insufficiency, seizures, bleeding, and pulmonary sepsis, which eventually led to death. Subsequent implantations of this artificial heart have been performed as a bridge to transplantation (18). These cases offer considerable insight into the potential application of the artificial heart. Since 1985, a registry of mechanical VADs used in conjunction with heart transplantation has been compiled (19). Of the 400 patients who required circulatory support, 178 received the TAH and 128 (71.9%) eventually had a heart transplantation. In the majority, anticoagulation with heparin and dipyridamole was initiated when mediastinal drainage decreased (usually 8 h). Intravenous heparin was administered at 500 U/h to maintain the partial thromboplastin time between 2 and 2.5 times control. Dipyridamole 75 mg was administered every 8 h.

Major device-related complications included postoperative bleeding, mediastinal infection, renal failure, and multisystem organ failure. Thromboembolic complications have been reported in two large series, one from Pittsburgh and the other from La Pitié Hospital in

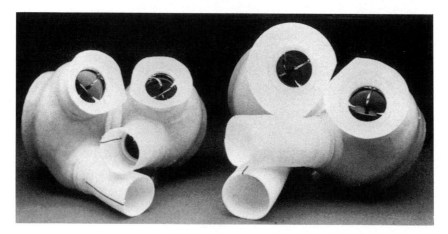

Figure 11   The Jarvik 70 and 7 total artificial hearts. (From Baumgartner W, ed. Heart and heart-lung transplantation. Philadelphia: W.B. Saunders, 1990.)

France (20,21). In the Pittsburgh series, one patient had a cerebral embolism in spite of anticoagulation. The explanted devices showed deposition of small thrombi in the crevices between the valve rings and the housings (Fig. 4). The experience at La Pité Hospital has been informative. "Gelatine Resorcine Formal Glue" was used to assure hemostasis, thereby allowing an aggressive antithrombosis approach. The glue was applied to all vascular anastomoses and at suture lines, eliminating postoperative bleeding complications. The anticoagulation regimen included heparin, dipyridamole, aspirin, and pentoxifylline. There were no thromboembolic complications and no evidence of clots in any of the explanted devices.

VI. FUTURE CONSIDERATIONS

Further advances in mechanical circulatory support are dependent on the elimination of device-related complications such as infection and thromboembolic events, which are particularly devastating in this critically ill patient population. The development of biocompatible materials that are resistant to infection and thrombosis is crucial to the realization of this goal. When gelatin glue becomes available for clinical use in the United States, a more aggressive antithrombotic approach may be possible. Endothelialized prosthetic materials may also provide a thromboresistant surface. Each of these developments will benefit the growing number of patients who require mechanical circulatory support by minimizing thromboembolic complications.

REFERENCES

1. DeVries W, Anderson J, Joyce L, et al. Clinical use of the total artificial heart. N Engl J Med 1984; 310:273–8.
2. Hill JD. Polymer surfaces for prosthetic ventricles. In: Chin R, ed. Transformed muscle for cardiac assist and repair. Mount Kisco, New York: Futura, 1990, 299–309.
3. Farrar D, Litivak P, Lawson J, et al. In vivo evaluations of a new thromboresistant polyurethane for artificial heart blood pumps. J Thorac Cardiovasc Surg 1988; 95:191–200.
4. Dasse K, Chipman S, Sherman C, Levine A, Frazier O. Clinical experience with textured blood contacting surfaces in ventricular assist devices. ASA10, 1987; 10:418–25.
5. Pasche B, Kodoma K, Larm O, et al. Thrombin inactivation on surfaces with covalently bonded heparin. Thromb Res 1986; 44:739.
6. Griffith B. Interim use of the Jarvik-7 artificial heart: lessons learned at Presbyterian University Hospital of Pittsburgh. Ann Thorac Surg 1989; 47:158–66.
7. McGree M, Zillgitt, Trono R, et al. Retrospective analyses of the need for mechanical circulatory support (intraaortic balloon pump/abdominal left ventricular assist device or partial artificial heart) after cardiopulmonary bypass. Am J Cardiol 1980; 46:135–42.
8. Pennock J, Pierce W, Wisman C, Bull A, Waldhausen J. Survival and complications following ventricular assist pumping for cardiogenic shock. Ann Surg 1983; 198:469–78.
9. Park S, Liebler G, Burholder J, Maher T, et al. Mechanical support of the failing heart. Ann Thorac Surg 1986; 42:627–31.
10. Bolman R, Cox J, Marshall W, et al. Circulatory support with a centrifugal pump as a bridge to cardiac transplantation. Ann Thorac Surg 1989; 47:108–12.
11. Pennington DG, McBride L, Swartz M, et al. Use of the Pierce-Donachy ventricular assist device in patients with cardiogenic shock after cardiac operations. Ann Thorac Surg 1989; 47:130–5.
12. Termuhlen D, Swartz M, Pennington G, McBride L, et al. Thromboembolic complications with the Pierce-Donachy ventricular assist device. Trans Am Soc Artif Intern Organs 1989; 35:616–8.

13. Portner P, Oyer P, McGregor C, et al. First human use of an electrically powered implantable ventricular assist system. Artif Organs 1985; 9(A):36.

14. Portner P, Oyer P, Pennington D, et al. Implantable electrical left ventricular assist system: bridge to transplantation and the future. Ann Thorac Surg 1989; 47:142–50.

15. Nakatoni T, Frazier OH, McGee M, Parnis S, et al. Extended support prior to cardiac transplant using a left ventricular assist device with textured blood-contacting surfaces. Presented at the World Congress of the International Society for Artificial Organs, Oct 1–4, 1989.

16. Frazier D, Cooley D. Use of cardiac assist devices as bridges to cardiac transplantation. Review of current status and report of the Texas Heart Institute's experience. In: Unger F, ed. Assisted circulation. Berlin: Springer-Verlag, 1989:2467–259.

17. Frazier OH, Wampler RK, Duncan M, Dean WE, Macris MP, Parnis SM, Fuqua JM. First human use of the hemopump, a catheter-mounted ventricular assist device. Ann Thorac Surg 1990; 49:299–304.

18. Copeland J, Smith R, Jcenogle T, et al. Orthotopic total artificial heart bridge to transplantation: preliminary results. J Heart Transplant 1989; 8:124–38.

19. Miller C, Pae W, Pierce W. Combined registry for the clinical use of mechanical ventricular assist pumps and the total artificial heart in conjunction with heart transplantation. Fourth official report—1989. J Heart Transplant 1990; 9:453–8.

20. Griffith B. Temporary use of the Jarvik-7 artificial heart—the Pittsburgh experience. In Unger F, ed. Assisted circulation. Berlin: Springer-Verlag, 1989:269–81.

21. Muneretto C, Rabago G Jr, Pavie A, Leger P, Gandjbakhch I, Sasako Y, Tedy G, Bors V, Desruennes M, Szefner J, et al. Mechanical circulatory support as a bridge to transplantation: current status of total artificial heart in 1989 and determinants of survival. J Cardiovasc Surg 1990; 31:486–91.

Index